D1388221

EVIDENCE-BASED MEDICINE

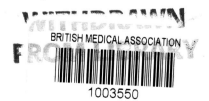

WITHDRAWN
BRITISH MEDICAL ASSOCIATION
FROM LIBRARY

1003550

Dedication

This book is dedicated to Dr. David L. Sackett.

EVIDENCE-BASED MEDICINE

HOW TO PRACTICE AND TEACH EBM

Fifth Edition

Sharon E. Straus, MD
Professor, Department of Medicine, University of Toronto, Ontario, Canada

Paul Glasziou, MRCGP, FRACGP, PhD
Professor, Faculty of Health Sciences and Medicine, Bond University, Australia

W. Scott Richardson, MD
Professor of Medicine and Campus Associate Dean for Medical Education, AU/UGA
Medical Partnership Campus, Athens, Georgia, USA

R. Brian Haynes, MD
Professor Emeritus of Health Research Methods, Evidence and Impact, McMaster
University, Hamilton, Ontario, Canada

With contributions by

Reena Pattani, MD MPH
Assistant Professor, Department of Medicine, St. Michael's Hospital, University of Toronto,
Toronto, Ontario, Canada

Areti Angeliki Veroniki, PhD
Banting Postdoctoral Fellow, Knowledge Translation Program, Li Ka Shing Knowledge
Institute of St. Michael's, Toronto, Ontario, Canada

> **For additional online content visit** http://ebm-tools
> .knowledgetranslation.net/

ELSEVIER

Edinburgh   London   New York   Oxford   Philadelphia   St. Louis   Sydney   2019

ELSEVIER

Copyright © 2019 Sharon E. Straus, Paul Glasziou, W. Scott Richardson and R. Brian Haynes.
Published by Elsevier Limited. All rights reserved.

First edition 1997
Second edition 2000
Third edition 2005
Fourth edition 2011
Fifth edition 2019

The right of Sharon E. Straus, Paul Glasziou, W. Scott Richardson and R. Bryan Haynes to be identified as authors of this work has been asserted by them in accordance with the Copyright, Designs and Patents Act 1988.

Chapter 4 was updated for this edition by Reena Pattani. Appendix 2 was originally written by Douglas G. Altman of the ICRF Medical Statistics Group and the Centre for Statistics in Medicine, Oxford, UK, and updated for this edition by Areti Angeliki Veroniki.

No part of this publication may be reproduced or transmitted in any form or by any means, electronic or mechanical, including photocopying, recording, or any information storage and retrieval system, without permission in writing from the publisher. Details on how to seek permission, further information about the Publisher's permissions policies and our arrangements with organizations such as the Copyright Clearance Center and the Copyright Licensing Agency, can be found at our website: www.elsevier.com/permissions.

This book and the individual contributions contained in it are protected under copyright by the Publisher (other than as may be noted herein).

Notices

Knowledge and best practice in this field are constantly changing. As new research and experience broaden our understanding, changes in research methods, professional practices, or medical treatment may become necessary.

Practitioners and researchers must always rely on their own experience and knowledge in evaluating and using any information, methods, compounds, or experiments described herein. In using such information or methods they should be mindful of their own safety and the safety of others, including parties for whom they have a professional responsibility.

With respect to any drug or pharmaceutical products identified, readers are advised to check the most current information provided (i) on procedures featured or (ii) by the manufacturer of each product to be administered, to verify the recommended dose or formula, the method and duration of administration, and contraindications. It is the responsibility of practitioners, relying on their own experience and knowledge of their patients, to make diagnoses, to determine dosages and the best treatment for each individual patient, and to take all appropriate safety precautions.

To the fullest extent of the law, neither the Publisher nor the authors, contributors, or editors, assume any liability for any injury and/or damage to persons or property as a matter of products liability, negligence or otherwise, or from any use or operation of any methods, products, instructions, or ideas contained in the material herein.

ISBN: 978-0-7020-6296-4

Printed in China
Last digit is the print number: 9 8 7 6 5 4 3 2 1

Content Strategist: Pauline Graham
Content Development Specialist: Fiona Conn
Project Manager: Janish Ashwin Paul
Design: Ashley Miner/Brian Salisbury
Illustration Manager: Karen Giacomucci
Marketing Manager: Deborah Watkins

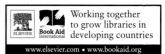

Working together
to grow libraries in
developing countries

www.elsevier.com • www.bookaid.org

Contents

Preface   ix

Acknowledgements   xii

Introduction   1

Asking answerable clinical questions   19   **1**

Acquiring the evidence: How to find current best evidence and have current best evidence find us   35   **2**

Appraising the evidence   67   **3**

Therapy   71   **4**

Diagnosis and screening   153   **5**

Prognosis   185   **6**

Harm   201   **7**

Evaluation   223   **8**

Teaching evidence-based medicine   237   **9**

Appendix 1: Glossary   299
Appendix 2: Confidence intervals (ebook only)   e1
Index   309

Contents of EBM Toolbox

Tools to accompany this book are available at
http://ebm-tools.knowledgetranslation.net/

- Critical appraisal worksheets
- Educational prescription
- Pocket cards
- EBM calculator
- NNT/LR tables
- CQ log
- Links to teaching curricula (medportal)

Index of Teaching Moments

Teaching the asking of answerable clinical questions   28

Validity criteria   85

Learning and teaching with CATs   177

Tips for teaching around diagnostic tests   181

Evaluations of strategies for teaching the steps of EBM   232

Preface

This book is for clinicians, at any stage of their training or career, who want to learn how to practise and teach evidence-based medicine (EBM). It's been written for the busy clinician, and thus, it's short and practical. The book emphasizes direct clinical application of EBM and tactics to practise and teach EBM in real time. Those who want, and have time for, more detailed discussions of the theoretical and methodological bases for the tactics described here should consult one of the longer textbooks on clinical epidemiology.*

The focus of the book has changed with the continuing clinical experiences of the authors. For Sharon Straus, the ideas behind the ongoing development of the book have built on her experiences as a medical student on a general medicine ward, when she was challenged by a senior resident to provide evidence to support her management plans for each patient she admitted. This was so much more exciting than some previous rotations, where the management plan was learned by rote and was based on whatever the current consultant favoured. After residency, Sharon undertook postgraduate training in clinical epidemiology, and this further stimulated her interest in EBM, leading to a fellowship with Dave Sackett in Oxford, UK, where her enthusiasm for practising and teaching EBM continued to grow. She continues to learn from colleagues, mentors, and trainees, using many of their teaching tips! Sharon hopes that this has led to improved patient care and to more fun and challenge for her students and residents, from whom she's learned so much.

For Paul Glasziou, the first inkling of another way began when, as a newly qualified and puzzled doctor, he was fortunate enough to stumble on a copy of Henrik Wulff's *Rational Diagnosis and Treatment*. After a long journey of exploration (thanks Arthur, Jorgen, John, and Les), a

---

*We suggest: Haynes RB, Sackett DL, Guyatt GH, Tugwell P. *Clinical Epidemiology: How to Do Clinical Practice Research*. Philadelphia, PA: Lippincott Williams & Wilkins; 2006.

serendipitous visit by Dave Sackett to Sydney in the late 1980s led him to return to clinical work. A brief visit to McMaster University in Hamilton, Canada, with Dave Sackett convinced him that research really could be used to improve care. Feeling better armed to recognize and manage the uncertainties inherent in clinical consultations, he continues to enjoy general practice and teaching others to record and answer their own clinical questions. He remains awed by the vast unexplored tracts of clinical practice not visible from the eyepiece of a microscope. Rather than write "what I never learned at medical school," he is delighted to contribute to this book.

For Scott Richardson, the ideas for this book began coming together very slowly. As a beginning clinical clerk in the 1970s, one of his teachers told him to read the literature to decide what to do for his patients, but then said, "Of course, nobody really does that!" During residency, Scott tried harder to use the literature but found few tools to help him do it effectively. Some of the ideas for this book took shape for Scott when he came across the notions of clinical epidemiology and critical appraisal in the late 1970s and early 1980s, and he began to use them in his practice and in his teaching of students and postgraduates at the University of Rochester, New York. On his journeys in Rochester; Hamilton, Canada; Oxford, UK; San Antonio, California; Dayton, Ohio; and Athens, Greece, Scott has worked with others in EBM (including these coauthors), fashioning those earlier ideas into clinician-friendly tools for everyday use. Scott continues to have big fun learning from and teaching with a large number of EBM colleagues around the world, all working to improve the care of patients by making wise use of research evidence.

Brian Haynes started worrying about the relationship between evidence and clinical practice during his second year of medical school when a psychiatrist gave a lecture on Freud's theories. When asked, "What's the evidence that Freud's theories were correct?" the psychiatrist admitted that there wasn't any good evidence and that he didn't believe the theories, but he had been asked by the head of the department "to give the talk." This eventually led him to a career combining clinical practice (in internal medicine) with research (in clinical epidemiology) to "get the evidence"— only to find that the evidence being generated by medical researchers around the world wasn't getting to practitioners and patients in a timely and dependable way. Sabbaticals permitted a career shift into medical informatics to look into how knowledge is disseminated and applied and how practitioners and patients can use and benefit from "current best evidence." This led to the development of several evidence-based information resources, including the *ACP Journal Club*, *Evidence-Based Medicine*, *Evidence-Based Nursing*, and *Evidence-Based Mental Health*, in both print and electronic versions, to make it easier for practitioners to get at the best current evidence, as described in detail in chapter 2. He continues to devise ever more devious ways to get evidence into practice, including making high-quality evidence so inexpensive and available that less refined evidence won't stand a chance in competing for practitioners' reading materials, computers, or brains. They also say that he's a dreamer …

A note about our choice of words: We'll talk about "our" patients throughout this book, not to imply any possession or our control of them but to signify that we have taken on an obligation and responsibility to care for and serve each of them.

We're sure that this book contains several errors—when you find them, please go to our website (http://ebm-tools.knowledgetranslation.net/) and tell us about them. Similarly, because some of the examples used in this book will be out of date by the time you're reading this, the website will provide updates and new materials, so we suggest that you check it periodically. It will also be a means of contacting us and letting us know where we've gone wrong and what we could do better in the future.

For the contents of this book to benefit patients, we believe that clinicians must have a mastery of the clinical skills including history taking and physical examination, without which we can neither begin the process of EBM (by generating diagnostic hypotheses) nor end it (by integrating valid, important evidence with our patient's values and expectations). We also advocate continuous, self-directed, lifelong learning. T.H. White wrote in *The Once and Future King*, "Learning is the only thing which the mind can never exhaust, never alienate, never be tortured by, never fear or distrust, and never dream of regretting." By not regarding knowledge with humility and by denying our uncertainty and curiosity, we risk becoming dangerously out of date and immune to self-improvement and advances in medicine. Finally, we invite you to add the enthusiasm and irreverence to endeavour, without which you will miss the fun that accompanies the application of these ideas!

SES, PG, WSR, RBH

Acknowledgements

If this book is found to be useful, much of the credit for it goes to Muir Gray and David L. Sackett, who created and led, respectively, the NHS R&D Centre for Evidence-based Practice at Oxford, UK, which provided a home and working retreat for all of the authors at various times. They provided the authors with great mentorship and advice, including the following: "If you can dream it, you can do it." And we thank them for encouraging us to dream and for helping us to realize many of those dreams.

We thank our colleagues for their infinite patience and our families for their loving support. Sharon Straus gives special thanks to all the students, fellows, and residents for their inspiration and fun; to Reena Pattani, who took on the authorship of Chapter 4 on Therapy for this edition and represents the bright future of academic medicine; to Jessie McGowan, for developing some of the searches that informed this book; to Argie Veroniki, who updated Appendix 2 on Confidence Intervals (available online) and is an emerging leader in biostatistics internationally; to Barbara and Dave Sackett, for their friendship and mentorship; and, to her family for always supporting and encouraging her. Paul Glasziou thanks Arthur Elstein, Jorgen Hilden, John Simes, Les Irwig, and Dave Sackett for their mentorship and friendship. Scott Richardson gives special thanks to Sherry Parmer and Alexandra Richardson and to his many teachers and colleagues, who have taught by example and who have given him both intellectual challenge and personal support so generously. Brian Haynes thanks the American College of Physicians and the BMJ Publishing Group for leading the way in providing opportunities to create and disseminate many of the "evidence-based" information resources featured in this book.

We're still seeking better ways of explaining the ideas mentioned in this book and their clinical applications and will acknowledge readers' suggestions in subsequent editions of this book. In the meantime, we take cheerful responsibility for the parts of the current edition that are still fuzzy, wrong, or boring. We thank those who provided comments on previous editions of this book and helped us strengthen its contents.

Introduction

What is evidence-based medicine?

Evidence-based medicine (EBM) requires the integration of the best research evidence with our clinical expertise and our patient's unique values and circumstances.

- By *best research evidence,* we mean clinically relevant research, sometimes from the basic sciences of medicine, but especially from patient-centred clinical research into the accuracy and precision of diagnostic tests (including the clinical examination), the power of prognostic markers, and the efficacy and safety of therapeutic, rehabilitative, and preventive strategies.

- By *clinical expertise,* we mean the ability to use our clinical skills and past experience to rapidly identify each patient's unique health state and diagnosis, his or her individual risks and benefits of potential interventions/exposures/diagnostic tests, and his or her personal values and expectations. Moreover, clinical expertise is required to integrate evidence with patient values and circumstances.

- By *patient values,* we mean the unique preferences, concerns, and expectations that each patient brings to a clinical encounter and that must be integrated into shared clinical decisions if they are to serve the patient; by *patient circumstances,* we mean the patient's individual clinical state and the clinical setting.

Why the interest in EBM?

Interest in EBM has grown exponentially since the coining of the term[1] in 1992 by a group led by Gordon Guyatt at McMaster University, Hamilton, Canada, from one Medline citation in 1992 to over 119,000 in December 2016. A search using the term "evidence-based medicine" retrieves almost 40 million hits and more than 1.5 million hits in Google and Google Scholar, respectively. We encourage interested readers to review "An oral history of EBM" by Dr. Richard Smith published in 2014 in the *Journal of the American Medical Association* (*JAMA*) and the *British Medical Journal* (*BMJ*).[2] This online resource outlines the origins and development of EBM, including discussions with Drs. David Sackett, Brian Haynes, and Gordon Guyatt. We also recommend taking a look at the James Lind Library, which provides a more detailed history of the development of "fair tests of treatments in health care," including many of the seminal moments in the history of EBM.[3] As a teaching tip, we use many of the resources provided in the James Lind Library, such as the story of James Lind's 1753 "Treatise of the scurvy" and the randomized trial of streptomycin treatment for pulmonary tuberculosis, published in 1948.[4] These are great articles to engage learners and stimulate interest in EBM, while highlighting that EBM isn't a new concept but instead one that builds on a solid foundation, the work of countless people worldwide who have been interested in using evidence to support decision making!

Evidence-based practice has become incorporated into many health care disciplines, including occupational therapy, physiotherapy, nursing, dentistry, and complementary medicine, among many others. Indeed, we've been told by one publisher that adding "evidence-based" to the title of a book can increase sales—alas, regardless of whether or not the book is evidence based! Similarly, its use has spilled over into many other domains, including justice, education, and policymaking. When we first started working in this area, although we were looking for the day when politicians would talk freely about using research evidence to inform their decision making, we did not anticipate it happening so soon or across so many countries![5,6]

Because of the recognition that EBM is critical for decision making, the focus of professional organizations and training programs for various health care providers has moved from *whether* to teach EBM to *how* to teach it, resulting in an explosion in the number of courses, workshops, and seminars offered in this practice. Similarly, EBM educational interventions for the public, policymakers, and health care managers have grown. Colleagues have extended training on critical appraisal to primary and secondary school students, highlighting that everyone should develop the ability to understand research evidence and use it in their own decision making, thus enhancing health literacy.[7-9] The format for teaching EBM to these diverse audiences has also grown, placing less emphasis on didactic sessions and more on interactive, case-based discussion, opportunistic teaching, and use of different media, including online platforms and social media.[10,11] Indeed, we hope that this ebook stimulates interest in sharing content and curricula worldwide and developing collaborative educational opportunities, such as Twitter journal clubs and massive online courses (MOCs).

Although champions and opinion leaders have facilitated the rapid spread of EBM over the last 25 years, its dissemination over this period has arisen from several realizations:

1. Our daily clinical need for valid and quantitative information about diagnosis, prognosis, therapy, and prevention (up to five times per inpatient[12] and twice for every three outpatients[13])

2. The inadequacy of traditional sources for this information because they are out of date (traditional textbooks[14]), frequently wrong (experts[15]), ineffective (didactic continuing medical education[16]), or too overwhelming in their volume and too variable in their validity for practical clinical use (medical journals[17])

3. The disparity between our diagnostic skills and clinical judgement, which increase with experience, and our up-to-date knowledge[18] and clinical performance,[19] which decline over time

4. Our inability to afford more than a few seconds for each patient to find and assimilate this evidence[20] or to set aside more than half an hour per week for general reading and practice reflection[21]

5. The gaps between evidence and practice (including overuse and underuse of evidence) leading to variations in practice and quality of care.[22-24] This issue, in particular, has gained increasing recognition, including a recent series of articles in the *Lancet* on research waste highlighting the inadequate return on investment in research.[25,26] Recognition of this issue has created moral and financial imperatives for funders, clinicians, researchers, and policymakers to try to bridge these evidence-to-practice gaps.

All of the above challenges have given rise to innovations to facilitate the practice of EBM:

1. The development of strategies for efficiently tracking down and appraising evidence (for its validity and relevance)

2. The creation and explosion in development of evidence synopsis and summary services, which allow us to find and use high-quality preappraised evidence[27]

3. The creation of information systems for bringing these evidence resources to us within seconds,[20] including "meta-search" engines that search across multiple resources

4. The development of innovative strategies for integrating evidence with electronic health records (creating both pull and push strategies for evidence)

5. The identification and application of effective strategies for lifelong learning and for improving our clinical performance[28]

6. The engagement of other stakeholders, including patients, the public, and policymakers, in seeking and applying evidence.

This book is devoted to describing some of these innovations, demonstrating their application to clinical problems and showing how they can be learned and practised by clinicians who are able to devote just 30 minutes per week for their continuing professional development.

Why the need for a new edition of this book?

First, new resources have become available for finding, organizing, and utilizing evidence in clinical practice, and we wanted to bring this book up to date. Second, many challenges to successfully translating evidence into practice persist, and we wanted to outline them and consider and describe possible solutions. We sent an e-mail survey to 40 colleagues worldwide to ask them: "What do you see as the challenges facing EBM practitioners and teachers now and in the next 5 years?" They identified a number of issues that we will attempt to tackle in this book. We encourage readers to offer their own tips to overcoming these challenges to include in future editions of this book.

How do we practise EBM?

The complete practice of EBM comprises five steps, and this book addresses each in turn:

- Step 1—converting the need for information (about prevention, diagnosis, prognosis, therapy, causation, etc.) into an answerable question (Chapter 1, pp. 19 to 34)

- Step 2—tracking down the best evidence with which to answer that question (Chapter 2, pp. 35 to 65)

- Step 3—critically appraising that evidence for its validity (closeness to the truth), impact (size of the effect), and applicability (usefulness in our clinical practice) (Chapters 4 through 7, pp. 71 to 222)

- Step 4—integrating the critical appraisal with our clinical expertise and with our patient's unique biology, values, and circumstances (Chapters 4 through 7, pp. 71 to 222)
- Step 5—evaluating our effectiveness and efficiency in executing steps 1 to 4 and seeking ways to improve them both for next time (Chapter 8, pp. 223 to 237).

When we examine our practice and that of our colleagues and trainees in this five-step fashion, we identify that clinicians can incorporate evidence into their practices in three ways. The first is the "doing" mode, in which at least the first four steps above are completed. The second is the "using" mode, in which searches are restricted to evidence resources that have already undergone critical appraisal by others, such as evidence summaries (thus skipping step 3). The third is the "replicating" mode, in which the decisions of respected opinion leaders are followed (abandoning at least steps 2 and 3). All three of these modes involve the integration of evidence (from whatever source) with our patient's unique biology, values, and circumstances of step 4, but they vary in the execution of the other steps. For the conditions we encounter every day (e.g., acute coronary syndrome [ACS] and venous thromboembolism [VTE]), we need to be "up to the minute" and very sure about what we are doing. Accordingly, we invest the time and effort necessary to carry out both steps 2 (searching) and 3 (critically appraising), and operate in the "doing" mode; all the chapters in this book are relevant to this mode. For the conditions we encounter less often (e.g., salicylate overdose), we conserve our time by seeking out critical appraisals already performed by others who describe (and stick to!) explicit criteria for deciding what evidence they selected and how they decided whether it was valid. We omit the time-consuming step 3 (critically appraising) and carry out just step 2 (searching) but restrict the latter to sources that have already undergone rigorous critical appraisal (e.g., *ACP Journal Club*). Only the third portions ("Can I apply this valid, important evidence to my patient?") of Chapters 4 through 7 (pp. 71 to 222) are strictly relevant here, and the growing database of preappraised resources (described in Chapter 2) is making this "using" mode more and more feasible for busy clinicians.

For the problems we're likely to encounter very infrequently in our own practices (e.g., graft-versus-host disease [GvHD] in a bone marrow transplant recipient), we "blindly" seek, accept, and apply the recommendations we receive from authorities in the relevant branch of medicine. This "replicating" mode also characterizes the practice of medical students and clinical trainees when they haven't yet been granted independence and have to carry out the orders of their consultants. The trouble with the "replicating" mode is that it is "blind" to whether the advice received from the experts is authoritative (evidence based, resulting from their operating in the "appraising" mode) or merely authoritarian (opinion based). We can sometimes gain clues about the validity of our expert source (Do they cite references?). If we tracked the care we give when operating in the "replicating" mode into the literature and critically appraised it, we would find that some of it was effective, some useless, and some harmful. But in the "replicating" mode, we'll never be sure which.

We don't practise as EBM doers all of the time, and we find that we move between the different modes of practising EBM, depending on the clinical scenario, the frequency with which it arises, and the time and resources available to address our clinical questions. Although some clinicians may want to become proficient in practising all five steps of EBM, many others would instead prefer to focus on becoming efficient users (and knowledge managers) of evidence. This book tries to meet the needs of these various end users. For those readers who are teachers of EBM, including those who want to be primarily users or doers of EBM, we try to describe various ways in which the learning needs of the different learners can be achieved.

Can clinicians practise EBM?

Surveys conducted among clinicians and students from various disciplines and from different countries have found that clinicians are interested in learning the necessary skills for practising EBM.[28-32] One survey of UK general practitioners (GPs) suggests that many clinicians already practise in the "using" mode, using evidence-based summaries generated by others (72%) and evidence-based practice guidelines or protocols (84%).[18] Far fewer claimed to understand (and to be able to explain) the "appraising" tools of numbers needed to treat (NNTs) (35%) and confidence intervals (CIs) (20%). Several studies have found that participants' understandings of EBM concepts are quite variable and that substantial barriers to its practice persist.[33-38]

If clinicians have the necessary skills for practising EBM, can it be done in real time? One of the first studies showing how this could be accomplished was conducted on a busy (180+ admissions per month) inpatient medical service. Electronic summaries of evidence previously appraised either by team members (critically appraised topics [CATs]) or by synopsis resources were brought to working rounds, and it was documented that, on average, the former could be accessed in 10 seconds and the latter in 25 seconds.[19] Moreover, when assessed from the viewpoint of the most junior member of the team caring for the patient, this evidence changed 25% of their diagnostic and treatment suggestions and added to a further 23% of them. This study has been replicated in other clinical settings, including an obstetrical service.[39] Finally, clinical audits from many practice settings have found that there is a significant evidence base for the primary interventions that are encountered on these clinical services.[40-47]

What's the "E" in EBM?[48-67]

There is an accumulating body of evidence relating to the impact of EBM on health care providers from systematic reviews of training in the skills of EBM[68] to qualitative research describing the experience of EBM practitioners.[69] Indeed, since the last edition of this book was published, there has been an explosion in the number of studies evaluating EBM educational interventions targeting primary school and secondary school students, undergraduates, postgraduates, and practising clinicians. However, these studies on the effect of teaching and practising EBM are challenging to conduct. In many studies, the intervention has been difficult to define. It's unclear what the appropriate "dose" or "formulation" should be. Some studies use an approach to clinical practice, whereas others use training in one of the discrete "microskills" of EBM, such as performing a Medline search[70-72] or a critical appraisal.[73] Studies have evaluated online, in-person, small-group, and large-group educational interventions.[74] Learners have different learning needs and styles, and these differences must be reflected in the educational experiences provided.

Just as the intervention has proven difficult to define, evaluating whether the intervention has met its goals has been challenging. Effective EBM interventions will produce a wide range of outcomes. Changes in knowledge and skills are relatively easy to detect and demonstrate. Changes in attitudes and behaviours are harder to confirm. Randomized studies of EBM educational interventions have shown that these interventions can change knowledge and attitudes.[75] Similarly, randomized trials have shown that these interventions can enhance EBM skills.[48,74,76,77] A study has shown that a multifaceted EBM educational intervention (including access to evidence resources and a seminar series using real clinical scenarios) significantly improved evidence-based practice patterns in a district general hospital.[78] Still more challenging is detecting changes in clinical outcomes. Studies of undergraduate and postgraduate educational interventions have shown limited impact on ongoing behaviour or clinical outcomes.[74,79] Studies demonstrating better patient survival when practice is evidence based (and worse when it isn't) are limited to outcomes research.[80,81] There hasn't been a trial conducted whereby access to evidence is withheld from control clinicians. Finally, it is also important to explore the impact on all of these various outcomes over time.[53,65]

Along with the interest in EBM, there has been growing interest in evaluating EBM and developing evaluation instruments.[54,67] Several instruments are available for evaluating EBM educational interventions, including those that assess attitudes[55,82-84] knowledge and skills. We encourage interested readers to review the systematic review that addresses this topic; however, note that this hasn't been updated since it was published in 2006, so it should serve only as a starting point.[85] For any educational intervention, we encourage teachers and researchers to keep in mind that it is necessary to consider changes in performance and outcomes over time because EBM requires lifelong learning, and this is not something that can be measured over the short term.

By asking about the "E" in EBM, are we asking the right question? It has been recognized that providing evidence from clinical research is a necessary, but not sufficient, condition for the provision of optimal care. This has created interest in knowledge translation, the scientific study of the methods for closing the knowledge-to-practice gap, and the analysis of barriers and facilitators inherent in this process.[86] (As a side note here, although in Canada and Australia we call this *knowledge translation*, we know other terms are used in other countries, including *implementation science* in the United Kingdom and *dissemination* and *implementation* in the United States).[87] Proponents of knowledge translation have identified that changing behaviour is a complex process that requires comprehensive approaches directed toward patients, physicians, managers, and policy-makers and that provision of evidence is but one component. In this edition, we'll touch briefly on knowledge translation, which focuses on evidence-based implementation. This is not the primary focus of the book, which, instead, targets the practice of individual clinicians, patients, and teachers.

What are the limitations of EBM?

Discussion about the practice of EBM naturally engenders negative and positive reactions from clinicians. Some of the criticisms focus on misunderstandings and misperceptions of EBM, such as the concerns that it ignores patient values and preferences and promotes a "cookbook" approach (for interested readers, we refer you to an early systematic review of the criticisms of EBM and editorial discussing these[88,89]). We have noted that discussion of these same criticisms bubbles up periodically in the literature. An examination of the definition and steps of EBM quickly dismisses these criticisms. Evidence, whether strong or weak, is never sufficient to make clinical decisions. Individual values and preferences must balance this evidence to achieve optimal shared decision making and highlight that the practice of EBM is not a "one size fits all" approach. Other critics have expressed concerns that EBM will be hijacked by managers to promote cost cutting. However, it is not an effective cost-cutting tool because providing evidence-based care directed toward maximizing patients' quality of life often increases the costs of their care and raises the ire of some health economists.[90] The self-reported employment of the "using" mode by a great majority of frontline GPs dispels the contention that EBM is an "ivory tower" concept, another common criticism. Finally, we hope that the rest of this book will put to rest the concern that EBM leads to therapeutic nihilism in the absence of randomized trial evidence. Proponents of EBM would acknowledge that several sources of evidence inform clinical decision making. The practice of EBM stresses finding the best available evidence to answer a question, and this evidence may come from randomized trials, rigorous observational studies, or even anecdotal reports from experts. Hierarchies of evidence have been developed to help describe the quality of evidence that may be found to answer clinical questions. Randomized trials and systematic reviews of randomized trials provide the highest quality evidence—that is, the lowest likelihood of bias, and thus the lowest likelihood to mislead because they establish the effect of an intervention. However, they are not usually the best sources for answering questions about diagnosis, prognosis, or the harmful impact of potentially noxious exposures.

This debate has highlighted limitations unique to the practice of EBM that must be considered. For example, the need to develop new skills in seeking and appraising evidence cannot be underestimated. The need to develop and apply these skills within the time constraints of our clinical practice must be also addressed.

This book attempts to tackle these limitations and offers potential solutions. For example, EBM skills can be acquired at any stage in clinical training, and members of clinical teams at various stages of training can collaborate by sharing the searching and appraising tasks. Incorporating the acquisition of these skills into grand rounds, as well as postgraduate and undergraduate seminars, integrates them with the other skills being developed in these settings. These strategies are discussed at length on pages 239–300. Important developments to help overcome the limited time and resources include the growing numbers of evidence-based journals and evidence-based summary services. These are discussed throughout the book and in detail on pages 35–65. Indeed, one of the goals of this edition of the book is to provide tips and tools for practising EBM in "real time." We encourage readers to use the website to let us know about ways in which they've managed to meet the challenges of practising EBM in real time.

How is this resource organized?

The overall package is designed to help practitioners from any health care discipline learn how to practise evidence-based health care. Thus, although the book is written within the perspectives of internal medicine and general practice, the website provides clinical scenarios, questions, searches, critical appraisals, and evidence summaries from other disciplines, permitting readers to apply the strategies and tactics of evidence-based practice to any health discipline.

To those of you who want to become more proficient "doers" of EBM, we'd suggest that you take a look at Chapters 1 through 9 (pp. 19 to 300). To readers who want to become "users" of EBM, we'd suggest tackling Chapters 1 and 2 (pp. 19 to 65), focusing on question formulation, and matching those questions to the various evidence resources. We have also provided tips on practising EBM in real time throughout the book. With the move to an ebook, we have been able to incorporate many of the tools/tips/strategies directly in the discussion where they are relevant. We hope this makes it easier for you to use the materials, and we encourage you to use the online forum to let us know your thoughts and how this book can be more user friendly. Finally, for those interested in teaching the practice of EBM, we have dedicated Chapter 9 (pp. 239 to 300) to this topic.

The chapters and appendices that comprise this book constitute a traditional way of presenting our ideas about EBM. It offers the "basic" version of the model for practising EBM. To those who want more detailed discussion, we'd suggest you review some other resources.[91]

References

1. Evidence-based Medicine Working Group. Evidence-based medicine. A new approach to teaching the practice of medicine. JAMA 1992;268: 2420–5.

2. The Jama Network. Evidence Based Medicine: An Oral History 2014 [December 2016]. Available from: http://ebm.jamanetwork.com/.

3. The James Lind Library. Illustrating the development of fair tests of treatments in health care 2003 [December 2016]. Available from: http://www.jameslindlibrary.org/.

4. The James Lind Library. Search results for "streptomycin and tuberculosis" [December 2016]. Available from: http://www .jameslindlibrary.org/?s=streptomycin+and+tuberculosis.

5. Edwards P. 'A cabinet that looks like Canada:' Justin Trudeau pledges government built on trust. Toronto Star Newspaper; 2015 [December 2016]. Available from: https://www.thestar.com/news/canada/ 2015/11/04/new-government-to-be-sworn-in-today.html.

6. Malterud K, Bjelland AK, Elvbakken KT. Evidence-based medicine – an appropriate tool for evidence-based health policy? A case study from Norway. Health Res Policy Syst 2016;14(1):15.

7. Steckelberg A, Hulfenhaus C, Kasper J, Muhlhauser I. Ebm@school–a curriculum of critical health literacy for secondary school students: results of a pilot study. Int J Public Health. 2009;54(3):158–65.

8. Austvoll-Dahlgren A, Danielsen S, Opheim E, Bjorndal A, Reinar LM, Flottorp S, et al. Development of a complex intervention to improve health literacy skills. Health Info Libr J 2013;30(4):278–93.

9. Oxman A. Teaching children unbiased testing. Can Professor Fair help? Nuffield Department of Medicine; 2016 [December 2016]. Available from: http://www.ndm.ox.ac.uk/andy-oxman-teaching -children-unbiased-testing.

10. Spot On. Social Media for Science Outreach – A Case Study: A Twitter Journal Club. Springer Nature; 2013 [December 2016]. Available from: http://www.nature.com/spoton/2013/04/social-media-for-science -outreach-a-case-study-a-twitter-journal-club/.

11. BMJ Blogs. EBN Twitter Journal Club – How to participate 2016 [December 2016]. Available from: http://blogs.bmj.com/ebn/ebn -twitter-journal-club/.

12. Covell DG, Uman GC, Manning PR. Information needs in office practice: are they being met? Ann Intern Med 1985;103:596–9.

13. Antman EM, Lau J, Kupelnick B, Mosteller F, Chalmers TC. A comparison of results of meta-analyses of randomised control trials and recommendations of clinical experts. JAMA 1992;268:240–8.

14. Oxman A, Guyatt GH. The science of reviewing research. Ann N Y Acad Sci 1993;703:125–34.

15. Davis D, O'Brien MA, Freemantle N, et al. Impact of formal continuing medical education. JAMA 1999;282:867–74.

16. Haynes RB. Where's the meat in clinical journals [editorial]. ACP J Club 1993;119:A–22–3.

17. Evans CE, Haynes RB, Birkett NJ, et al. Does a mailed continuing education program improve clinician performance? Results of a randomised trial in antihypertensive care. JAMA 1986;255:501–4.

18. Sackett DL, Haynes RB, Taylor DW, Gibson ES, Roberts RS, Johnson AL. Clinical determinants of the decision to treat primary hypertension. Clin Res 1977;24:648.

19. Sackett DL, Straus SE. Finding and applying evidence during clinical rounds: the "evidence cart." JAMA 1998;280:1336–8.

20. Sackett DL. Using evidence-based medicine to help physicians keep up-to-date. Serials 1997;9:178–81.

21. Shah BR, Mamdani M, Jaakkimainen L, Hux JE. Risk modification for diabetic patients. Can J Clin Pharmacol 2004;11:239–44.

22. Pimlott NJ, Hux JE, Wilson LM, et al. Educating physicians to reduce benzodiazepine use by elderly patients. CMAJ 2003;168:835–9.

23. Kennedy J, Quan H, Ghali WA, Feasby TE. Variations in rates of appropriate and inappropriate carotid endarterectomy for stroke prevention in 4 Canadian provinces. CMAJ 2004;171:455–9.

24. Haynes RB, Cotoi C, Holland J, et al. Second-order peer review of the medical literature for clinical practitioners. JAMA 2006;295:1801–8.

25. Glasziou P, Altman DG, Bossuyt P, Boutron I, Clarke M, Julious S, et al. Reducing waste from incomplete or unusable reports of biomedical research. Lancet 2014;383(9913):267–76.

26. Macleod MR, Michie S, Roberts I, Dirnagl U, Chalmers I, Ioannidis JP, et al. Biomedical research: increasing value, reducing waste. Lancet 2014;383(9912):101–4.

27. Effective practice and organization of care group. The Cochrane Library. Wiley; 2009.

28. McAlister FA, Graham I, Karr GW, Laupacis A. Evidence-based medicine and the practicing clinician: a survey of Canadian general internists. J Gen Intern Med 1999;14:236–42.

29. McColl A, Smith H, White P, Field J. General practitioners' perceptions of the route to evidence-based medicine: a questionnaire survey. BMJ 1998;316:361–5.

30. Parve S, Ershadi A, Karimov A, Dougherty A, Ndhlovu CE, Chidzonga MM, et al. Access, attitudes and training in information technologies and evidence-based medicine among medical students at University of Zimbabwe College of Health Sciences. Afr Health Sci 2016;16(3): 860–5.

31. Shehata GM, Zaki A, Dowidar NL, El Sayed I. Critical thinking and attitude of physicians toward evidence-based medicine in Alexandria, Egypt. J Egypt Public Health Assoc 2015;90(3):115–20.

32. Hisham R, Liew SM, Ng CJ, Mohd Nor K, Osman IF, Ho GJ, et al. Rural Doctors' Views on and Experiences with Evidence-Based Medicine: The FrEEDoM Qualitative Study. PLoS ONE 2016;11(3): e0152649.

33. Young JM, Glasziou P, Ward J. General practitioners' self ratings of skills in evidence based medicine: validation study. BMJ 2002;324: 950–1.

34. Sekimoto M, Imanaka Y, Kitano N, et al. Why are physicians not persuaded by scientific evidence? BMC Health Serv Res 2006;6:92.

35. Rashidbeygi M, Sayehmiri K. Knowledge and attitudes of physicians towards evidence based medicine in Ilam, Iran. Iran Red Crescent Med J 2013;15(9):798–803.

36. Ulvenes LV, Aasland O, Nylenna M, Kristiansen IS. Norwegian physicians' knowledge of and opinions about evidence-based medicine: cross-sectional study. PLoS ONE 2009;4(11):e7828.

37. Heselmans A, Donceel P, Aertgeerts B, Van de Velde S, Ramaekers D. The attitude of Belgian social insurance physicians towards evidence-based practice and clinical practice guidelines. BMC Fam Pract 2009; 10:64.

38. Hisham R, Ng CJ, Liew SM, Hamzah N, Ho GJ. Why is there variation in the practice of evidence-based medicine in primary care? A qualitative study. BMJ Open 2016;6(3):e010565.

39. Deshpande N, Publicover M, Gee H, Khan KS. Incorporating the views of obstetric clinicians in implementing evidence-supported labour and delivery suite ward rounds: a case study. Health Info Libr J 2003; 20(2):86–94.

40. Ellis J, Mulligan I, Rowe J, Sackett DL. Inpatient general medicine is evidence based. Lancet 1995;346:407–10.

41. Geddes JR, Game D, Jenkins NE, Peterson LA, Pottinger GR, Sackett DL. In-patient psychiatric care is evidence-based. Proceedings of the Royal College of Psychiatrists Winter Meeting, Stratford, UK, January 23–25, 1996.

42. Howes N, Chagla L, Thorpe M, McCulloch P. Surgical practice is evidence based. Br J Surg 1997;84:1220–3.

43. Kenny SE, Shankar KR, Rintala R, Lamont GL, Lloyd DA. Evidence-based surgery: interventions in a regional paediatric surgical unit. Arch Dis Child 1997;76:50–3.

44. Gill P, Dowell AC, Neal RD, Smith N, Heywood P, Wilson AE. Evidence based general practice: a retrospective study of interventions in one training practice. BMJ 1996;312:819–21.

45. Moyer VA, Gist AK, Elliott EJ. Is the practice of pediatric inpatient medicine evidence-based? J Paediatr Child Health 2002;38:347–51.

46. Waters KL, Wiebe N, Cramer K, et al. Treatment in the pediatric emergency department is evidence based: a retrospective analysis. BMC Pediatr 2006;6:26.

47. Lai TY, Wong VW, Leung GM. Is ophthalmology evidence based? Br J Ophthalmol 2003;87:385–90.

48. Ilic D, Nordin RB, Glasziou P, Tilson JK, Villanueva E. A randomised controlled trial of a blended learning education intervention for teaching evidence-based medicine. BMC Med Educ 2015;15:39.

49. Cheng HM, Guo FR, Hsu TF, Chuang SY, Yen HT, Lee FY, et al. Two strategies to intensify evidence-based medicine education of undergraduate students: a randomised controlled trial. Ann Acad Med Singapore 2012;41(1):4–11.

50. Ilic D, Hart W, Fiddes P, Misso M, Villanueva E. Adopting a blended learning approach to teaching evidence based medicine: a mixed methods study. BMC Med Educ 2013;13:169.

51. Johnston JM, Schooling CM, Leung GM. A randomised-controlled trial of two educational modes for undergraduate evidence-based medicine learning in Asia. BMC Med Educ 2009;9(1):63. doi:10.1186/1472-6920-9-63.

52. Sanchez-Mendiola M, Kieffer-Escobar LF, Marin-Beltran S, Downing SM, Schwartz A. Teaching of evidence-based medicine to medical students in Mexico: a randomized controlled trial. BMC Med Educ 2012;12:107.

53. Ilic D, Maloney S. Methods of teaching medical trainees evidence-based medicine: a systematic review. Med Educ 2014;48(2):124–35.

54. Walczak J, Kaleta A, Gabrys E, Kloc K, Thangaratinam S, Barnfield G, et al. How are "teaching the teachers" courses in evidence based medicine evaluated? A systematic review. BMC Med Educ 2010;10:64.

55. Ahmadi N, McKenzie ME, Maclean A, Brown CJ, Mastracci T, McLeod RS. Teaching evidence based medicine to surgery residents-is journal club the best format? A systematic review of the literature. J Surg Educ 2012;69(1):91–100.

56. Ilic D, Nordin RB, Glasziou P, Tilson JK, Villanueva E. Development and validation of the ACE tool: assessing medical trainees' competency in evidence based medicine. BMC Med Educ 2014; 14:114.

57. Maloney S, Nicklen P, Rivers G, Foo J, Ooi YY, Reeves S, et al. A Cost-Effectiveness Analysis of Blended Versus Face-to-Face Delivery of Evidence-Based Medicine to Medical Students. J Med Internet Res 2015;17(7):e182.

58. Ilic D, Tepper K, Misso M. Teaching evidence-based medicine literature searching skills to medical students during the clinical years: a randomized controlled trial. J Med Libr Assoc 2012;100(3): 190–6.

59. Kulier R, Gulmezoglu AM, Zamora J, Plana MN, Carroli G, Cecatti JG, et al. Effectiveness of a clinically integrated e-learning course in evidence-based medicine for reproductive health training: a randomized trial. JAMA 2012;308(21):2218–25.

60. Rohwer A, Young T, van Schalkwyk S. Effective or just practical? An evaluation of an online postgraduate module on evidence-based medicine (EBM). BMC Med Educ 2013;13:77.

61. Bradley P, Oterholt C, Herrin J, Nordheim L, Bjorndal A. Comparison of directed and self-directed learning in evidence-based medicine: a randomised controlled trial. Med Educ 2005;39(10):1027–35.

62. Ahmadi SF, Baradaran HR, Ahmadi E. Effectiveness of teaching evidence-based medicine to undergraduate medical students: a BEME systematic review. Med Teach 2015;37(1):21–30.

63. Khader YS, Batayha W, Al-Omari M. The effect of evidence-based medicine (EBM) training seminars on the knowledge and attitudes of medical students towards EBM. J Eval Clin Pract 2011;17(4):640–3.

64. Al Achkar M, Davies MK. A small group learning model for evidence-based medicine. Adv Med Educ Pract 2016;7:611–15.

65. Lewis LK, Wong SC, Wiles LK, McEvoy MP. Diminishing Effect Sizes with Repeated Exposure to Evidence-Based Practice Training in Entry-Level Health Professional Students: A Longitudinal Study. Physiother Can 2016;68(1):73–80.

66. Friederichs H, Marschall B, Weissenstein A. Practicing evidence based medicine at the bedside: a randomized controlled pilot study in undergraduate medical students assessing the practicality of tablets, smartphones, and computers in clinical life. BMC Med Inform Decis Mak 2014;14(1):113.

67. Young T, Rohwer A, Volmink J, Clarke M. What are the effects of teaching evidence-based health care (EBHC)? Overview of systematic reviews. PLoS ONE 2014;9(1):e86706.

68. Parkes J, Hyde C, Deeks J, Milne R. Teaching critical appraisal skills in health care settings. Cochrane Database Syst Rev 2001;(3):Art. No.: CD001270, doi:10.1002/14651858.CD001270.

69. Greenhalgh T, Douglas HR. Experiences of general practitioners and practice nurses of training courses in evidence-based health care: a qualitative study. Br J Gen Pract 1999;49:536–40.

70. Rosenberg W, Deeks J, Lusher A, et al. Improving searching skills and evidence retrieval. J R Coll Physicians Lond 1998;328:557–63.

71. Agoritsas T, Iserman E, Hobson N, Cohen N, Cohen A, Roshanov PS, et al. Increasing the quantity and quality of searching for current best evidence to answer clinical questions: protocol and intervention design of the MacPLUS FS Factorial Randomized Controlled Trials. Implement Sci 2014;9:125.

72. Bath-Hextall F, Wharrad H, Leonardi-Bee J. Teaching tools in evidence based practice: evaluation of reusable learning objects (RLOs) for learning about meta-analysis. BMC Med Educ 2011;11:18.

73. Taylor RS, Reeves BC, Ewings PE, Taylor RJ. Critical appraisal skills training for health care professionals: a randomised controlled trial. BMD Med Educ 2004;4:30.

74. Bradley P, Oterhold C, Herrin J, et al. Comparison of directed and self-directed learning in evidence-based medicine: a randomised controlled trial. Med Educ 2005;39:1027–35.

75. Johnston J, Schooling CM, Leung GM. A randomised controlled trial of two educational modes for undergraduate evidence-based medicine learning in Asia. BMC Med Educ 2009;9:63.

76. Shnval K, Berkovits E, Netzer D, et al. Evaluating the impact of an evidence-based medicine educational intervention on primary care

doctors' attitudes, knowledge and clinical behaviour: a controlled trial and before and after study. J Eval Clin Pract 2007;13:581–98.

77. Dizon JM, Grimmer-Somers K, Kumar S. Effectiveness of the tailored Evidence Based Practice training program for Filipino physical therapists: a randomized controlled trial. BMC Med Educ 2014; 14:147.

78. Straus SE, Ball C, Balcombe N, Sheldon J, McAlister FA. Teaching evidence-based medicine skills can change practice in a community hospital. J Gen Intern Med 2005;20(4):340–3.

79. Kim S, Willett LR, Murphy DJ, et al. Impact of an evidence-based medicine curriculum on resident use of electronic resources. J Gen Intern Med 2008;23:1804–8.

80. Mitchell JB, Ballard DJ, Whisnant JP, Ammering CJ, Samsa GP, Matchar DB. What role do neurologists play in determining the costs and outcomes of stroke patients? Stroke 1996;27:1937–43.

81. Wong JH, Findlay JM, Suarez-Almazor ME. Regional performance of carotid endarterectomy appropriateness, outcomes and risk factors for complications. Stroke 1997;28:891–8.

82. Kersten HB, Frohna JG, Giudice EL. Validation of an Evidence-Based Medicine Critically Appraised Topic Presentation Evaluation Tool (EBM C-PET). J Gradu Med Educ 2013;5(2):252–6.

83. Tilson JK. Validation of the modified Fresno test: assessing physical therapists' evidence based practice knowledge and skills. BMC Med Educ 2010;10:38.

84. Lewis LK, Williams MT, Olds TS. Development and psychometric testing of an instrument to evaluate cognitive skills of evidence based practice in student health professionals. BMC Med Educ 2011;11:77.

85. Shaneyfelt T, Baum KD, Bell D, et al. Instruments for evaluating education in evidence-based practice. JAMA 2006;296:1116–27.

86. Straus SE, Tetroe J, Graham ID. Defining knowledge translation. CMAJ 2009;181:165–8.

87. McKibbon KA, Lokker C, Wilczynski NL, Ciliska D, Dobbins M, Davis DA, et al. A cross-sectional study of the number and frequency of terms used to refer to knowledge translation in a body of health literature in 2006: a Tower of Babel? Implement Sci 2010;5:16.

88. Straus SE, McAlister FA. Evidence-based medicine: a commentary on common criticisms. CMAJ 2000;163:837–41.

89. Straus SE, Glasziou P, Haynes RB, Dickersin K, Guyatt GH. Misunderstandings, misperceptions and mistakes. ACP J Club 2007;146:A8.

90. Maynard A. Evidence-based medicine: an incomplete method for informing treatment choices. Lancet 1997;349:126–8.

91. Guyatt G, Rennie D, Meade M, Cook DJ, editors. Users' guides to the medical literature. A manual for evidence-based clinical practice. 3rd ed. Chicago: AMA Press; 2015.

1 Asking answerable clinical questions

As noted in the Introduction, as we care for patients, we will often need new health care knowledge to inform our decisions and actions.[1-4] Our learning needs can involve several types of useful knowledge and can range from simple and readily available to complex and much harder to find. In this chapter, we describe strategies for the first step in meeting these knowledge needs: asking clinical questions that are answerable with evidence from clinical care research. We will start with a patient encounter to remind us how clinical questions arise and to show how they can be used to initiate evidence-based clinical learning. We will also introduce some teaching tactics that can help us coach others to develop their questioning skills.

Clinical scenario

You've just begun a month as the attending physician supervising residents and students on a hospital medicine inpatient service. You join the team on rounds after they've finished admitting a patient. The patient is a 36-year-old woman admitted for episodes of chest discomfort and fatigue with exertion over the last several months. She has not seen a doctor after the birth of her second child 17 years ago, and she knows of no prior health conditions. Examination shows striking central cyanosis; pronounced clubbing of all fingers and toes; late systolic heave of right sternum; a loud, widely split S2; and a grade III/VI midsystolic murmur over the pulmonic area. Tests show elevated levels of blood hemoglobin and decreased oxygen partial pressure and saturation. Echocardiography shows a 7-mm secundum defect in the interatrial septum, with enlarged right atrium and ventricle, and signs of severe pulmonary hypertension and right-to-left shunting.

You ask your team for their questions about important pieces of medical knowledge they'd like to have to provide better care for this patient. What do you expect they would ask? What questions occur to you about this patient? Write the first three of your questions in the boxes on the next page:

1.

2.

3.

The team's medical students asked several questions, including these three:

a. What normal developmental process has gone awry to cause this patient's septal defect?

b. How does cyanosis develop in patients with hypoxemia?

c. What is clubbing, and what are its possible causes?

The team's house officers also asked several questions, including these three:

a. Among adults found to have atrial septal defect, does the presence of the right-to-left shunt and Eisenmenger syndrome portend a worse prognosis, compared with patients in whom this has not occurred?

b. For adults found to have atrial septal defect complicated by Eisenmenger syndrome, is surgical repair of the septal defect associated with enough improvement in symptoms, health-related quality of life, disease measures, or mortality to be worth its potential harmful effects and costs?

c. For adults with severe hypoxemia and secondary polycythemia resulting from cyanotic congenital heart disease, is long-term supplementation with low-flow oxygen associated with enough improvement in symptoms, health-related quality of life, disease measures (e.g., blood counts), or mortality to be worth its potential adverse effects and costs?

Background and foreground questions

Note that the students' questions concern general knowledge that would help them understand cyanosis or clubbing as a finding or atrial septal defect as a disorder. Such "background" questions can be asked about any disorder or health state, a test, a treatment or intervention, or other aspect of health care and can encompass biological, psychological, or sociologic phenomena.[5] When well formulated, such background questions usually have two components (Box 1.1):

a. A question root (who, what, when, where, how, why) with a verb.

b. An aspect of the condition or thing of interest.

Note that the house officers' questions concern specific knowledge that could directly inform one or more "foreground" clinical decisions they face with this patient, including a broad range of biological, psychological, and sociologic issues. When well built, such foreground questions usually have four components[6,7] (see Box 1.1):

a. The patient situation, population, or problem of interest.

b. The main intervention, defined very broadly, including an exposure, a diagnostic test, a prognostic factor, a treatment, a patient perception, and so forth

c. A comparison intervention or exposure (also defined very broadly), if relevant.

d. The clinical outcome(s) of interest, including a time horizon, if relevant.

Go back to the three questions you wrote down about this patient. Are they background questions or foreground questions? Do your background questions specify two components (root with verb and condition), and do your foreground questions contain three or four components (patient/problem, intervention, comparison, and outcomes)? If not, try rewriting them to include these components, and consider

---

Box 1.1 Well-built clinical questions

"Background" questions

Ask for general knowledge about a condition, test, or treatment
  Have two essential components:
1. A question root (who, what, where, when, how, why) and a verb.
2. A disorder, test, treatment, or other aspect of health care.

Examples:

"How does heart failure cause pleural effusions?"
"What causes swine flu?"

"Foreground" questions

Ask for specific knowledge to inform clinical decisions or actions
  Have four essential components:
1. P: Patient, population, predicament, or problem.
2. I: Intervention, exposure, test, or other agent.
3. C: Comparison intervention, exposure, test, and so on, if relevant.
4. O: Outcomes of clinical importance, including time, when relevant.

Example:

"In adults with heart failure and reduced systolic function, would adding the implantation of an electronic resynchronization device to standard therapy reduce morbidity or mortality enough over 3 to 5 years to be worth the potential additional harmful effects and costs?"

---

whether these revised questions come closer to asking what you really want to know.

As clinicians, we all have needs for both background and foreground knowledge, in proportions that vary over time and that depend primarily on our experience with the particular disorder at hand (Fig. 1.1). When our experience with the condition is limited, as at point "A" (like a beginning student), the majority of our questions (shown in the figure by the vertical dimension) might be about background knowledge. As we grow in clinical experience and responsibility, such as at point "B" (like a house officer), we'll have increasing proportions of questions about the foreground of managing patients. Further experience with the condition puts us at point "C" (like a consultant), where most of our questions will be foreground questions. Note that the diagonal line is placed to show that we're never too green to learn foreground knowledge, nor too experienced to outlive the need for background knowledge.

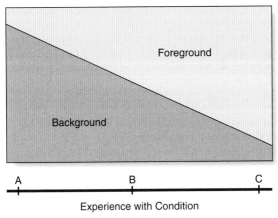

Fig. 1.1 Knowledge needs depend on experience with condition.

Our reactions to knowing and to not knowing

Clinical practice demands that we use large amounts of both background and foreground knowledge, whether or not we're aware of their use. These demands and our awareness come in three combinations we'll examine here. First, our patient's predicament may call for knowledge we know we already possess, so we will experience the reinforcing mental and emotional responses termed "cognitive resonance" as we apply the knowledge in clinical decisions. Second, we may realize that our patient's illness calls for knowledge we don't possess, and this awareness brings the mental and emotional responses termed "cognitive dissonance" as we confront what we don't know but need. Third, our patient's predicament might call upon knowledge we don't have, yet these gaps may escape our attention, so we don't know what we don't know, and we carry on in undisturbed ignorance. (We'll return to this third situation in Chapter 2, where we'll introduce strategies to regularly strengthen and update our knowledge of current best evidence.)

Reflect for a moment on how you've learned to react to the first two situations noted above. When teachers asked questions to which you knew the answers, did you learn to raise your hand to be called upon to give the answers? We did, and so did virtually all of our learners, and

23

in the process, we've learned that teachers and examinations reward us for already knowing the answer. When teachers asked questions to which you didn't know the answers, did you learn to raise your hand to be called upon and say, "I don't know this, but I can see how useful it would be to know, and I'm ready to learn it today"? Didn't think so, and neither did we or our learners, so in the process, we've all learned that teachers and examinations do not reward us for showing our ignorance and being ready and willing to learn. And although in the short run, hiding our ignorance in the classroom may have proved useful, in the long run, it becomes maladaptive in clinical practice if we continue to try to hide our knowledge gaps from ourselves and avoid learning, for it will be our patients who will pay the price.

These situations of cognitive dissonance (we know that we don't know) can become powerful motivators for learning, if handled well, such as by celebrating the finding of knowledge needs and by turning the "negative space" of knowledge gaps into the "positive space" of well-built clinical questions and learning how to find the answers.[8,9] Unfortunately, if handled less well, our cognitive dissonance might lead us to less adaptive behaviours, such as trying to hide our deficits, or by reacting with anger, fear, or shame.[10] By developing awareness of our knowing and thinking, we can recognize our cognitive dissonance when it occurs, recognize when the knowledge we need would come from clinical care research, and articulate the background or foreground questions we can use to find the answers.

Where and how clinical questions arise

Over the years, we've found that most of our foreground questions arise around the central issues involved in caring for patients (Box 1.2). These groupings are neither jointly exhaustive (other worthwhile questions can be asked) nor mutually exclusive (some questions are hybrids, asking about both prognosis and therapy, for example). Still we find it useful to anticipate that many of our questions will arise from common locations on this "map": clinical findings, etiology and risk, differential diagnosis, diagnostic tests, prognosis, therapy, prevention, patient experience and meaning, and self-improvement. We keep this list handy and use it to help locate the source of our knowledge deficits when we recognize the "stuck" feelings of our cognitive dissonance. Once we've recognized our knowledge gaps, articulating the questions can be done quickly, usually in 15 to 30 seconds.

Box 1.2 Central issues in clinical work, where clinical questions often arise

---

1. **Clinical findings**: how to properly gather and interpret findings from the history and physical examination.
2. **Etiology/risk**: how to identify causes or risk factors for disease (including iatrogenic harms).
3. **Clinical manifestations of disease**: knowing how often and when a disease causes its clinical manifestations and how to use this knowledge in classifying our patients' illnesses.
4. **Differential diagnosis**: when considering the possible causes of our patient's clinical problems, how to select those that are likely, serious, and responsive to treatment.
5. **Diagnostic tests**: how to select and interpret diagnostic tests, to confirm or exclude a diagnosis, based on considering their precision, accuracy, acceptability, safety, expense, and so on.
6. **Prognosis**: how to estimate our patient's likely clinical course over time and anticipate likely complications of the disorder.
7. **Therapy**: how to select treatments to offer our patients that do more good than harm and that are worth the efforts and costs of using them.
8. **Prevention**: how to reduce the chance of disease by identifying and modifying risk factors and how to diagnose disease early by screening.
9. **Experience and meaning**: how to empathize with our patients' situations, appreciate the meaning they find in the experience, and understand how this meaning influences their healing.
10. **Improvement**: how to keep up to date, improve our clinical and other skills, and run a better, more efficient clinical care system.

Over the years, we've also found that many of our knowledge needs occur around, or during, our clinical encounters with patients.[11,12] Although they often arise first in our heads, just as often they are voiced, at least in part, by our patients. For instance, when our patients ask, "What is the matter?" this relates to questions about diagnosis that are in our minds. Similarly, "What will this mean for me?" conjures both prognosis, and experience and meaning questions, whereas "What should be done?" brings up issues of treatment and prevention. No matter who initiates the questions, we count finding relevant answers as one of the ways we serve our patients, and to indicate this responsibility we call these questions "ours." When we can manage to do so, we find it helpful to negotiate explicitly with our patients about which questions should be addressed, in what order, and by when. And, increasingly, our patients want to work with us on answering some of these questions.

Practising evidence-based medicine in real time

Since our patients' illness burdens are large and our available time is small, we find that we usually have many more questions than time to answer them. For this circumstance, we'll recommend three strategies: capturing or saving, scheduling, and selecting.

First, because unsaved questions become unanswered questions, it follows that we need practical methods to rapidly capture and save questions for later retrieval and searching. Having just encouraged you to articulate your questions fully, it may surprise you that we recommend using very brief notations when recording questions on the run, using shorthand that makes sense to you. For instance, when we jot down "S3 DxT HF," we mean "Among adults presenting with dyspnea, how accurate is the clinical finding S3 gallop in confirming or excluding the diagnosis of congestive heart failure, compared with a reference standard?" Note that while the shorthand often has the P, I, C, and O (see Box 1.1) elements visible within it, it needn't always, as long as it reminds you what your question really was.

But how best to record these questions? Over the years, we've tried or heard of others trying several solutions:

1. Jotting brief notes on a blank letter—or A4—sized page with four columns predrawn, labelled "P," "I," "C," and "O," for each of the elements of foreground questions; this can be used by itself, or along with a separate sheet for questions about background knowledge (see Box 1.1).

2. Keying brief notes into a similarly arrayed electronic file on a desktop computer.

3. Jotting concise questions onto actual prescription blanks (and trying to avoid giving them to the patient instead of their actual prescriptions!).

4. Jotting shorthand notes onto blank 3 by 5 cards kept in our pocket.

5. Opening a smartphone app and writing or dictating our questions.

First, whenever we've timed ourselves, we find it takes us about 15 seconds to record our questions with an early generation handheld device,[13] about 5 to 15 seconds when recording on paper, and 4 to 10 seconds when dictating a question.

Second, by scheduling, we mean deciding by when we need to have our questions answered, in particular considering when the resulting decisions need to be made. Although integrated clinical care and information systems may improve to the point where our questions will be answerable at the time they arise, for most of us, this is not yet the case, and we need to be realistic in planning our time. With a moment of reflection, you can usually discern the few questions that demand immediate answers from the majority that can be scheduled to be answered later that day or at the next scheduled appointment.

Third, by selecting, we mean deciding which one or few of the many questions we asked, or could have asked, should be pursued. This decision requires judgement and we'd suggest you consider the nature of the patient's illness, the nature of your knowledge needs, the specific clinical decisions in which you'll use the knowledge, and your role in that decision process. Then, try this sequence of filters:

1

a. Which question is most important to the patient's well-being, whether biological, psychological, or sociologic?

b. Which question is most relevant to your/your learners' knowledge needs?

c. Which question is most feasible to answer within the time you have available?

d. Which question is most interesting to you, your learners, or your patient?

e. Which question is most likely to recur in your practice?

With a moment of reflection with these explicit criteria, you can usually select one or two questions that best pass these tests and will best inform the decisions at hand.

Why bother formulating questions clearly?

Our own experiences suggest that well-formulated questions can help in seven ways:

1. They help us focus our scarce learning time on evidence that is directly relevant to our patients' clinical needs.

2. They help us focus our scarce learning time on evidence that directly addresses our particular knowledge needs, or those of our learners.

3. They can suggest high-yield search strategies.

4. They suggest the forms that useful answers might take.

5. When sending or receiving a patient in referral, they can help us communicate more clearly with our colleagues.

6. When teaching, they can help our learners to better understand the content of what we teach while also modelling some adaptive processes for lifelong learning.

7. When our questions get answered, our knowledge grows, our curiosity is reinforced, our cognitive resonance is restored, and we can become better, faster, and happier clinicians.

In addition, the research we've seen so far suggests that clinicians who are taught this structured approach ask more specific questions,[14] undertake more searches for evidence,[15] use more detailed search methods, and find more precise answers.[16,17] In addition, when family doctors include a clinical question that is clearly articulated when they "curbside consult" with their specialty colleagues, they are more likely to receive an answer.[18] Some groups have begun to implement and evaluate answering services for their clinicians, with similarly promising initial results.[19,20] A randomized trial of one such service found that providing timely answers to clinical questions had a highly positive impact on decision making.[21]

Teaching the asking of answerable clinical questions

Good questions are the backbone of both practising and teaching evidence-based medicine (EBM), and patients serve as the starting point for both. Our challenge as teachers is to identify questions that are both patient based (arising out of the clinical problems of this real patient under the learner's care) and learner centred (targeting the learning needs of this learner). As we become more skilled at asking questions ourselves, we should also become more skilled in teaching others how to do so.

As with other clinical or learning skills, we can teach question asking powerfully by role modelling the formation of good questions in front of our learners. Doing this also lets us model admitting that we don't know everything, identifying our own knowledge gaps, and showing our learners adaptive ways of responding to the resulting cognitive dissonance. Once we've modelled asking a few questions, we can stop and describe explicitly what we did, noting each of the elements of good questions, whether background or foreground.

The four main steps in teaching clinical learners how to ask good questions are listed in Box 1.3. If we are to recognize potential questions in learners' cases, help them select the "best" question to focus on, guide

---

Box 1.3 Key steps in teaching how to ask questions for evidence-based medicine

1. **Recognize**: how to identify combinations of a patient's needs and a learner's needs that represent opportunities for the learner to build good questions.
2. **Select**: how to select from the recognized opportunities the one (or few) that best fits the needs of the patient and the learner at that clinical moment.
3. **Guide**: how to guide the learner in transforming knowledge gaps into well-built clinical questions.
4. **Assess**: how to assess the learner's performance and skill at asking pertinent, answerable clinical questions for practising EBM.

---

them in building that question well, and assess their question-building performance and skill, we need to be proficient at building questions ourselves. Moreover, we need several general attributes of good teaching, such as good listening skills, enthusiasm, and a willingness to help learners develop to their full potential. It also helps to be able to spot signs of our learners' cognitive dissonance, to know when and what they're ready to learn.

Teaching questions for EBM in real time

Note that teaching question-asking skills can be integrated with any other clinical teaching, right at the bedside or other site of patient care, and it needn't take much additional time. Modelling question asking takes less than a minute, whereas coaching learners on asking a question about a patient usually takes 2 to 3 minutes.

Once we have formulated an important question with our learners, how might we keep track of it and follow its progress toward a clinically useful answer? In addition to the methods for saving questions we mentioned earlier, one tactic we've used for teaching questions is the Educational Prescription, shown in Figure 1.2. This helps both teachers and learners in five ways:

1. It specifies the clinical problem that generated the questions.

2. It states the question with all of its key elements.

3. It specifies who is responsible for answering it.

4. It reminds everyone of the deadline for answering it (taking into account the urgency of the clinical problem that generated it).

5. Finally, it reminds everyone of the steps of searching, critically appraising, and relating the answer back to the patient.

R℞ Educational Prescription

| Patient's Name | Learner: |

3-part Clinical Question

Target Disorder:

Intervention (+/– comparison):

Outcome:

Date and place to be filled:

Presentations will cover:
1. search strategy;
2. search results;
3. the validity of this evidence;
4. the importance of this valid evidence;
5. can this valid, important evidence be applied to your patient;
6. your evaluation of this process.

Fig. 1.2 Educational Prescription form.

How might we use the Educational Prescription in our clinical teaching? The number of ways is limited only by our imagination and our opportunities for teaching. For instance, Educational Prescriptions have been incorporated into undergraduate medical education settings, particularly within clinical clerkships.[22,23] As we'll reinforce in the chapter on teaching (Chapter 9), Educational Prescriptions can be incorporated into familiar inpatient teaching settings from work rounds and attending/consultant rounds to morning report and noon conferences. They can also be used in outpatient teaching settings, such as ambulatory morning report.

Will you and your learners follow through on the Educational Prescriptions? You might, if you build the writing and "dispensing" of them into your everyday routine. One tactic we use is to make specifying clinical questions an integral part of presenting a new patient to the group. For example, we ask learners on our general medicine inpatient clinical teams, when presenting new patients, to tell us "31 things in 3 minutes" about each admission, although only the first 21 at the bedside. As shown in Box 1.4, the final element of their presentation is the specification of an important question to which they need to know the answer and don't. If the answer is vital to the immediate care of the patient, it can be provided at once by another member of the clinical team, perhaps by accessing some of the evidence synopsis resources you will learn more about in Chapter 2. Most of the time the answer can wait a few hours or days, so the question can serve as the start of an Educational Prescription.

Finally, we can ask our learners to write Educational Prescriptions for us. This role reversal can help in four ways:

1. The learners must supervise our question building, thereby honing their skills further.

2. The learners see us admitting our own knowledge gaps and practising what we preach.

3. It adds fun to rounds and sustains group morale.

4. Our learners begin to prepare for their later roles as clinical teachers.

Like most clinical skills, learning to ask answerable questions for EBM takes time, coaching, and deliberate practice.[24] Our experience suggests that after a brief introduction, it takes supervising our learners' practice and giving them specific feedback on their questions to help them develop proficiency. Others have found that providing a brief introduction alone may not be sufficient for learners to show proficiency.[25]

Box 1.4 A bedside patient presentation that includes an Educational Prescription

---

1. The patient's surname.
2. The patient's age.
3. When the patient was admitted.
4. The illness or symptom(s) that led to admission. For each symptom, mention:
   a. Where in the body it is located.
   b. Its quality.
   c. Its quantity, intensity, and degree of impairment.
   d. Its chronology: when it began, constant/episodic, progressive.
   e. Its setting: under what circumstances did it/does it occur.
   f. Any aggravating or alleviating factors.
   g. Any associated symptoms.
5. Whether a similar problem had happened previously. If so:
   a. How it was investigated.
   b. What the patient was told about its cause.
   c. How the patient had been treated for it.
6. Pertinent past history of other conditions that are of diagnostic, prognostic, or pragmatic significance and would affect the evaluation or treatment of the present illness.
7. How those other conditions have been treated.
8. Family history, if pertinent to present illness or hospital care.
9. Social history, if pertinent to present illness or hospital care.
10. The condition on admission:
    a. Acutely and/or chronically ill.
    b. Severity of complaints.
    c. Requesting what sort of help.
11. The pertinent physical findings on admission.

And, after leaving bedside and moving to a private location, finish with:

12. The pertinent diagnostic test results.
13. Your concise, one-sentence problem synthesis statement.
14. What you think is the most likely diagnosis ("leading hypothesis").
15. What few other diagnoses you're pursuing ("active alternatives").
16. The further diagnostic studies you plan to confirm the leading hypothesis or exclude active alternatives.
17. Your estimate of the patient's prognosis.
18. Your plans for treatment and counselling.
19. How you will monitor the treatment in follow-up.
20. Your contingency plans if the patient doesn't respond to initial treatment.
21. The Educational Prescription you would like to write for yourself, to better understand the patient's disorder (background knowledge), or how to care for the patient (foreground knowledge) so that you can become a better clinician.

That concludes this chapter on the first step in practising and teaching EBM: asking answerable clinical questions. Because you and your learners will want to move quickly from asking questions to finding their answers, our next chapter will address this second step in practising and teaching EBM.

References

1. Smith R. What clinical information do doctors need? BMJ 1996;313: 1062–8.

2. Dawes M, Sampson U. Knowledge management in clinical practice: a systematic review of information seeking behaviour in physicians. Int J Med Inf 2003;71(1):9–15.

3. Case DO. Looking for information: a survey of research on information seeking, needs, and behaviour. San Diego, CA: Academic Press; 2002.

4. Del Fiol G, Workman TE, Gorman PN. Clinical questions raised by clinicians at the point of care: a systematic review. JAMA Intern Med 2014;174(5):710–18.

5. Richardson WS. Ask, and ye shall retrieve [EBM Note]. Evid Based Med 1998;3:100–1.

6. Oxman AD, Sackett DL, Guyatt GH, for the Evidence-Based Medicine Working Group. Users' guides to the medical literature. I. How to get started. JAMA 1993;270:2093–5.

7. Richardson WS, Wilson MC, Nishikawa J, Hayward RSA. The well-built clinical question: a key to evidence-based decisions [Editorial]. ACP J Club 1995;123:A12–13.

8. Neighbour R. The inner apprentice: an awareness-centred approach to vocational training for general practice. Newbury, UK: Petroc Press; 1996.

9. Schon DA. Educating the reflective practitioner. San Francisco, CA: Jossey-Bass; 1987.

10. Claxton G. Wise-up: the challenge of lifelong learning. New York, NY: Bloomsbury; 1999.

11. Sackett DL, Straus SE. Finding and applying evidence during clinical rounds: the "Evidence Cart." JAMA 1998;280:1336–8.

12. Straus SE, Eisinga A, Sackett DL. What drove the Evidence Cart? Bringing the library to the bedside. J R Soc Med 2016;109(6):241–7.

13. Richardson WS, Burdette SD. Practice corner: Taking evidence in hand [Editorial]. ACP J Club 2003;138(1):A9–10.

1

14. Villanueva EV, Burrows EA, Fennessy PA, Rajendran M, Anderson JN. Improving question formulation for use in evidence appraisal in a tertiary care setting: a randomized controlled trial. BMC Med Inform Decis Mak 2001;I:4.

15. Cabell CH, Schardt C, Sanders L, Corey GR, Keitz SA. Resident utilization of information technology. J Gen Intern Med 2001;16(12): 838–44.

16. Booth A, O'Rourke AJ, Ford NJ. Structuring the pre-search interview: a useful technique for handling clinical questions. Bull Med Libr Assoc 2000;88(3):239–46.

17. Rosenberg WM, Deeks J, Lusher A, Snowball R, Dooley G, Sackett D. Improving searching skills and evidence retrieval. J R Coll Physicians Lond 1998;32(6):557–63.

18. Bergus GR, Randall CS, Sinift SD, Rosenthal DM. Does the structure of clinical questions affect the outcome of curbside consultations with specialty colleagues? Arch Fam Med 2000;9:541–7.

19. Brassey J, Elwyn G, Price C, Kinnersley P. Just in time information for clinicians: a questionnaire evaluation of the ATTRACT project. BMJ 2001;322:529–30.

20. Jerome RN, Giuse NB, Gish KW, Sathe NA, Dietrich MS. Information needs of clinical teams: analysis of questions received by the Clinical Informatics Consult Service. Bull Med Libr Assoc 2001;89(2):177–84.

21. McGowan J, Hogg W, Campbell C, Rowan M. Just-in-time information improved decision-making in primary care: a randomized trial. PLoS ONE 2008;3(11):e3785.

22. Nixon J, Wolpaw T, Schwartz A, Duffy B, Menk J, Bordages G. SNAPPS-Plus: An educational prescription for students to facilitate formulating and answering clinical questions. Acad Med 2014;89(8): 1174–9.

23. Umscheid CA, Maenner MJ, Mull N, Veesenmeyer AF, Farrar JT, Goldfarb S, et al. Using educational prescriptions to teach medical students evidence-based medicine. Med Teach 2016;38(11):1112–17.

24. Ericsson KA. Deliberate practice and the acquisition and maintenance of expert performance in medicine and related domains. Acad Med 2004;79(10):S1:S70–81.

25. Wyer PC, Naqvi Z, Dayan PS, Celentano JJ, Eskin B, Graham ML. Do workshops in evidence-based practice equip participants to identify and answer questions requiring consideration of clinical research? A diagnostic skill assessment. Adv Health Sci Educ Theory Pract 2009; 14:515–33.

2 Acquiring the evidence: How to find current best evidence and have current best evidence find us*

My students are dismayed when I say to them, "Half of what you are taught as medical students will in 10 years have been shown to be wrong. And the trouble is, none of your teachers knows which half."

Dr. Sydney Burwell, Dean of Harvard Medical School[1]

As Dr. Burwell's quote from over half a century ago (in 1956) indicates, medical knowledge evolves quite rapidly. In the past 2 decades, the pace has greatly accelerated because of the maturation of the spectrum of methods for biomedical research (from bench to bedside), and huge new investments in health care research of over US$120 billion per year.

Fortunately, the ways and means for clinicians to efficiently find current best evidence for clinical decisions have also advanced rapidly—so much so, that this chapter has had to be extensively rewritten, based on the innovations that occurred during the past 6 years since its predecessor. This is great news for us as clinicians and the patients we care for. Working through this chapter will bring us up to speed for becoming informed users of evidence-based resources—*resources for which much of the critical appraisal of evidence has already been done for us.*

One solution for the inherent problem of obsolescence of professional education is "problem-based learning" or "learning by inquiry." That is, when confronted by a clinical question for which we are unsure of the current best answer, we must develop the habit of looking for the current best answer as efficiently as possible. (Literary critics will point out the redundancy of the term "current best"—we risk their scorn to emphasize that last year's best answer may not be this year's.)

The success of learning by inquiry depends heavily on being able to find the current best evidence to manage pressing clinical problems, a task that can be either quick and highly rewarding or time consuming and frustrating. Which of these it is depends on several factors that we

---

*Disclaimer: The lead author for this chapter is Brian Haynes, who developed or contributed to many of the resources described herein.

can control or influence, including which questions we ask, how we ask these questions (see Ch. 1), how well we use information resources (the subject of this chapter), and how skilled we are in interpreting and applying these resources (detailed in the chapters that follow). We can learn a great deal about current best evidence sources from librarians and other experts in health informatics and should seek hands-on training from them as an essential part of our clinical education. This chapter provides adjunctive strategies for clinicians to use to find evidence quickly—including some that we may not learn from librarians—as well as to deal with evidence that finds us, bidden or unbidden.

Here, we consider finding preappraised evidence to help solve clinical problems about the treatment or prevention, diagnosis and differential diagnosis, prognosis and clinical prediction, cause, and economics of a clinical problem. "Preappraised evidence" resources for clinical decisions are built according to an explicit process that values research according to both its scientific merit ("hierarchy of evidence") and its readiness for use for clinical decisions ("Evidence-Based Health Care [EBHC] Pyramid 5.0," described within). The term "preappraised evidence" is emphasized here for three key reasons: if we (1) don't know how to critically appraise research evidence, (2) don't consistently apply the criteria, or (3) don't have the time to do our own detailed critical appraisal, then the best we can do is to look for answers in preappraised evidence resources. Only if we can't find what we want there would we need to tackle the harder task of searching larger bibliographic databases, such as MEDLINE, and applying the critical appraisal skills that are taught in this book.

This chapter provides an orientation to the types of preappraised evidence sources that exist today, followed by "raw" unappraised evidence services (e.g., MEDLINE). Then we'll track down the best evidence-based answers to specific clinical problems.

Orientation to evidence-based information resources: where to find the best evidence

Treat traditional textbooks as if they were long past their "best before" date

We begin with traditional medical textbooks (whether in print or online), only to dismiss them. If the pages of textbooks smelled like decomposing garbage when they became outdated, the nonsmelly bits could be useful because textbooks are often well organized for clinical review and much of their content could be current at any one time. Unfortunately, in traditional texts, there's often no way to tell what information is up to date and what is not or whether the information is evidence based or simply expertise based. Expertise is essential in authoring recommendations for clinical care, but it does not ensure that the recommendations are also "evidence based"—this chapter provides ways to determine whether the text we're reading is also evidence based. So, although we may find some useful information in texts about "background questions" (see p. 21), such as the pathophysiology of clinical problems, it is best not to use texts for seeking the answers to "foreground questions," such as the causal (risk) factors, diagnosis, prognosis, prevention, or treatment of a disorder, unless they are also transparently evidence based and up to date.

Here's a simple two-stage screening test to determine whether a text is likely to be evidence based and up to date:

2

Stage 1. A text that provides recommendations for patient care must cite evidence, with "in line" references that support each of its key recommendations about the diagnosis, treatment, or prognosis of patients.

Stage 2. If the text does indicate specific references for its recommendations, check the date of publication of the references; if the most recent is more than 2 to 3 years old, we will need to check whether more recent studies require a change in recommendation.

Texts that fail these two screens should be used for background reading only, no matter how eminent their authors.

Table 2.1 provides a more detailed set of guides for the ideal text resource for clinical practice. Note that these guides should be applied only to texts that are available online. Printed texts that include recommendations for tests and treatments simply cannot be reliably up to date because print production processes are too lengthy to keep pace with advancement of medical knowledge. Typically, it takes a year or more for print preparation before books begin shipping, and then the book continues to rot until the renewal process begins again, usually 2 to 5 years later.

That's not to say that online texts are current either, let alone reliably evidence based. Check out your favourites with the guides in Table 2.1. A text that scores less than 5 is definitely not "evidence based" and should be used, at most, for "background" information. Table 2.2 provides an evaluation of online medical texts in 2012, illustrating that a few texts exhibit a favourable profile. A second study assessed the top four texts from the 2012 study for the proportion of 200 topics that appeared

Table 2.1 Guides for judging whether an online clinical text is evidence based and current

Criterion	Rating	
"In-line references" for treatment recommendations	0	1
In line = references that are in the text next to individual declarations	None or few	Usually or always
"In-line references" for diagnostic recommendations	0	1
	None or few	Usually or always
Policy indicating steps by the editors/authors to find new evidence	0	1
Likely to be found in the "About" information concerning the text	Absent	Present
Policy indicating the quality rating of research evidence ("levels of evidence")	0	1
	Absent	Present
Policy indicating the grading of strength of recommendations ("grades of recommendations")	0	1
	Absent	Present
Date stamping of individual chapters	0	1
Should be at the beginning or end of each chapter	Absent	Present
Indication of a schedule for updating chapters	0	1
Should be at the start of each chapter or in "About"	Absent	Present
"New evidence" tabs for individual chapters/topics	0	1
Could be called "updates," "best new evidence," etc.	Absent	Present
User alerts for new evidence according to user discipline	0	1
	Absent	Present
Can users sign up for alerts for updates for specific disciplines (e.g., primary care; cardiology)?	0	1
	Absent	Present
User alerts for new evidence according to individual topic	0	1
	Absent	Present
Can users sign up for new evidence alerts for specific topics (e.g., diabetes; warts; hypertension)?	0	1
	Absent	Present
Metasearch of content and external evidence source	0	1
	Absent	Present
Simultaneous search of several identified evidence-based sources	0	1
	Absent	Present

© Health Information Research Unit, McMaster University. Contact: Brian Haynes, e-mail: bhaynes@mcmaster.ca.

to be out of date, that is, with newer studies available that had conclusions different from the recommendations in the text. The potential for updates (with 95% confidence interval [CI]) varied significantly with *DynaMed* having the fewest topics in arrears, at 23% (17% to 29%), then *UpToDate* at 52% (45% to 59%), and *Best Practice* at 60% (53% to 66%).[2]

Table 2.2 Evaluation* of online clinical texts

Text	Timeliness	Breadth	Quality
DynaMed	1	3	2
UpToDate	5	1	2
Micromedex	2	8	2
Best Practice	3	4	7
Essential Evidence Plus	7	7	2
First Consult	9	5	2
Medscape Reference	6	2	9
Clinical Evidence	8	10	1
ACP PIER	4	9	7
PEPID	N/A	6	10

Numbers in the table are ranks from 1 to 10, with 1 being the best.
*Prorok JC, Iserman EC, Wilczynski NL, Haynes RB. Quality, breadth, and timeliness of content updating of ten online medical texts: an analytic survey. *J Clin Epidemiol.* 2012 Dec;65(12):1289–95, with permission.

2

Any burning questions at this point? Here are three that you might have.

First, what about authority? If we added that as a criterion for rating a text, it could go along these lines: "Does the publication include a list of distinguished editors who are older white males with endowed chairs at prestigious institutions?" Just joking—but high-fidelity, explicit processes for finding, evaluating, incorporating, and updating evidence concerning the diagnosis, course, cause, prevention, treatment, and rehabilitation of health problems are more important than named academic chairs. It's not that expertise isn't important, but even if named chairs do connote expertise at some time in a person's career, the chair-holder is more likely to be renowned for the research he or she had done than for the care he or she provides currently or will be so subspecialized and out of touch with level of care provided by most frontline clinicians that his or her advice is likely to be of dubious value for handling all but the most complicated and arcane cases, which we would need to refer to a specialist in any event. We need to look at what's under the hood, not at the ornaments atop it. Authority must come from an explicit, robust evidence process.

Second, should traditional textbooks really be treated like garbage? They should—and not even recycled—they should be handled as dangerous waste. At this point, our publisher is probably getting edgy about where this discussion is heading, considering all the journals and textbooks it publishes, including this one. Fear not, any money saved from not purchasing traditional textbooks can be spent on ongoing subscriptions to evidence-driven sources of current best knowledge for clinical practice, so publishers will be rewarded if they invest in creating these.

Third, what's the alternative to traditional, expertise-based textbooks of medicine? Answer: Evidence-based, regularly updated, online texts and preappraised evidence services. Read on, as we head into the "EBHC Pyramid 5.0" (P5) territory of evidence-based resources.[3]

Take a "P5" approach to evidence-based information access

We can help ourselves to current best evidence for clinical questions and decisions by recognizing and using the most evolved evidence-based information services for the topics of interest to us and our patients. Figure 2.1 provides a five-level hierarchical structure ("EBHC Pyramid 5.0"), with original preappraised *studies* at the base, followed by *syntheses* or systematic reviews on the first higher level, *systematically derived recommendations* (guidelines), *synthesized summaries for clinical reference* (i.e., frequently updated online clinical texts), and, at the pinnacle, *systems* that link evidence-based recommendations with individual patients.

We should begin our search for best evidence by looking at the highest-level resource available for the problem that prompts our search. Typically, because systems are scarce and limited in scope at present, the first stop would be an evidence-driven, online textbook that meets many, preferably all, of the criteria in Table 2.1, so meriting the title of a synthesized summary for clinical reference. The details of why and how to go about this follow.

Systems

The ideal

A perfect evidence-based clinical information *system* would integrate and concisely summarize all relevant and important research evidence about a clinical problem and would automatically link, through an electronic medical record, a specific patient's circumstances to the relevant information. The information contained in the system would be based on an explicit review process for finding and evaluating new evidence as it is published and then reliably and promptly updating whenever important new, high-quality, and confirmatory or discordant research evidence becomes available. We would then consult—indeed, be prompted by—the system whenever the patient's medical record is reviewed.

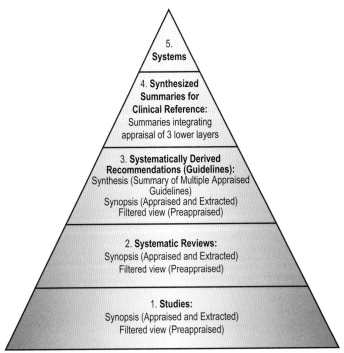

Fig. 2.1 Evidence-Based Health Care Pyramid 5.0 for finding preappraised evidence and guidance. (From Alper BS, Haynes RB. EBHC pyramid 5.0 for accessing preappraised evidence and guidance. *Evid Based Med*. 2016;21:123–125, with permission.)

Clinician and patient decisions would thereby always have the benefit of the current best evidence.

It is important to note that such a system would not tell the decision makers what to do. These judgements need to integrate the system's evidence with the patient's circumstances and wishes via their clinician's expertise.[4] The system's role would be to ensure that the cumulative research evidence concerning the patient's problem is immediately at hand. Further, to maximize speed of use, our first point of interaction would be a short *synopsis,* but links to *syntheses* and then to original *studies* would be provided so that we could drill down as deeply as needed to verify the accuracy, currency, applicability, and details of the synopsis.

The present state of evolution

Current systems don't reach this level of perfection as yet, but production models exist for parts of such systems. Electronic medical record systems with computerized decision support rules have been shown in randomized trials to improve the process and sometimes the outcomes of care.[5] Evidence-Based Medicine electronic Decision Support (EBMeDS) is now implemented at sites in several European countries and represents an operational prototype, assessed for process in a randomized controlled trial (RCT)[6] but as yet not evaluated for clinical impact. However, most systems cover a very limited range of clinical problems, are not consistently hard wired to current best evidence, and are mainly "homebuilt"; thus, they are not easily transferred to other practice settings. Further, more recent studies have suggested unanticipated adverse events associated with their implementation, highlighting the complexity of this issue. Thus, the jury is still out as to whether computerized decision support will be a panacea or even a net benefit for evidence-based care.

Synthesized summaries for clinical reference (online, evidence-driven, clinical textbooks)

Several robust *synthesized summaries of evidence* for individual clinical problems appear in Table 2.2. These have varying combinations of both background information and foreground evidence for clinical practice. Thus, they include information on the nature of the condition, the evidence concerning its management, and guidelines from various interested groups, along with the clinical expertise of the author of each topic. Ideally, their evidence will be up to date as readily verified by the date stamp at the top of each topic page and the dates of the articles that are cited, and fairly based on the evidence from the lower levels of the pyramid.

Twenty-two "evidence-based" texts were recently evaluated.[7] We look forward to many more such texts soon; but beware, these texts are in transition. It is important to check whether the systematic consideration of evidence promised in the title and introduction of these clinical references is actually delivered in the content. Unfortunately, the term "evidence-based" has been coopted to increase sales by many publishers and authors without the savvy or scruples to deliver honest evidence-based content. Thus, our first task in seeking synthesized summaries is to look for texts and websites that pass the screening tests above and the majority of the guides in Table 2.1, some of which are evaluated in Table 2.2.

Some Internet-based "aggregators" provide special "Pyramid 5.0" services for evidence-based information, with a single search running through multiple layers of the pyramid simultaneously. Look for these "meta-search" services toward the end of this chapter.

The *summary* publications mentioned here are but a few of those available today. If your discipline or clinical question isn't covered by them, consult with colleagues or check the Internet, putting "evidence-based" in the search line followed by your discipline (e.g., evidence-based surgery) or the clinical problem you are researching (e.g., evidence-based warts). Try it!

2

Systematically derived recommendations (evidence-based guidelines)

Systematically derived recommendations are similar to synthesized summary texts, but with a much narrower and sharper focus, for example, a single disease condition or even a special problem within a disease condition, such as diabetic nephropathy. Just as with summary texts, the principles of Table 2.1 can be applied. Most important, specific recommendations should cite the evidence in support, via systematic reviews conducted to address the specific questions that gave rise to the guidelines. Further, each recommendation should include a statement of the strength of the recommendation, for example, "strong" (most patients should receive the treatment) or "conditional" (clinicians should help patients decide on treatment concordant with their values), and the graded quality of the evidence on which this recommendation is made (e.g., "very low," "low," "moderate," or "high") in support. The evidence should be not only gathered systematically, but it should be graded systematically, for example, according to the GRADE process (Grading of Recommendations, Assessment, Development, and Evaluation; more about GRADE in Chapter 4 on Therapy).[8]

When conducted and reported this way, the strength of recommendations and the quality of evidence are often found to be "strange bedfellows." For instance, the recent American College of Rheumatology guidelines for therapy of rheumatoid arthritis[9] made 10 "strong" recommendations for treatment based on only "low" or at best "moderate" evidence. How could this be? The GRADE Working Group recommends that this not be done.[10] The arthritis experts made strong recommendations anyway. We seem to be in a transitional phase at present, where the experts and evidence are often not on common ground. Blame can be shared. The experts need to feel less empowered to make strong recommendations based on weak evidence. However, assuming that they did a thorough job of finding all strong evidence, there would appear to be many aspects of treating rheumatoid arthritis that researchers haven't reached yet. Indeed, given the complexity of current treatments for rheumatoid arthritis, it may be that researchers will never get to testing more than a fraction of them. This is a useful reminder of the limitations of both experts and evidence at present. Of importance, providing recommendations, each transparently connected with the best current evidence, is essential for informed, shared decision making.

Systematic reviews (syntheses)

If clinical summaries and guidelines have clearly and consistently addressed our clinical question, there is no need to look further. However, it takes time following publication of original articles to prepare clinical summaries and guidelines, and neither provides full details. So, if we want to be sure that the summary or guideline is up to date and complete enough in its details, then we'll need to look for more recent *systematic reviews* (aka syntheses) and original *studies.* Syntheses are based on exhaustive searches for evidence, explicit scientific reviews of the studies uncovered in the search, and systematic assembly of the evidence, often including meta-analysis, to provide as clear a signal as the accumulated evidence will allow about the effects of a health care intervention, diagnostic test, or clinical prediction guide. The Cochrane Collaboration provides the largest single source of syntheses, but only about 30% to 40% of the world's supply. Cochrane Reviews have mainly focused on preventive or therapeutic interventions to date, but the Cochrane Collaboration also summarizes diagnostic test evidence.

A key single source of preappraised syntheses is *EvidenceAlerts* (http://plus.mcmaster.ca/evidencealerts), a free service sponsored by EBSCO Health. *EvidenceAlerts* includes all Cochrane Reviews and systematic reviews from over 120 leading clinical journals. Another ready source of syntheses is Ovid's *Evidence-Based Medicine Reviews* (EBMR) service.

Additional reviews not available in the preceding sources are typically of lower quality and can be found in bibliographic databases, such as PubMed and EMBASE. For both of these, searches are likely to be more productive, with less "junk," using the "Clinical Queries" search strategy for "reviews." When articles are obtained by this route, the searcher must take on the responsibility for critical appraisal of the retrieved articles (as described in the rest of this book). More about this in the example later in this chapter.

Studies

It takes time to summarize new evidence; summaries, guidelines, and syntheses necessarily follow the publication of original *studies,* usually by at least 6 months, and sometimes by years. If every other "S" fails (i.e., no systems, summaries, systematically derived recommendations, or syntheses exist with clear answers to your question), then it's time to look for original studies.

Looking for scientifically sound and clinically relevant studies in full-text print journals (the classic way of keeping up-to-date) is generally hopeless, but preappraised studies can be retrieved relatively efficiently on the Internet in several ways. For example, several "evidence refinery" services are available. Most of these journal article critical appraisal services are organized according to a targeted range of clinical disciplines, such as general practice (*Essential Evidence Plus,* www.essentialevidenceplus.com; requires a subscription); primary care, internal medicine and subspecialties (*ACP Journal Wise,* http://journalwise.acponline.org/, a membership benefit of the American College of Physicians); general medicine and major specialties (*EvidenceAlerts*); nursing (*Nursing PLUS,* http://plus.mcmaster.ca/np, sponsored by the Health Information Research Unit, McMaster University); and rehabilitation sciences (*Rehab PLUS,* http://plus.mcmaster.ca/rehab, sponsored by the School of Rehabilitation Science, McMaster University). These services also provide "alerts" for newly published evidence according to the user's clinical discipline. Alerts are an important complement to searching for evidence: They help fill the gaps of "what you don't know and didn't think to ask" and "what you know that ain't so." Our recommendation is to subscribe and get to know the services that best match your professional evidence needs.

Synopsis

Closer inspection of Figure 2.1 reveals a subheading within the lower three levels of the pyramid: Synopsis. A synopsis is a somewhat rare but valuable, independently written abstract of a highly rated original study, synthesis, or guideline, and most readily available at present in *ACP*

Journal Club in *Annals of Internal Medicine, ACP JournalWise,* and Ovid's EBMR service.

Synopses of guidelines and syntheses are higher in the hierarchy (see Fig. 2.1) because guidelines and syntheses review all pertinent studies concerning an intervention, diagnostic test, prognosis, or etiology, whereas original studies describe just one research project.

Evidence-based meta-search services

It can be tedious and time consuming to work through texts and journal article services in sequence, so how about a service that runs our query through multiple sources and levels of evidence simultaneously? In fact, several online services offer various versions of one-stop shopping for evidence-based online texts, guidelines, syntheses, preappraised studies, synopses, and the broader medical literature. ACCESSSS (http://plus.mcmaster.ca/accessss) is based on the Pyramid 5.0 model and also provides simultaneous searching of PubMed via Clinical Queries, as well as PubMed using only the user's search terms. It also provides alerts of newly published evidence according to the user's clinical interests, for physicians, nurses, and rehab specialists (occupational/physical therapists [OT/PT]). Essential Evidence Plus (http://www.essentialevidenceplus.com/) and TRIP Database (https://www.tripdatabase.com/) provide variations on this theme.

General search engines

> **Warning**: we are now entering "do it yourself" appraisal territory!

For original publish-ahead-of-print (PAP) articles and reviews, MEDLINE is freely available (www.ncbi.nlm.nih.gov/PubMed), and the Clinical Queries (CQ) screen (available as a menu item on the main PubMed screen or directly at www.ncbi.nlm.nih.gov/entrez/query/static/clinical .html) provides detailed search filters that home in on clinical content for therapy, diagnosis, prognosis, clinical prediction, etiology, economics, and systematic reviews. Complex search strategies are embedded in the Clinical Queries screen, so we don't need to remember them. We can use the "sensitive" or "broad" search strategy if we want to retrieve every article that might be fit to bear on our question. Or we can use the "specific" or "narrow" search strategy if we want "a few good references" and don't have time to sort out the citations that are tainted or aren't on target. In either case, although the CQ filters improve the yield of high-quality, clinically relevant evidence, we must do our own critical appraisal of individual articles.

These search strategies can also be run in proprietary systems that include the MEDLINE database, such as Ovid and EBSCO, and in EMBASE. A complete listing of the search strategies for various access routes and databases appears on: http://hiru.mcmaster.ca/hiru/HIRU_Hedges_home.aspx.

If we still have no luck and the topic is, say, a new treatment (that one of our patients has asked about but we don't yet know much about …), then we can try Google (www.google.com). We can retrieve a product monograph in a few milliseconds … in which we'll find what the manufacturer of the treatment claims it can do along with detailed information on currently known adverse effects, contraindications, and prescribing. We can also retrieve open access summaries, for example, from Medscape's eMedicine, but these are not reliably evidence based or up to date. Many original studies and syntheses are also available via Google and Google Scholar, but the quick retrieval times for millions of documents is trumped by the burden of appraisal that is required to determine which of these documents accurately represents current best evidence. That said, Google is also the fastest way to get to almost any service on the Internet that we haven't "bookmarked" for our web browser, including all the ones named in this article that are web accessible: We just type in their proper names, and we'll likely "get lucky."

We end this section with two warnings. First, beware of "federated" or "enterprise" search engines provided by large publishers. These promote the publishers' products and have few or no markers for quality. Their prime "virtue" is retrieving a hoard of references instantly: Quantity is the enemy of quality in efficient evidence-based decision making.

Second, one of our colleagues, Ann McKibbon, found in a small study that it was not uncommon for physicians to change from a correct decision to a wrong decision about a clinical scenario following completion of a search—this was associated with the search engine used—in particular, Google was a likely contributor to wrong answers.

Organize access to evidence-based information services

It's worth emphasizing that all the resources just reviewed are available on the Internet. The added value of accessing these services on the Internet is considerable, including links to full-text journal articles, patient information, and complementary texts. To be able to do this, we need

47

to be in a location, such as a medical library, hospital or clinic, where all the necessary subscription licences have been obtained or, better still, have proxy server permission or remote access to a local computer from whatever organizations we belong to, whether it be a university, hospital, or professional organization, so that we can use these services wherever we access the Internet. A typical package of services for health professionals might include *Best Practice, Clinical Evidence, DynaMed, Evidence-Based Medicine Guidelines* (from Duodecim), and *UpToDate,* backed up by an Ovid collection of full-text journals and their Evidence-Based Medicine Reviews service.

Ask your university, professional school, hospital, or clinical librarian about which digital library licences are available and how you can tap into them. If you lack local institutional access, you may still be in luck, depending on the region in which you live. For example, some countries have national health libraries and have licensed access to the Cochrane Library. In addition, many professional societies provide access to some of the resources as membership benefits or at reduced rates.

Unfortunately, it isn't safe to assume that our institutions or professional societies will make evidence-based choices about the publications and services they provide. We should decide which services we need for our clinical work and then check to see if these have been chosen by our institution. If not, we'll need to consult with the librarian to make a case for the resources we want. When we do so, we'll need to be prepared to indicate what our library could give up, to keep its budget balanced. The easiest targets for discontinuation are high-priced, low-impact-factor journals, and it will be perceived as a whole lot less self-serving if we target publications in our own clinical discipline that are at the bottom end of the evidence-based ladder of evolution, rather than the high-priced favourite journals of our colleagues in other disciplines. A guide for which journals to select for several disciplines appears in an article by Ann McKibbon et al.[11]

If you live in a country with low resources, don't despair! The Health Internetwork Access to Research Information program (HINARI, www.healthInternetwork.net/) provides institutional access to a wide range of journals and texts at no or low cost, and *EvidenceAlerts* provides a free service to search for the best articles.

If you are on your own, have no computer, can't afford to subscribe to journals, but have access to a public library with a computer linked to the Internet, you're still in luck. Free access to high-quality evidence-based information abounds on the Internet, beginning with *EvidenceAlerts* for pre-appraised evidence, TRIP, and SUMsearch for metasearches (simultaneous searches of multiple evidence-based resources); and open-access journals, such as the *BMJ*, BioMed Central (www.biomedcentral.com/), and the Public Library of Science (www.PLOS.org/). Beware, however, that using free Internet services requires a commitment to finding and appraising information unless using the preappraised services. Free, high-quality evidence-based information is in much lower supply and concentration on the Internet than in the specialized, evidence preappraisal resources mentioned above. The reason is simple: It is much easier and cheaper to produce low-quality, rather than high-quality, information.

Is it time to change how you seek best evidence?

Compare the Pyramid 5.0 approach with how you usually seek evidence-based information. Is it time to revise your tactics? It may surprise you that MEDLINE (PubMed) is not listed as a resource for P5. This is because articles retrieved via PubMed are not "preappraised" for quality and clinical relevance, and searches typically retrieve many more "false" hits than true ones. Resources for finding preappraised evidence are a lot quicker and more satisfying for answering clinical questions if the features of your quest match those of one of the evolved services.

This is not to say MEDLINE is obsolete. MEDLINE continues to serve as a premier access route to the studies and reviews that form the foundation for all the other more specialized databases reviewed above, but the sound, clinically relevant articles in MEDLINE are a very tiny fraction of the mix. MEDLINE includes both the wheat and chaff of the health care scientific process, most of which is not ready for clinical consumption. Evidence-based clinical resources separate the wheat from the chaff (level 1 of P5) and bake "foods for thought" that are increasingly digestible and nourishing for clinical decisions as we find them higher on the pyramid.

Another way to think of organizing our information needs, proposed by Muir Grey, is "prompt, pull, push." "Prompt" corresponds to the highest P5 level *systems.* When we interact with an electronic patient record or an evidence-based diagnostic or pharmacy service, it ought to prompt us if a feature of our patient corresponds to an evidence-based care guideline that we haven't already incorporated into their care plan. As indicated above, such systems are not widely available at present, although this is beginning to change. "Pull" corresponds to the lower four levels of the P5 approach: We go searching to "pull" the evidence we need from available resources. "Push" refers to having evidence sent to us; controlling this is the subject of the next section.

To embrace the principles of evidence-based medicine, we need an operational plan for the regular use of *both* "push" and "pull" resources that are tailored as closely as possible to our own clinical discipline needs.

How to deal with the evidence that finds US ("push" evidence): keeping up to date efficiently

Cancel our full-text journal subscriptions

Trying to keep current with the knowledge base that is pertinent to our clinical practice by reading full-text journals is a hopeless task. From an evidence-based perspective, for a broad discipline, such as general practice or any major specialty (internal medicine, pediatrics, gynaecology, psychiatry, surgery), the number of articles we need to read to find just one article that meets basic criteria for quality and relevance ranges from 86 to 107 for the top five full-text general journals.[11] At, say, 2 minutes per article, that's about 3 hours to find one article ready for clinical action, and then the article may cover old ground or provide "me-too" evidence of yet-another statin or not be useful to us because of the way we have specialized our practice. We should trade in (traditional) journal subscriptions. That will save time but won't necessarily save money because we will need to invest in better resources for keeping current.

Invest in evidence-based journals and online evidence services

During the past few years, the Health Information Research Unit at McMaster University has collaborated with professional organizations and publishers to create several online services that "push" new, pre-appraised evidence to subscribers. Most of these services also archive evidence that can be "pulled" to provide best evidence concerning specific clinical questions. These services include *ACP Journal Wise*, *EvidenceAlerts*, *Nursing PLUS*, and *Rehab PLUS*, as well as, for more specialized interests, the *Optimal Aging Portal*, *Pain PLUS*, *Obesity PLUS*, and *Clot PLUS*, to name a few. For each of these, users sign up according to their clinical interests and then receive alerts to new studies that have been preappraised for scientific merit and clinical relevance. Relevance assessments are made by a voluntary international panel of physicians, nurses, and rehab practitioners. (If you are in independent clinical practice in medicine, nursing, or rehabilitation, you may wish to sign up as a rater: send an e-mail to: more@mcmaster.ca.) Similar services exist for other disciplines, and by other providers; use the Table 2.1 guides 3, 4, 9, and 10 to judge their credentials.

Periodicals, such as *ACP Journal Club*, summarize the best studies in traditional journals, making selections according to explicit criteria for scientific merit, providing structured abstracts and expert commentaries about the context of the studies and the clinical applicability of their findings.

For the most part, these evidence-based synopsis journals are targeted for generalists. However, subspecialty evidence-based journal clubs and books are sprouting on the web, such as *PedsCCM Evidence Based Journal Club* (http://pedsccm.org/journal-club.php) for pediatrics and a Twitter journal club for geriatrics (@GeriMedJC). Googling "evidence-based [your discipline or topic of choice]" is a way to find these resources. But don't forget to check the evidence-based credentials and currency of whatever you find with the appropriate items in Table 2.1.

2

Walking the walk: searching for evidence to solve patient problems

As in swimming, bicycle riding, alligator wrestling, and flame eating, the use of evidence-based information resources is best learned by examples and practice, not by didactic instruction alone. Commit yourself to paper on these matters for the problem below before you move on to the rest of the chapter:

1. The key question to seek an answer for (using the PICO(T) guidelines from pp. 19–29).

2. The best answer to the clinical problem that you currently have stored in your brain (being as quantitative as possible).

3. The evidence resources (both traditional and evolved) that you would consult to find the best current answers.

Clinical scenario

Mrs. JS, an accountant, is an overweight, 56-year-old white woman. She visits you in a somewhat agitated state. Her 54-year-old sister has recently died of a heart attack. Mrs. JS had missed her previous appointment 6 months ago ("tax time") and has not been at the clinic for

---

Continued

Clinical scenario—continued

over a year. Mrs. JS found some information on the Internet that allows her to calculate her own risk of having a heart attack in the future but she lacks some of the information needed to do the calculation, including her cholesterol levels and current blood pressure. She asks for our help in completing the calculation and our advice about reducing her risk.

She is currently trying to quit her smoking habit of 25 years. She is on a prescribed regimen of a calorie-restricted diet (with no weight loss in the past year) and exercise (she states about 20 minutes of walking once or twice a week, hampered by her osteoarthritis). Mrs. JS is accompanied by her husband on this visit, and he interjects that she is also taking vitamin E and beta-carotene to lower her risk for heart disease, based on a "health advisory" that Mr. JS read on the Internet. She has no other physical complaints at present but admits to being depressed since her sister's death. She specifically denies a previous heart attack or stroke.

On examination, Mrs. JS weighs 98 kg (216 lb), and her height is 172 cm (5′ 8″). Her blood pressure is 156/92 mm Hg measured on the left arm with a large adult cuff and repeated. The rest of her examination is unremarkable.

Looking through her previous visit notes, you observe that her blood pressure had been mildly elevated. You ask her about the risk calculator she found on the Internet, and she shows you the web page that she had printed out (http://www.cvriskcalculator.com/). You tell her that you will check out the web page as soon as you get a moment.

She warns you that she is not keen to consume prescription medications, preferring "natural remedies," but states that she is open to discussion, especially in view of her sister's death. She wants to know her risk of having a heart attack or stroke and just how much benefit she can expect from anything she can do for herself.

You enthusiastically recommend a heart-heathy diet, weight reduction, increased exercise, and especially quitting smoking. You tell her that you will be pleased to help her get the answers to her questions but will need to update her laboratory tests and have her return in 2 weeks to recheck her blood pressure, review her tests, and see how she is making out with your lifestyle recommendations. She is not very pleased about having to wait that long for her risk estimate but accepts your explanation.

Heeding a recent dictum from your clinic manager, you order a "lean and mean" minimalist set of laboratory tests: hemoglobin A_{1c}, lipid profile, creatinine, and electrocardiogram (ECG). These investigations show that Mrs. JS has an A_{1c} of 5.5% (normal range 4–6%); dyslipidemia, with total cholesterol 6.48 mmol/L (250 mg/dL; target <5.2 mmol/L, 200 mg/dL for primary prevention), low-density lipoprotein (LDL) 3.4 mmol/L (131 mg/dL), high-density lipoprotein (HDL) 0.9 mmol/L (34.7 mg/dL), and triglycerides 3.9 mmol/L (345 mg/dL; <1.7 mmol/L (150 mg/dL) desirable); and a normal ECG.

Write down the key questions that identify the evidence needed to give Mrs. JS clear answers about the cardiovascular risks from her condition and benefits from its treatments. Then indicate your best answers before searching (stick your neck out!), and select evidence resources that you feel will provide current best evidence to support your answers suited to this patient.

Questions:

Your initial answers:

Your proposed evidence resources:

2

At this point, you should have written down the key question(s), your top-of-the-head answer(s), and the evidence resources that you feel are best suited to answer these questions. Now would be a good time to try your hand at finding the answers by the routes you've selected, keeping track of how much time you spent, ease/aggravation, and money the searches cost, and how satisfied you are in the end. Put yourself under some time pressure: Summarize the best evidence you can find in 30 minutes or less for each question. (You may be thinking about skipping this exercise, hoping that the rest of this chapter will teach you how to do it effortlessly. But there is wisdom in the maxim "no pain, no gain." Invest at least 30 minutes of your time on at least one of the questions before you press on.)

As a teaching tip here, sometimes we give each member of our team a different evidence resource to search for the answer to the same clinical question. We find this to be an efficient and fun way of comparing and contrasting search strategies and evidence resources.

What follows is based on the general approach, described earlier in this chapter, to identifying and using key evidence-based resources. It is important to note that there may be more than one good route (not to mention a myriad of bad routes) and that as this book ages, better routes will certainly be built. Indeed, many improved resources have become available since publication of the fourth edition of this book in 2011, and such resources as *Best Practice, DynaMed,* and *UpToDate* have greatly matured. Thus, one of the foundations of providing efficient, evidence-based health care is keeping tabs on the availability, scope, and quality of new resources that are directly pertinent to our own professional practice.

If you have tried to search for evidence on these problems, compare what you did and what you found with our methods, reported below. If you haven't tried to search yet, we issue you a challenge: See if you can find better answers than we did (we searched in mid-2016, but we will applaud you for a better answer that you found after this time; we hope and expect that the evidence will keep improving).

Carrying out the searching steps

Basic steps for acquiring the evidence to support a clinical decision are shown in Figure 2.2. We've supplied the clinical problem and ask you to take the first step, defining the questions to be answered, following the lead on pages 19–29. Have a go at it if you haven't done so already.

Here's our try for the example above.

Problems

Hypertension, dyslipidemia, smoking, and related cardiovascular risk.

Asking answerable questions

On the basis of the information at hand, we posed several questions. First, from the patient's primary motivation for visiting, "In a 56-year-old female smoker with elevated blood pressure and dyslipidemia, but no history of coronary artery disease or stroke, what is the evidence concerning increased risk for cardiovascular complications?" Second, "Among such patients, do any medical interventions to control blood pressure and

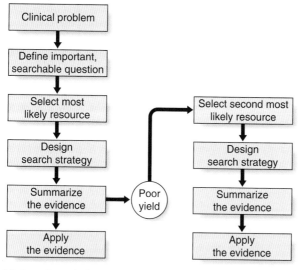

Fig. 2.2 General search strategy.

cholesterol or for smoking cessation reduce subsequent morbidity and mortality, compared with lesser levels of control?" Third, "Compared with placebo or no intervention, what is the evidence that beta-carotene and vitamin E supplements reduce cardiovascular risk among people who are at elevated cardiovascular risk but have not experienced cardiovascular events (i.e., primary prevention)?"

Selecting an evidence resource

Such a patient would often be seen in primary care and internal medicine specialties, so the focus of our search should be on the best and quickest evidence-based information sources for these clinical disciplines.

The first piece of information to consider in this case falls into the general category of "evidence that finds us." As in our case, patients often find information that they want us to comment on, and we need an efficient approach to evaluating the pedigree and evidence base for claims they encounter on the Internet or other media. This patient brought along a web page (http://www.cvriskcalculator.com/) that she had found through Google, so it was easy to examine this source. This website has an easy-to-use risk calculator and appears to have good credentials, combining recent evidence-based guidelines sponsored by the American College of Cardiology (ACC)/American Heart Association (AHA), the US Preventive Services Task Force (USPSTF), and the 2014 Joint National Commission evidence-based guidelines on the management of high blood pressure in adults. Online links are provided by the website to recently published, full-text, evidence-based reports from each of these organizations. This is not to say that the information on the website is necessarily either accurate or up to date, but it is more likely to be so than websites that lack these features. You breathe a sigh of relief for such an easy search.

According to the cardiovascular risk calculator, Mrs. JS has a substantial absolute risk (13.7%) of experiencing coronary heart disease (CHD) or stroke during the coming decade. The calculator allows us to modify the figures, monitoring our patient's status over time as test results change, and estimating the effect of interventions that alter the laboratory results and blood pressure. At this level of risk, the website recommends aspirin 81 mg daily for at least 10 years, a moderate to high intensity statin, and a thiazide diuretic, angiotensin-converting enzyme (ACE) inhibitor or calcium blocker. There is no recommendation about vitamin E or beta-carotene. Surprisingly, although smoking is included in her risk calculation, the treatment recommendations don't include stopping smoking, let alone any medical interventions to help do so.

Keeping our skeptic's hat on, we quickly checked *EvidenceAlerts* and found a study comparing five risk calculators, including the ACC/AHA risk calculator that the website is mainly based on.[12] In a cohort of people of mixed ethnicity followed for more than 10 years, all calculators overestimated the observed cardiovascular event rates, with the overestimates ranging from 25% to 115%! The authors speculate that this could be caused by the calculators being derived from ancient cohorts, such as Framingham, when fewer treatments were available for hypertension and dyslipidemia. In other words, it seems that the calculators are out of date. But if so, Mrs. JS isn't on any "modern treatments," so the risk calculation might apply. In any event, we should be careful in telling her about her calculated risk, while we look elsewhere for evidence to support intervention with the treatments recommended by the website, as well as for smoking.

Where to find the best evidence on interventions

The intervention question we posed was: "Among such patients, do medical interventions for high blood pressure and cholesterol and to stop smoking reduce subsequent morbidity and mortality?" Using the

Pyramid 5.0 approach, we began with a simple search in ACCESSSS, a "meta-" search engine that simultaneously searches multiple evidence-based resources, ordered according to the P5 hierarchy.

Executing the search strategy

Using ACCESSSS (http://plus.mcmaster.ca/accessss), a search using the term "cardiovascular risk reduction" retrieves information from all P5 levels, except *Systems* (which would require integration of research-based evidence and individual patient information within an electronic medical record—an EMR is available at our institution, but integration with evidence-based guidelines for care is very limited at present). Note that we could have chosen other search terms (e.g., "hypertension or dyslipidemia or smoking cessation") and can easily modify the terms if the search doesn't retrieve what we're looking for. The key principles are to choose words that we think will retrieve what we want, keep the search terms simple, and modify, if needed. Knowledge of complex search logic is neither needed nor desirable for the relatively small databases that incorporate current best evidence.

Here's a brief survey of what we found. *At the Summaries level* (presented in alphabetical order by publication title):

BMJ Best Practice (http://bestpractice.bmj.com)

Best Practice (BP) does not appear to have a matching topic for our particular search terms. We can move on to another resource, which would be reasonable to do here. But for the sake of completeness, we try different search terms within BP, for the individual risk factors, hypertension, hypercholesterolemia, and smoking cessation. As for all P5 resources, the BP topics are date-stamped. For example, the most recent updates for hypercholesterolemia and smoking cessation in BP were 7 months before the time of search. Only one risk calculator is offered, the ACC/AHA calculator for atherosclerotic cardiovascular disease (ASCVD), without discussion of the options or evidence concerning performance. The text within topics is well organized and includes step-by-step instructions for treatment options, in order of levels of evidence, in point form, with little narrative.

DynaMed Plus

For *DynaMed Plus*, our "cardiovascular risk reduction" search yields a closely matching topic, "Cardiovascular disease prevention overview," and this topic was updated just 12 days before our search. *DynaMed Plus* presents its information in point form, including current recommendations and their respective levels (strength) of evidence (http://www.dynamed .com/home/content/levels-of-evidence) according to evidence-based guidelines from various professional organizations and agencies, for diet, exercise, smoking cessation, hypertension, and dyslipidemia, as well as for aspirin for primary prevention. Evidence is also presented favouring supplements of omega-3 fatty acids and specifically advising against vitamin E (useless) and beta-carotene (harmful, especially in smokers).

Following the *DynaMed Plus* recommendations, Mrs. JS could be offered diet changes, smoking cessation help, an exercise program, and medications for blood pressure control and dyslipidemia that are consistent with those recommended by the cardiovascular risk calculator. Options for smoking cessation are also outlined, but in a different section. Unfortunately, no recommendations are offered concerning how to assist Mrs. JS to adhere to such a comprehensive regimen. However, the levels of evidence are higher for medications and against vitamins, than for diet and exercise, which could be used to prioritize our approach when discussing the recommendations for our patient.

An option at this point would be to stop searching, as further searching will take more time and presumably have diminishing returns. However, we'll describe the findings for the remaining resources for the sake of illustration (especially as we are reviewing the Summary resources in alphabetical order!).

EBM Guidelines

As with *Best Practice,* our search of *EBM Guidelines* does not yield a topic that unifies recommendations for reduction of cardiovascular risk for primary prevention but does provide recommendations for management of individual risks, including hypertension, dyslipidemia, and smoking cessation. Recommendations are annotated with evidence levels and links to references and given in point form and tables. A step-by-step guide to diagnosis and management geared to primary care is provided. Comprehensive cardiovascular risk estimation is not covered, but there are comments in separate topics summarizing, for example, the quantitative effect of stopping smoking on cardiovascular risk. Mrs. JS, an accountant, might be interested! The topic, "Treatment of dyslipidemias," was updated about 2 years before our search, smoking cessation 6 weeks ago, and hypertension about 18 months ago. The *EBM Guidelines* recommendations are consistent with those in the other texts.

UpToDate (www.uptodate.com)

Our search in *UpToDate* retrieves two topics of direct interest: "Estimation of cardiovascular risk in an individual patient without known cardiovascular disease" and "Prevention of cardiovascular disease events in those with established disease or at high risk," both updated about 4 months before our search. The risk assessment topic is an extensive narrative on studies of risk estimation published from 1998 to 2015, pointing out their strengths and limitations. The treatment recommendations are consistent with those in *Best Practice, DynaMed,* and *EBM Guidelines* and include smoking cessation evidence and guidelines, a section that was updated less than a month ago. If this resource had come up first on searching, it would be appropriate to stop here. (ACCESSSS is ecumenical and posts results from the summary level according to how many text references are retrieved from the source.)

Searching note: It took about 15 minutes to review these four summary resources, and the results appear to be consistent and impressive from an evidence-based perspective—certainly better than what was available when we prepared the fourth edition of this book 5 years ago. *DynaMed Plus* and *UpToDate* were most recently updated for this topic and *DynaMed Plus* was both comprehensive and succinct on this topic. *UpToDate* was comprehensive and provided much more narrative, which can be better or worse, depending on how much background information you need and have time for. *Best Practice* and *EBM Guidelines* were not as well organized for this particular topic, but it didn't take long to piece together the components.

We surveyed the findings of four leading Summary resources in alphabetical order and found that their recommendations were consistent, but that doesn't mean that all these clinical reference texts are equal for a given question. What they offer may differ in content coverage, organization, quality, and currency. These are important reasons for comparing their recommendations as efficiently as possible. For example, a test of three of these resources found that *DynaMed Plus* topics were more up to date, by a substantial margin, compared with the same topics in *UpToDate* or *Best Practice.*[2] Unfortunately, currency varies from topic to topic in these resources, so no evidence-driven text has a "lock" on current best evidence.

Again, it would be reasonable to stop the search at this point and apply the findings in decisions with Mrs. JS. However, it will be instructive to continue the search to see whether additional information is available and supplementary from the lower levels of the pyramid.

*Systematically derived recommendations
(evidence-based guidelines)*

We get a quick hit on the systematically derived recommendations level of our search, with complementary guidelines on the benefits and harms of aspirin for the primary prevention of cardiovascular disease. With aspirin doses of 100 mg or less per day, the absolute risk reduction in nonfatal myocardial infarction (MI) ranged from 0.15 to 1.43 events per 1000 person-years, with older, higher-risk individuals benefitting in the higher end of this range.[13] On the downside, estimated excess major bleeding events were 1.39 (CI 0.70–2.28) per 1000 person-years for gastrointestinal (GI) bleeding, and 0.32 (CI –0.05 to 0.82) for hemorrhagic stroke per 1000 person-years of aspirin exposure, using baseline bleeding rates from a community-based observational sample. A 14% reduction in nonfatal stroke benefit was also noted.[14] As we'll see in Ch. 4 on Therapy, these figures translate to a number needed to treat (NNT) for 5 years of about 200 people to prevent one event, with an offsetting number needed to harm (NNH) over 5 years for one additional adverse event of 143 for GI bleeding, and of 625 for hemorrhagic stroke. These NNT–NNH dyads are often not provided in the same article, so this is a "gem" retrieved from our plunge into the lower P5 levels and shows that the benefits and risks are a trade-off, with the balance depending on how you value nonfatal MI and nonfatal stroke, and major bleeding events, including intracerebral hemorrhage.

The search also provides a guideline from the AHA on the prevention of cardiovascular disease specifically for women![15] This is a little dated (2011), but covers each of Mrs. JS's problems, including smoking, hypertension, dyslipidemia, and use of nonhelpful vitamins.

Bonus: As with many guidelines, the full text of these three articles is free, so if we didn't have full-text access to the subscription-based Summary resources, this is a very helpful fallback.

Systematic reviews ("Syntheses") are the next stop on the evidence tour.

Again, our search is rewarding at the Systematic Review level, with recent reviews on the efficacy of the Mediterranean diet, multiple risk factor interventions for primary prevention of cardiovascular disease, the (lack of) effectiveness of Tai Chi for this purpose, and other relevant topics.

Studies

This lowest level of P5, original studies, is large and less wieldy, requiring more sorting and appraisal by the user. However, it is worth recalling that it takes time for studies to be digested by the higher levels of the pyramid, and this can take weeks to months to years, depending on the resource and the evidence. In most cases, new studies will not provide a strong enough discordant signal to change the message of the syntheses and summaries at higher levels, but "landmark" studies can be published at any time, and nonlandmark studies can also attract a lot of press coverage, with patients as their primary audience. Thus, it is helpful for practitioners to be able to access current, preappraised studies, and our ACCESSSS search includes them. One article includes a nuance that is relevant for our patient. It reports that aspirin was cost-effective for primary prevention of cardiovascular events in older women at moderate risk.[16]

The base of P5 is preappraised studies, but ACCESSSS also takes us two levels deeper—in descending order of clinical usefulness: (1) articles retrieved via CQ from MEDLINE, and (2) articles retrieved via PubMed using just our search terms, "cardiovascular risk reduction." The number of articles retrieved increases dramatically at these lowest levels, and the amount of appraisal we will need to do increases accordingly. Nevertheless, it is easy and reasonably safe to discard many of the articles just on the basis of their titles, and some digging may yield a few nuggets. Intriguing titles that might be of interest for our patient include a systematic review of published "phase 3 trial" data on anti-PCSK9 monoclonal antibodies in patients with hypercholesterolemia, and a study of "triple combination therapy for global cardiovascular risk: atorvastatin, perindopril, and amlodipine," but these both turn out to be pharma studies promoting new products.

What about traditional textbooks of medicine?

If you don't use traditional medical texts, you've already correctly addressed this question. If you do use traditional texts in print or online, please check to see if they provide the detailed, up-to-date, evidential basis for care that we've just surveyed. Send us the name of any text that you feel merits a score of 6 or more (passing grade) on the 11-point scale in Table 2.1. Any that don't should not be used to support health care decisions, although they might be remarkable for "background" information.

If you would like more information and demonstrations of using ACCESSSS and its twin, McMaster PLUS Federated search (MPFS), use these YouTube video links:

ACCESSSS: Herbert Wertheim College of Medicine, South Florida
  https://www.youtube.com/watch?v = n-V2_wH5cik

https://www.youtube.com/watch?v=n-V2_wH5cik; T Shaneyfelt,
University of Alabama at Birmingham

MPFS

https://www.youtube.com/playlist?list=PL3xOBJ7f7CkVmW0VkEIIZ
luL7olCvd8u4

Examining the evidence

We've quickly assembled the summary, systematic guideline, systematic review, and study level preappraised information needed to inform evidence-based decisions for Mrs. JS. Her blood pressure and lipids are not well controlled, she is overweight, and she continues to smoke. She is worried about cardiovascular consequences, given her sister's premature demise, and her cardiovascular risk score is high, but that may be overestimating her actual risk, especially if her risk factors are lowered. Thus, the list of targets for which validated, beneficial interventions can be offered includes dyslipidemia, high blood pressure, and smoking. Should she decide to deal with her smoking, the P5 is well populated by validated interventions, from the summaries level on down. The easiest-to-implement, high-payoff interventions, however, are likely to be a daily statin and an ACE inhibitor, and pharmacologic support to help her quit smoking, as well as daily low-dose aspirin. She should be advised that there is evidence that omega-3 fatty acids could be advantageously substituted for her vitamin E and beta-carotene.

Applying the evidence

Evidence can build a strong foundation for helping Mrs. JS with her problems, including gaining an accurate prognosis, determining current best methods for reducing her risks for adverse cardiovascular outcomes, and providing her with information concerning nonprescription treatments she is taking. However, it is important to observe that "evidence does not make decisions."[4] Other key elements are her clinical circumstances and her wishes. It is important to note that her circumstances include a number of medical problems: untreated hypertension, dyslipidemia, and smoking, to begin with, and then obesity and low physical activity. Dealing with all these problems simultaneously is unlikely to occur because of the heavy behavioural demands of the complex regimen that would be required to treat them all successfully. (If you doubt this for an instant, try following the "ideal prescription" that you would prescribe for Mrs. JS— substituting candies for pills, and losing weight, increasing exercise, and quitting the favourite habit (smoking). Our prediction: Mrs. JS won't make it through a day without failing on one or more of your instructions, and there's a 50% chance that she will quit altogether in the first month.) We will need to carefully negotiate priorities with Mrs. JS to find the best match between the evidence and her wishes, then incorporate current best evidence concerning interventions to help her follow the treatments that she has agreed to accept.[17] Thus, the evidence we have accumulated in this chapter will get us only part of the way toward the decisions that Mrs. JS and we will need to make, but at least our decisions will be informed by the best available evidence concerning her risks and the interventions that will reduce or, in the case of beta-carotene, increase them. We'll discuss the application of evidence about therapy in further detail on pages 101–112.

Other ways to find evidence

The ACCESSSS search engine provides a focused, one-stop-shop approach to tracking down evidence for clinical decisions that will serve well for most clinical problems. A fallback would be getting to know each of the resources ACCESSSS searches and selecting the appropriate resources to search one at a time for the question(s) you are addressing until you find a credible answer.

Don't forget to subscribe to a "push" publication that suits your needs and allows you to tailor alerts to your area(s) of clinical interest.

References

1. Pickering GW. The purpose of medical education. BMJ 1956;2:113–16.

2. Jeffery R, Navarro T, Lokker C, Haynes RB, Wilczynski NL, Farjou G. How current are leading evidence-based medical texts? An analytic survey of four online textbooks. J Med Internet Res 2012;14(6):e175.

3. Alper BS, Haynes RB. EBHC pyramid 5.0 for accessing preappraised evidence and guidance. Evid Based Med 2016;doi:10.1136/ebmed -2016-110447.

4. Haynes RB, Devereaux PJ, Guyatt GH. Clinical expertise in the era of evidence-based medicine and patient choice. ACP J Club 2002; 136(2):A11A13.

5. Garg AX, Adhikari N, McDonald H, et al. Effects of computerized clinical decision support systems on practitioner performance and patient outcomes: a systematic review. JAMA 2005;293(10):1323–38.

6. Kortteisto T, Raitanen J, Komulainen J, Kunnamo I, Mäkelä M, Rissanen P, et al.; EBMeDS (Evidence-Based Medicine electronic Decision Support) Study Group. Patient-specific computer-based decision support in primary healthcare–a randomized trial. Implement Sci 2014;9:15. doi:10.1186/1748-5908-9-15.

7. Kwag KH, González-Lorenzo M, Banzi R, Bonovas S, Moja L. Providing doctors with high-quality information: an updated evaluation of web-based point-of-care information summaries. J Med Internet Res 2016;18(1):e15.

8. Alonso-Coello P, Oxman AD, Moberg J, Brignardello-Petersen R, Akl EA, Davoli M, et al.; GRADE Working Group. GRADE Evidence to Decision (EtD) frameworks: a systematic and transparent approach to making well informed healthcare choices. 2. BMJ 2016;353:i2089. doi:10.1136/bmj.i2089.

9. Singh JA, Saag KG, Bridges SL Jr, et al. 2015 American College of Rheumatology guideline for the treatment of rheumatoid arthritis. Arthritis Rheumatol 2016;68:1–26.

10. Alexander PE, Brito JP, Neumann I, Gionfriddo MR, Bero L, Djulbegovic B, et al. World Health Organization strong recommendations based on low-quality evidence (study quality) are frequent and often inconsistent with GRADE guidance. J Clin Epidemiol 2016;72:98–106.

11. McKibbon KA, Wilczynski NL, Haynes RB. What do evidence-based secondary journals tell us about the publication of clinically important articles in primary healthcare journals? BMC Med 2004;2:33.

12. DeFilippis AP, Young R, Carrubba CJ, et al. An analysis of calibration and discrimination among multiple cardiovascular risk scores in a modern multiethnic cohort. Ann Intern Med 2015;162(4):266–75. doi:10.7326/M14-1281. (Original) PMID: 25686167.

13. Guirguis-Blake JM, Evans CV, Senger CA, et al. Aspirin for the primary prevention of cardiovascular events: a systematic evidence review for the U.S. Preventive services task force. Ann Intern Med 2016;164(12): 804–13. doi:10.7326/M15-2113. Epub 2016 Apr 12.

14. Whitlock EP, Burda BU, Williams SB, et al. Bleeding risks with aspirin use for primary prevention in adults: a systematic review for the U.S. preventive services task force. Ann Intern Med 2016;164(12):826–35. doi:10.7326/M15-2112. Epub 2016 Apr 12.

15. Mosca L, Benjamin EJ, Berra K, et al. Effectiveness-based guidelines for the prevention of cardiovascular disease in women–2011 update: a guideline from the American Heart Association. Circulation

2011;123(11):1243–62. doi:10.1161/CIR.0b013e31820faaf8. Epub 2011 Feb 14.

16. Pignone M, Earnshaw S, Pletcher MJ, Tice JA. Aspirin for the primary prevention of cardiovascular disease in women: a cost-utility analysis. Arch Intern Med 2007;167:290–5.

17. Tierney WM. Review: evidence on the effectiveness of interventions to assist patient adherence to prescribed medications is limited. [Abstract for McDonald HP, Garg AX, Haynes RB. Interventions to enhance patient adherence to medication prescriptions: scientific review. JAMA. 2002;288(22):2868–2879.]. ACP J Club 2002;139(1):19.

2

3 Appraising the evidence

We've finished our literature search, and we've identified some evidence. Now, we need to decide if it's valid and important before we can apply the evidence to our patients. The order in which we consider validity and importance depends on individual preference. We could start by appraising its validity, arguing that if it isn't valid, who cares whether it appears to show a huge effect? Alternatively, we could determine its clinical importance, arguing that if the evidence doesn't suggest a clinically important impact, who cares if it's valid? We can start with either question, as long as we remember to follow up one favourable answer with the other question, and to move on if one answer is unfavourable.

There are many sources of potential bias (defined as systematic deviation from the truth) that can affect the validity of studies and thus affect whether we believe their results. We're not going to describe all of the potential sources of bias here (we refer you to some classic readings listed at the end of this section). Instead, in subsequent chapters, we'll address some of the key sources of bias in different study types that we need to consider so that we can become effective consumers of the literature.

Some features are common to appraisal of most studies of therapy, diagnosis, prognosis, and etiology/harm. Paul Glasziou has suggested we consider a race analogy to illustrate these commonalities. First, was there a fair start? This would include consideration of what was the population of interest. How was it identified? Was the population appropriately selected? Was assignment to the intervention or exposure appropriate? Second, was the race fair? Specifically, were the study participants treated the same throughout? Did they all complete the study? Third, was it a fair finish? Was there an appropriate measurement of outcomes, namely, blind and/or objective? Was the analysis of results appropriate? We'll review these concepts in more detail in subsequent chapters.

Note that instead of the racing analogy, we could use the PICO format from page 21 when we consider validity. First, what is the Population (who are the patients), which requires consideration of how they were recruited and whether an appropriate target population was identified. Second, what was the Intervention, exposure, or test that they were subjected to? Third, what was the Comparison, or Control, group, and how were the participants selected or allocated? Fourth, were clinically important Outcomes measured in a blind and/or objective fashion, and were they measured at an appropriate time from a clinical perspective? We'll discuss each of these issues (and potential sources of bias) in subsequent chapters.

As mentioned on page 44, when we're performing a literature search, rather than seeking the results from a single study, we should seek a knowledge synthesis that systematically searches for and combines evidence from all studies relevant to the topic because this will provide us with a more reliable answer to our clinical question. Knowledge syntheses or systematic reviews of the literature are most commonly found for therapy topics, and we'll review them in detail on page 112. Over the past 10 years, the publication of systematic reviews has exploded; new types of reviews and analyses, such as "network met-analysis," have emerged; and new targets of review, such as clinical prediction guides, have been tackled. Whether we are considering systematic reviews of prognosis, therapy, diagnostic test accuracy, or harm, concerns about validity are common to all of these systematic reviews.

1. Was the literature search comprehensive? This question includes consideration of whether the authors included studies from appropriate electronic databases; whether they used additional sources for identifying studies, such as by hand searching journals or contacting experts in the field; and whether the authors placed any language restrictions on their search results.

2. Was the quality of the individual studies assessed? We would like to see that the investigators critically appraised the individual studies for validity (using criteria similar to those which we describe in subsequent chapters) and that they provided an explicit methodology for this.

In subsequent chapters, after a discussion on the validity of the studies (whether individual studies or systematic reviews), we'll consider whether their results are important. This discussion will include a consideration of the magnitude and precision of the results. For systematic reviews, we also want to consider heterogeneity—how consistent are the results from study to study?

Many different critical appraisal worksheets and checklists can be used when considering the validity of individual studies. We have provided one format in this book, but there are others you might want to review, including the GATE assessment tool, developed by Rod Jackson

(https://www.fmhs.auckland.ac.nz/en/soph/about/our-departments/
epidemiology-and-biostatistics/research/epiq/evidence-based-practice
-and-cats.html), and the CASP tools (http://www.casp-uk.net/#!casp-tools
-checklists/c18f8). There is no one way of critically appraising a study
or of teaching critical appraisal (indeed, we're only limited by our
imagination!), and we encourage you to find strategies that work for
you and your colleagues and learners.

For now, sit back and relax, and let's see how the race to the finish
unfolds!

Further reading

Guyatt G, Rennie D, Meade M, Cook DJ, editors. Users' guides to the
medical literature. A manual for evidence-based clinical practice. 3rd ed.
Chicago, IL: AMA Press; 2015.

Haynes RB, Sackett DL, Guyatt GH, Tugwell P. Clinical epidemiology: how
to do clinical practice research. Philadelphia, PA: Lippincott Williams &
Wilkins; 2006.

Sackett DL. Bias in analytic research. J Chronic Dis 1979;32:51–63.

3

4 Therapy

In this chapter, we're going to tackle the critical appraisal of therapy articles. We will start by considering individual trials because a lot of the strategies that we use in appraising individual trials can be applied to the evaluation of other types of studies. However, individual trials are not the best-quality evidence that we can find about the effects of therapy unless the trials are large, high-quality randomized trials. There are many reasons for this. On the one hand, individual trials may not be internally valid; in other words, there may be methodological flaws. On the other hand, the methods may be sound, but they may not be externally valid; that is, they are not generalizable to our clinical context. The reason could be that the population under study in the trial was too narrowly defined and selected. There are other factors that can help us determine the validity of an individual trial, which will be described later in this chapter.

After we build some basic principles and tools to appraise individual studies, we will use them to develop skills to appraise systematic reviews (SRs) and meta-analyses (MAs). MAs pool the results from individual studies quantitatively. SRs may include MAs but may also limit synthesis to a narrative description. In the hierarchy of evidence quality, these reviews are of higher quality compared with individual trials because they identify whether the findings in a single study are consistent across several studies, creating greater faith in the results.

After describing individual trials and reviews, we will briefly examine qualitative studies and the issue of adherence. Qualitative studies are increasingly contributing to the evidence base because they offer methods to address clinical questions that cannot be readily answered by using standard quantitative methods. They make use of interviews and focus groups, to name but a few methodologies, to describe the values, goals, and experiences of patients or other individuals.

Sometimes we will want to expand our search to support our decision making, looking outside of individual trials, SRs, and qualitative studies. For example, perhaps there is a trade-off between the benefits and harms of the intervention. In this case, we may want to capture a clinical decision analysis (CDA) in our literature search. In this chapter's review of clinical decision analyses, we will describe how a tool called a *decision tree* can be used to evaluate a variety of possible therapies and their potential outcomes. This leads naturally into a discussion about economic analyses, studies that combine the tools of decision analyses with economics to examine cost minimization, cost effectiveness, cost benefit, or cost utility.

We will close by appraising literature that is at the most macroscopic level—clinical practice guidelines (CPGs). These summarize the evidence for a particular target disorder across various aspects of care, including making the diagnosis, establishing the prognosis, and recommending the appropriate therapy. This will be followed by the studies that are at the most microscopic of levels—n-of-1 trials. We use these types of studies in situations in which we may not be able to track down evidence that clearly answers a question about therapy posed by our patients or ourselves. These studies are best used for chronic diseases without a solid evidence base. In these cases, we might set up a study in which our patient serves as his or her own control, crossing over between interventions (to which we are both, preferably, blinded), to determine which management strategy helps control symptoms or reduce exacerbations.

At each step of the way throughout this chapter, we will ask ourselves to determine whether studies are valid, important, and applicable to our situation.

Reports of individual studies

We begin with individual trials. To illustrate our discussion, let's consider a scenario:

> We are seeing a 62-year-old woman in clinic for evaluation of her cardiac risk. She is previously healthy, known only for being mildly overweight with an increased waist-to-hip ratio of 0.84. She has no known diabetes, hypertension, or dyslipidemia. She is concerned because her father died at the age of 50 years following a heart attack. She does not take any medications or have any allergies to medications. She does not smoke, drink alcohol, or use drugs. She eats a balanced diet and exercises regularly. She inquires if there is any role for taking cholesterol-lowering medications, akin to what her brother is taking, to reduce her risk of a heart attack.

Based on this scenario, we posed the following question, "In a patient at intermediate risk of coronary artery disease, does cholesterol lowering decrease the risk of myocardial infarction?" Recall from page 43 that we can use search engines, such as PubMed Clinical Queries, and tools, such as the *ACP Journal Club*, to find the evidence that answers our question. We use the search terms "cholesterol lowering" and "myocardial infarction," and we identify a recent trial[1] that might help us answer this question. This trial specifically addresses the impact of statins on a composite primary endpoint of death from a cardiovascular cause, nonfatal myocardial infarction (MI), and nonfatal stroke, but it also offers data on each of the individual components of the composite outcome.

When we are appraising individual studies, we can take a systematic approach to determine whether the results are valid (Box 4.1). By asking the questions enumerated below, you can very quickly determine whether a study is worth reviewing to answer your particular clinical question. Given the exponential growth in evidence, the Consolidated Standards of Reporting Trials (CONSORT) Guidelines were established to ensure that investigators reported the results of randomized controlled trials (RCTs) in a transparent and standardized way to help evidence consumers reliably appraise their findings.[2] Many journals have adopted the CONSORT

4

Box 4.1 Is this evidence about therapy (from an individual randomized trial) valid?

Was there a fair start?

1. Was the assignment of patients to treatment randomized?
2. Was the randomization concealed?
3. Were the groups similar at the start of the trial?

Was there a fair race?

1. Was follow-up of patients sufficiently long and complete?
2. Were all patients analyzed in the groups to which they were randomized?

Some finer points

1. Who was blinded: Were patients, clinicians, and study personnel kept blind to treatment?
2. Were groups treated equally, apart from the experimental therapy?

---

statement[a] for reporting, and this has made it easier for us to review articles for validity.

Are the results of this individual study valid?

1. Was the assignment of patients to treatment randomized?

It was believed previously that hormone replacement therapy (HRT) could decrease the risk of coronary artery disease (CAD) in postmeno-pausal women. This belief was based on data from several *observational studies* that found that women who used HRT had a decreased risk of having a cardiac event.[3] However, in a subsequent *experimental study* of postmenopausal women with established CAD (secondary prevention study), patients were randomized to receive either HRT or placebo and the investigators found that there was no reduction in the rate of cardiac events with HRT, much to the surprise of clinicians and patients![4] Subsequently, the Women's Health Initiative study found that HRT was not effective in the primary prevention of CAD either.[5] This was practice changing, to say the least, especially because HRT was simultaneously noted to increase the risk of certain cancers and venous thromboembolism. It also illuminated the limitations of observational studies—for example, cohort studies or case-control studies that look for patterns in data sets—and it highlighted the importance of trying to test hypotheses experimentally, using such study methods as the RCT.

There are many examples of randomized trials yielding surprising results, contradicting what was previously found in observational studies or even from outcomes that we might expect based on "first principles" of pathophysiology. For example, case series and case reports of extracranial–intracranial (EC/IC) arterial bypass suggested that this surgery could reduce the risk of ischemic stroke, but a randomized trial of EC/IC bypass compared with medical treatment (the standard of care) alone found no benefit with surgery.[6] Another noteworthy example comes from cardiology—ventricular arrhythmia after MI is a known risk factor for death. It was thought that if these arrhythmias were suppressed (with some agents, such as encainide and flecainide), mortality would be decreased in these patients. However, results from a randomized trial (Cardiac Arrhythmia Suppression Trial [CAST]) found more harm than

---

[a]Note that there have been various extensions to CONSORT and if readers are interested, they can be viewed on the equator network website at http://www.equator-network .org.

good resulted from these agents.[7] Indeed, it has been estimated that more Americans died as a result of receiving these agents than as a result of the Vietnam War over the same period![8]

Why is there such a difference between the results of observational and experimental studies? In observational studies, the patient's and/or clinician's preferences determine whether or not the patient receives the treatment. Often, such factors as the presence of comorbid illnesses, use of other medications, the individual's beliefs, and the severity of the disease and its symptoms influence the patient's and physician's therapeutic decision-making process. Patient factors, such as these, which are extraneous to the question being posed may be associated with other resources, attitudes, or behaviours that could independently influence the clinical outcome that we are trying to evaluate with the treatment. Moreover, such factors may be unevenly distributed between the intervention groups. These factors are called *confounders* because they "confound" our ability to determine causality between a certain treatment and the outcome of interest. Formally stated, a confounder is something that is associated with the exposure of interest and the outcome of interest but is not on the causal pathway. This means that it gives the semblance of causality between the exposure (e.g., treatment) and outcome (e.g., CAD), even though the relationship is merely one of association through these shared, unobserved factors. For example, many people believe that drinking a glass of red wine each day can help reduce the risk of cardiac events. Even though this assertion is based, in part, on an SR and an MA, the individual studies that were included in conducting this MA were all cohort studies (observational studies).[9] Critics of this theory have made the astute observation that these findings might be the result of confounding by socioeconomic status, specifically, drinking red wine is associated with a higher socioeconomic status. A higher socioeconomic status is itself associated with a reduced risk of having a cardiac event, likely because of all sorts of health-promoting factors, including being able to afford healthy foods or having the time and means to exercise. If we are evaluating socioeconomic status as a confounder, we must also confirm that it is not, itself, on the causal pathway. We can see that drinking red wine does not lead to a higher socioeconomic status, which would lead to a lower risk of cardiac events, so it satisfies this criterion. In short, it may not be the red wine but, rather, all the advantages conferred by a higher socioeconomic status that is mediating the reduction in cardiac events! Socioeconomic status might be a confounder! Unfortunately, we could never confirm these findings with an RCT because an ethics review board would be hard pressed to approve

4

a study that randomly assigns patients to drink alcohol—with all its attendant possible adverse health effects.

We can see that if these factors, or confounders, are unevenly distributed between the intervention groups, they may exaggerate, cancel, or even counteract the effects of therapy. For example, if these factors exaggerated the apparent effect of an otherwise ineffectual treatment, as might be the case with red wine and socioeconomic status, this could lead to the false-positive conclusion that the treatment was useful when in fact it was not. In contrast, if the confounder nullified or counteracted the effects of a truly efficacious treatment, this could lead to a false-negative conclusion that a useful treatment was useless or even harmful.

Although there are ways to mitigate the impact of confounding (exclusion, stratified sampling, matching, stratified analysis, standardization and multivariate modelling) they all require that the confounder be identified. However, sometimes when studying an outcome, all the prognostic factors for the disease are not yet known or they cannot be easily measured. In these cases, randomization can reduce confounding and help us draw conclusions about causality by balancing the intervention groups for the known and unknown prognostic factors. The assumption here is that if a group is large enough and patients are randomly assigned to each of the intervention groups, their traits and risk factors will be evenly distributed between the two groups. Of course, this conclusion takes a bit of a leap of faith and reminds us that we should always scan the "Table 1" of any study to check for ourselves that important clinical features and risk factors have been distributed evenly between both intervention groups. We should insist on random allocation to treatment because it comes closer than any other research design to creating groups of patients at the start of the trial who are identical in their risk of having the event that we are trying to prevent. From there, we can say that differences in the rates of the outcomes can be reasonably attributed to the single parameter that was different between the two groups, namely, the intervention. For instance, if we were to miraculously get approval to conduct an RCT comparing risk of MI among patients taking red wine versus patients taking a placebo, the act of randomizing would generate two groups that are likely balanced with regard to socioeconomic status, as well as other potential (and possibly unidentified) confounders. When we confirm randomization during our appraisal of a study, we should check that the investigators have described some method analogous to tossing a coin[b] to assign patients to treatment groups (e.g., the

---

[b]In practice, this should be done by computers, but the principle remains the same.

experimental treatment is assigned if the coin landed "heads" and a conventional, "control" or "placebo"[c] treatment is given if the coin landed "tails").

Randomization is something for investigators to be proud of, and often you will find it mentioned explicitly in the abstract (or the title!). If the study was not randomized, we would suggest that you stop reading it and go on to the next article in your search. Note that this can help you efficiently appraise the literature by scanning the abstract to determine whether a study is randomized—if it is not, move on. Only seek out the conclusions of observational studies if you cannot find any randomized trials. In these cases, if the only evidence that you have about a treatment is from nonrandomized observational studies, you have five options:

1. Check page 35–65 again, or get some help from a librarian to perform another literature search to see if you missed any randomized trials of the therapy.

2. Assess whether the treatment effect described in the nonrandomized trial is so huge that it would be unlikely to be a false-positive study. (This is very rare, and usually only satisfied when the prognosis of untreated patients is uniformly terrible; e.g., 100% mortality in bacterial meningitis without the use of antibiotics.) As a check, you may ask your colleagues whether they consider the candidate therapy so likely to be efficacious that they would consider it unethical to randomize a patient like yours into a study that includes a no-treatment or placebo group.

3. If the nonrandomized trial concluded that the treatment was useless or harmful, then it is usually safe to accept that conclusion.[d] False-positive conclusions from nonrandomized studies are far more common than false-negative ones. This makes sense when you consider that treatments are typically withheld from patients with the poorest prognoses. Furthermore, patients who faithfully take their medicine are destined for better outcomes, even when they are taking worthless treatments or placebos, further reducing the chance of a false-negative result.

---

[c]A placebo is a treatment that is similar to the active treatment in appearance, taste, and other features such that the patient, clinician, and study personnel cannot distinguish between the two.
[d]Note that if we are looking for evidence about harms from an intervention, this is often identified from observational studies; refer to Chapter 7 for more details.

4. Consider whether an "n-of-1" trial might make sense for you and your patient. These are useful in chronic disease management (and we describe them in detail a bit later).

5. Try to find evidence for an alternative management option.

> To answer our question about cholesterol-lowering and rates of MI, the abstract of the trial report by Yusuf et al. states that patients were randomly assigned to receive rosuvastatin 10 mg daily or placebo. The randomization was stratified by centre, a strategy that is useful because a health care centre might itself be a prognostic factor——if there are variations in practices across various centres (or even across countries). Because this study was conducted in 228 centres across 21 countries, this stratification procedure is of benefit. It also makes it easier to interpret the data if one centre happens to withdraw from the study because we can trust that the prognostic factors remain balanced across the remaining centres.

2. Was the randomization concealed?

Was randomization concealed from the clinicians and study personnel who entered patients into the trial and monitored them? If allocation was concealed, the clinicians will be unaware of which intervention the next patient will receive and they are thus unable, consciously or subconsciously, to distort the balance between the groups being compared. Knowledge of the assignments might lead to the exclusion of certain patients from one of the groups based on their prognosis—clinicians might avoid allocating some patients to a group that they perceive to be inappropriate, or without benefit. As with failure to use randomization, inadequate concealment of allocation can distort the apparent effect of treatment in either direction, causing the effect to seem larger or smaller than it is in reality.

Articles sometimes do not explicitly state whether the randomization list was concealed, but if randomization occurred through a system that is kept at a distance from the frontline (i.e., where patients are being entered into the trial), for example, via telephone or centralized computer, we can assume that there has been adequate concealment. Assignments should also be delivered one at a time, as each patient is enrolled, to prevent disruptions to randomization.

It has been shown that investigators report overcoming virtually every type of allocation concealment strategy—from holding an envelope to a bright light to ransacking office files of the principal investigator to find the allocation list![10] We can thus see that concealment is not as easy to attain as one might imagine!

> The "methods" section of the full text indicates that patients were randomized using a "central concealed randomization procedure."

3. Were the groups similar at the start of the trial?

We should check to see if the groups were similar in all prognostically important ways (except for receiving the treatment) at the start of the trial. As noted above, the benefit of randomization is that we can assume an equal distribution of potential confounders between the study groups. However, baseline differences between the study groups may be present as a result of chance. There is usually no value to providing p values in the table describing baseline characteristics of participants, and journals are encouraging authors to move away from providing these. These hypothesis tests assess the probability that differences observed between the two groups could result from chance, and in well-designed randomized trials, we can safely assume this to be true. Studies have shown that researchers who use hypothesis tests to compare baseline characteristics report fewer significant results than expected by chance. The reason may be that investigators may not report significant differences in baseline characteristics because of concern that this might impact the credibility of their results. If the groups aren't similar we must determine whether adjustment for these potentially important prognostic factors was carried out. Adjustments can be carried out using many different methodologies, including exclusion, stratified sampling, matching, stratified analysis, and standardization. It is reassuring if the adjusted and unadjusted analyses yield similar results.

> In the study by Yusuf et al., a scan of Table 1 reveals that there were no important differences between patients in the two groups. Also, there are no p values provided for the baseline characteristics.

4. Was follow-up of patients sufficiently long and complete?

Once we are satisfied that the study was randomized, we can look to see if all patients who were entered into the trial were accounted for at its conclusion. Determining this has become easier with the inclusion of flow diagrams, usually designated as a "Figure 1" in the study. Inclusion of a flow diagram is part of the CONSORT statement (http://www .consort-statement.org, which, as previously noted, aims to enhance the reporting accuracy of trials) (Fig. 4.1).[11]

Ideally, we would like to see that no patients were lost to follow-up because these patients may have had outcomes that would affect the

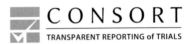

CONSORT 2010 Flow Diagram

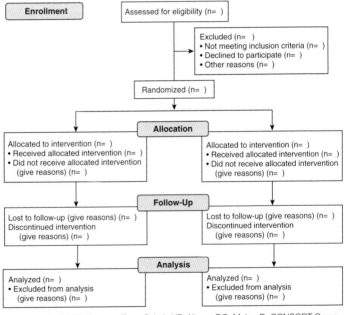

Fig. 4.1 CONSORT diagram. (From Schulz KF, Altman DG, Moher D, CONSORT Group. CONSORT 2010 Statement: Updated Guidelines for Reporting Parallel Group Randomised Trials. *PLoS Med.* 2010;7(3):e1000251, with permission.)

conclusions of the study. If, for example, patients receiving the experimental treatment dropped out because of adverse outcomes, their absence from the analysis would lead to an overestimation of the efficacy of the treatment (and underreporting of potential adverse events from the intervention).

What can we consider to be an acceptable loss? To be sure of a trial's conclusion, the investigators should be able to take all patients who were lost to follow-up, assign them to the worst-case outcome (assume that everyone lost from the group whose remaining members fared better had a bad outcome and assume that everyone lost from the group whose remaining members fared worse had a good outcome) and still be able to support their original conclusion. If this method doesn't change the study's conclusions, the loss to follow-up is not a threat to the study's validity. However, if the study result does change, its validity is threatened, and we must decide if the results derived from the worst-case method are plausible. It would be unusual for a trial to withstand a worst-case analysis if it lost more than 20% of its patients (but this depends on the number of outcomes observed—e.g., if there were only a few outcomes that were observed in a large study, the loss of 20% of patients could have a big impact on the results). The 20% cut-off is a good estimate for most large randomized studies, so much so that journals, such as the *ACP Journal Club*, won't publish trials with less than 80% follow-up.

We should also ensure that the follow-up of patients was sufficiently long to see a clinically important effect. For example, if our study assessing the use of a statin and the risk of an MI only followed up patients for 1 week or 1 month, we wouldn't find the results very helpful because that is too short a time interval to observe this clinical outcome. Given the nature of the target disorder, we would like to see a follow-up period of, ideally, many, many years. One of the challenges that we face as clinicians appraising the literature is that medications are often used for longer periods of time in real life than they are in the follow-up period of most studies. As with statin trials, for example, there is a lack of trials of serotonin reuptake inhibitors lasting more than just a handful of years for the treatment of depression, although these agents are often used for several years, if not a lifetime.[12] This is an issue we need to consider when deciding on the applicability of therapy studies. We need to ask ourselves if the follow-up period in the studies makes sense for the outcomes of interest based on what we know from other studies and from pathophysiology. A short follow-up period might be appropriate for a study evaluating the effect of antibiotics compared with placebo on the resolution of infectious symptoms, but it would not be appropriate for a study evaluating the impact of a chronic medication on such an outcome as death from a chronic disease.

We often see trials stopped early when a large benefit is seen. However, if this happens when the sample size and the number of outcomes are small, this can result in a dangerous overestimate of the treatment effect; the results of such a study should be interpreted with caution.[13,14] Sometimes, information about the follow-up is available in the study's abstract, but more often, we must turn to the results to obtain specific details.

In our study, the follow-up was 99.1% (this is remarkable!). The median follow-up was 5.6 years.

---

5. Were all patients analyzed in the groups to which they were randomized?

Anything that happens after randomization can affect the chance that a study patient has the outcome of interest. For example, a patient may engage in different health behaviours, acquire a new diagnosis of a relevant comorbidity, or have a change in socioeconomic factors that influence health for better or worse. Therefore, it is important that all patients, including those who fail to take their medicine or those that accidentally or intentionally receive the wrong treatment, are analyzed in the groups to which they were allocated. Once comparable groups are set up at the outset of the study, they should stay this way to preserve the benefits of randomization. It has been shown repeatedly that patients who "do" and "don't" take their study medicine have very different outcomes, even when the study medicine is a placebo. The study participants that leave a study or cross over into another treatment group may have a particular characteristic so that those remaining in the groups are no longer comparable as they were at study onset. To preserve the value of randomization, we should demand an "intention-to-treat analysis" whereby all patients are analyzed in the groups to which they were initially assigned, regardless of whether they received, or even actually took, their assigned treatment. We are therefore analyzing them "as intended." It is important that we not only look for the term "intention-to-treat analysis" in the "methods" section but also look at the results to ensure that this analysis was done.

In contrast to the superior method of intention-to-treat (ITT) analysis, per protocol (PP) analysis is a method that only analyzes patients that completed the treatment that they were originally assigned. This can lead to bias because there might be factors that compelled these patients to stick to their assigned protocols that may not be present in the average patient, thereby distorting how the therapy will work in the "real world."[15] Note that although this principle applies to superiority trials (trials demonstrating that one intervention is better than another), which are the types of studies with which we tend to be the most familiar, there is some controversy in the literature as to whether ITT analysis is required to the same extent in noninferiority studies (trials demonstrating that one intervention is no worse than another).

> The study by Yusuf et al. used an intention-to-treat (ITT) analysis.

6. Were patients, clinicians, and study personnel kept blind to treatment?

Blinding is necessary to avoid the patient's reporting of symptoms or the patient's adherence to treatment being affected by hunches about whether the treatment is effective. Similarly, a clinician or outcome assessor may be influenced by the perceived effectiveness of the study intervention, so blinding prevents how he or she *interprets* symptoms or reports outcomes during a study. Not surprisingly, blinding is particularly important when the outcome of interest is subjective, and judgement by the clinician or outcomes assessor is necessary.

When patients and clinicians cannot be kept blind (e.g., in surgical trials), often it is possible to have other blinded clinicians assess the medical records (purged of any mention of the assignment groups) to remove any bias in assessing outcomes that might be influenced by knowing the assignment. Another strategy is to use objective outcome measurements, such as death. For example, in the North American Symptomatic Carotid Endarterectomy Trial,[16] patients with symptomatic carotid artery stenosis were randomized to either carotid endarterectomy or medical therapy with aspirin. The patients in the surgical group (and the surgeons performing the procedure) could obviously not be blinded to the treatment. Instead, outcome events were assessed by four groups—the participating neurologist and surgeon; the neurologist at the study centre; "blinded" members of the steering committee; and "blinded" external adjudicators. These steps helped to mitigate the bias that might result from a lack of blinding of the clinician and the patient.

Clinicians interpret the term "double-blind" differently because there are many different players in studies, including patients, clinicians, and outcome adjudicators (who may or may not be the treating clinicians), that could be blinded. Ideally, an article should explicitly state who was blinded but it is rare to find articles that do this. Information about blinding may be present in the abstract or in the "methods" section, and sometimes in the title of the article.[17]

Initially, patients were placed on the medication in a single-blind run-in period, after which they were randomized if they were adherent and did not experience any serious adverse events (note that this means that the population of patients that underwent randomization may not be representative of the population-at-large, given that those who were nonadherent or suffered adverse consequences did not progress in the trial. This step may have introduced *selection bias*). Following randomization, patients were blinded to the treatment that they were receiving. Clinicians, also unaware of the treatment allocations, assessed the patients for cardiovascular outcomes at each of the follow-up visits. In the supplementary material provided, which included the detailed trial protocol, note is made that all primary and secondary outcomes were adjudicated by an Events Adjudication Committee, which was also blinded to the treatment allocation. The steering committee was also blinded. Thus, there were at least four levels of blinding in this study.

---

7. Were groups treated equally, apart from the experimental therapy?

Blinding of patients, clinicians, and study personnel can prevent them from adding any additional treatments (or "co-interventions"), apart from the experimental treatment, to just one of the groups. For example, both patients and clinicians may modify their behaviour or use adjunctive treatments that can affect the outcome. If clinicians know that their patient has been enrolled in the control group rather than the intervention group, and they believe that the intervention group will reap a benefit, they might differentially, or more aggressively, manage other risk factors in their patients to give their patients the best chance possible at averting the outcome. This would narrow the effect size that might be expected with the treatment because the control group might be treated more aggressively compared with the intervention group. Usually, we can find information about the use of co-interventions, intentional or unintentional, in the "methods" section and/or the "results" section of an article.

> In this study, clinicians identified patients in *both groups* with regard to individual lifestyle modifications that might be beneficial, and they tailored advice.

Putting it all together

If the study fails any of the criteria discussed above, we need to decide if the flaw is significant and threatens the validity of the study. If this is the case, we will need to look for another study. However, if we find that our article satisfies all the criteria, we can proceed to consider its importance.

> We believe that our study has satisfied all the major validity criteria, and we will look at its results. *Note:* How many validity criteria are mentioned in the abstract of the original article? In the study we identified, the abstract only mentions randomization and the median duration of follow-up. Although not all the validity criteria are mentioned, seeing these in the abstract helps us to assess the article more quickly. We can then move to the "methods" section to search for the other validity criteria.

Are the valid results of this individual study important?

In this section, we will discuss how to determine whether the potential benefits (or harms) of the treatment described in a study are important. We will refer to the guides in Box 4.2 for this discussion. Deciding whether we should be impressed with the results of a trial requires two steps. First, we try to determine the most useful clinical expression of these results—that is, does it make the most sense to report a result as a ratio, such as a relative risk (RR) or an odds ratio (OR), or is the result more meaningfully expressed as a difference, as with a risk difference

> **Box 4.2** Is this valid evidence about therapy (from an individual randomized trial) important?
>
> 1. What is the magnitude of the treatment effect?
> 2. How precise is the estimate of the treatment effect?

or absolute risk reduction? We will get into the computational "nitty gritty" in more detail as you read along. Second, we try to compare the results with other treatments for other target disorders. For example, the VA Cooperative Study was the first trial that compared aspirin with placebo to prevent death following acute coronary syndromes.[18] The combined outcome of death or acute myocardial infarction (AMI) was 5% in the aspirin group versus 10.1%, in the placebo group, a finding that was statistically significant with an unadjusted p value of 0.0005 (when adjusted for baseline characteristics, the p value became 0.0002). This amounts to an absolute risk reduction of 5.1% and a relative risk reduction (RRR) of 51% (we will explain how to do this math in detail below). The impressive findings led to an unequivocal uptake of aspirin use in the treatment of acute coronary syndromes! We rarely get results that are this compelling, but comparing the treatment effect that you see in your study to that of known treatments helps you determine whether it is clinically significant enough to warrant uptake.

1. What is the magnitude of the treatment effect?

Consideration of the magnitude of the results requires assessment of the outcomes that are included in the study. To date, we have limited the discussion to focus on the outcomes that were relevant to our patient. Sometimes, trials will report on surrogate outcomes, which are outcomes that are hypothesized to be linked to outcomes that might *actually* be of interest to patients. For example, in studies assessing the effectiveness of osteoporosis therapy, ideally the trials should include measurement of the impact of the intervention on fractures. However, bone mineral density (BMD) is a surrogate outcome that is often used in these studies. BMD has been shown to correlate with fracture risk, so it is an acceptable surrogate outcome. Surrogate outcomes can be acceptable if they are shown to be valid proxies for the clinically important outcomes. Therefore, when they are used, we need to think critically about their validity and not just assume that the investigators have chosen an outcome that is a reasonable approximation to what actually matters to patients and clinicians. Surrogate outcomes are often used because they can reduce sample size and follow-up time and thus may be more feasible to collect from a logistical or cost perspective.

Composite outcomes are also seen frequently in trials, and trials that use them must be assessed cautiously.[19] The benefit to the investigators of using a composite outcome is that it makes the trial more "efficient" in that more outcomes will occur within a reasonable time frame, making it less costly to conduct this study. This is important if the outcomes of interest take a long time to develop or if they are rare. The disadvantage is that the onus is on the reader to determine whether the benefit or harm seen in a composite outcome is being driven by all of its components or just by one of them, and whether or not all of the components trend in the same direction as the composite outcome. For example, in the ADVANCE (Action in Diabetes and Vascular Disease: Preterax and Diamicron MR Controlled Evaluation) trial, more than 11,000 patients with type 2 diabetes mellitus were randomized to intensive therapy (target A_{1C} of <6.5%) or standard therapy (target A_{1C} >6.5%).[20] The primary outcome was a composite outcome, including macrovascular (nonfatal MI or stroke or death from cardiovascular causes) or micro-vascular events (worsening nephropathy or retinopathy). Worsening nephropathy was defined as macroalbuminuria, doubling of serum creatinine, renal replacement therapy, or death from renal causes. A significant difference was seen in the composite outcome of macrovascular and microvascular events (Table 4.1). However, teasing these results apart, it is apparent that there was no significant difference in macro-vascular events. Microvascular events were significantly reduced with intensive therapy—however, the difference in macroalbuminuria is what drives this difference. Indeed, 1.2% of the overall risk difference of 1.9% is contributed by the reduction in macroalbuminuria alone.[21] Although a reduction in macroalbuminuria has been shown to have beneficial renal and cardiovascular effects, arguably it is not an outcome that matters to patients as much as macrovascular complications, such as MI or stroke! If we had not looked carefully at whether those macrovascular outcomes were also reduced with intensive therapy, we might have falsely assumed that the composite endpoint spoke for all of the individual endpoints!

4

> The study by Yusuf et al. makes use of two co-primary outcomes. The first co-primary outcome is a composite of death from cardiovascular causes, nonfatal MI, or nonfatal stroke. The second co-primary outcome is also a composite outcome; it adds revascularization, heart failure, and resuscitated cardiac arrest to the first co-primary outcome. Each of the individual components are also analyzed separately. It makes sense that these investigators would set up a composite outcome because they are looking at a patient population that is at intermediate risk of having cardiovascular events, so it will take them longer to develop one or more of the outcomes.

Table 4.1 Intensive versus standard glucose control to prevent vascular events in type 2 diabetes*

Outcomes at median 5 years	Intensive control	Standard control	RRR (95% CI)	NNT over 5 years (95% CI)
Macro- or microvascular event	18.1%	20%	9.6% (2.4%–16.3%)	51 (30–213)
Macrovascular event[†]	10.0%	10.6%	5.6% (−5.3% to 15.4%)	Not significant
Microvascular event[‡]	9.4%	10.9%	13.1% (2.9%–22.2%)	70 (39–333)
New or worsening nephropathy[§]	4.1%	5.2%	21.3% (6.8%–33.5%)	89 (53–303)
New-onset macroalbuminuria	2.9%	4.1%	29.3% (13.8%–42%)	83 (53–193)
New-onset microalbuminuria	23.7%	25.7%	8.1% (2%–13.9%)	47 (27–204)
Severe hypoglycemia	2.7%	1.5%	RRI 85.1% (41.6%–141.9%)	NNH 81 (56–141)

*Abbreviations are defined in the Glossary: RRR, RRI, NNT, NNH, and CI calculated from data in article.

[†]Nonfatal myocardial infarction (intensive vs standard, 2.7% vs 2.8%), nonfatal stroke (3.8% vs 3.8%), or death from cardiovascular causes (4.5% vs 5.2%).

[‡]New or worsening nephropathy or retinopathy (6.0% vs 6.3%).

[§]Macroalbuminuria, doubling of serum creatinine (1.2% vs 1.1%), and renal replacement therapy or death from renal causes (0.4% vs 0.6%).

From *ACP Journal Club.* 2008;149:JC3–JC6; The ADVANCE Collaborative Group. Intensive blood glucose control and vascular outcomes in patients with type 2 diabetes. *N Engl J Med.* 2008;358:2560–2572.

There are a variety of methods that we can use to describe results, and we have included the most important ones in Table 4.2, including the absolute risk reduction (ARR), RRR, and number needed to treat (NNT). We can use an analogy to understand the ARR and the RRR. Consider a sale at a retail store. If a clothing item were marked down from $25 to $20, this represents an absolute discount of $5 (similar to an ARR), but it can also be marketed as a discount of 20% (like the RRR).[22] We can see that the relative discount is more likely to catch a shopper's eye—which is why investigators (and journalists) often tend to report on the results of a study in terms of the RRR! It is up to us to determine whether research results are really as revolutionary as they seem, or if the use of the RRR is masking the fact that the absolute

Table 4.2 Measures of effect size

	Event rate ≡ Stroke (mean follow-up 5 years)		Relative risk reduction (RRR)	Absolute risk reduction (ARR)	Number needed to treat (NNT)
	Control event rate (CER)	Experimental event rate (EER)	|CER − EER|/CER	|CER − EER|	1/ARR
MRC trial	5.7%	4.3%	|5.7% − 4.3%|/5.7% ≡ 25%	|5.7% − 4.3%| ≡ 0.014 or 1.4%	1/1.4% ≡ 72
Hypothetical, trivial case	0.000057%	0.000043%	|0.000057% − 0.000043%|/0.000057% ≡ 25%	|0.000057% − 0.000043%| ≡ 0.000014%	1/0.000014% ≡ 7142857

4

treatment effect is small (in other words, there are small absolute numbers of outcomes in both groups).

We will illustrate these concepts with an example—a randomized trial of statins in patients at risk for stroke conducted by the Medical Research Council (referred to as MRC Trial). As you can see from the trial results reported in Table 4.2, at a mean of 5 years of follow-up, stroke occurred among 5.7% of patients randomized to the control group (we will call this the "control event rate" [CER]) and in 4.3% of the patients assigned to receive the intervention, statin therapy (we will call this the "experimental event rate" [EER]). This difference was statistically significant, but how can it be expressed in a clinically useful way? As previously noted, most often we see this effect reported in clinical journals and in the press as the RRR calculated as (|CER − EER|/CER). In this example, the RRR is (5.7% − 4.3%)/5.7% (i.e., 25%), and we can say that statin therapy decreased the risk of stroke by 25% relative to those who received placebo.

In a similar way, we can describe the situation in which the experimental treatment increases the risk of a good event as the "relative benefit increase" (RBI; also calculated as |CER − EER|/CER). If the treatment increases the probability of a bad event, we can use the same formulae to generate the "relative risk increase" (RRI). We can see that although the math stays the same, in each of these cases our frame of reference is shifting.

To make explicit the disadvantages of the RRR and the ways that it can be misleading, let's examine the hypothetical data outlined in the bottom row of Table 4.2. The RRR doesn't reflect the risk of the event without therapy (the CER, or baseline risk) and therefore cannot discriminate huge treatment effects from small ones. For example, if the stroke risk was trivial (0.000057%) in the control group and similarly trivial (0.000043%) in the experimental group, the RRR remains 25%!

One measure that overcomes this lack of discrimination between small and large treatment effects looks at the absolute arithmetic difference between the rates in the two groups. This is called *absolute risk reduction* (ARR) (or the risk difference), and it preserves the baseline risk. In the MRC trial, the ARR is 5.7% − 4.3% = 1.4%. In our hypothetical case where the baseline risk is trivial, the ARR is also trivial, at 0.000014%. Thus, the ARR is a more meaningful measure of treatment effects compared with the RRR. When the experimental treatment increases the probability of a good event, we can generate the absolute benefit increase (ABI), which is also calculated by finding the absolute arithmetic difference in event rates. Similarly, when the experimental treatment increases the probability of a bad event, we can calculate the absolute risk increase (ARI).

The inverse of the ARR (1/ARR) is a whole number and has the useful property of telling us the NNT with the experimental therapy for the duration of the trial to prevent one additional bad outcome. In our MRC trial example, the NNT is $1/1.4\% \equiv 72$, which means that we would need to treat 72 people with a statin (rather than placebo) for 5 years to prevent one additional person from suffering a stroke. Note that by convention, we always round up to the nearest whole number when describing the NNT. In our hypothetical example in the bottom row of Table 4.2, the clinical usefulness of the NNT is underscored; this tiny treatment effect means that we would have to treat over seven million patients for 5 years to prevent one additional bad event!

> The first co-primary outcome, which was the composite of death from cardiovascular causes, nonfatal MI, or nonfatal stroke, occurred in 3.7% of patients receiving rosuvastatin and 4.8% of patients receiving placebo, a finding that was statistically significant. These results yield an ARR of 1.1%, hazard ratio (HR) 0.76 (95% confidence interval [CI] 0.64–0.91). The individual outcomes[e] all trended in the same direction, and there was a statistically significant reduction in the occurrence of MI with ARR 0.4% and HR 0.65 (95% CI 0.44–0.94). There was a reduction in death from a cardiovascular cause with ARR 0.3% and HR 0.89 (95% CI 0.72–1.11), although as can be seen, this finding was not statistically significant. These results are listed in Table 2 of the paper.

4

What is a good NNT? We can get an idea by comparing an NNT we see in a study with NNTs for other interventions and durations of therapy, tempered by our own clinical experience and expertise. The smaller the NNT is, the more impressive is the result because we need to treat fewer patients to see a clinical benefit. However, we should also consider the seriousness of the outcome that we are trying to prevent. We've provided some examples of NNTs in Table 4.3. For example, we would only need to treat 63 people with hypertension with intensive therapy (versus

---

[e]The first co-primary outcome was the composite of death from cardiovascular causes, nonfatal MI, or nonfatal stroke. The second co-primary outcome was the composite of death from cardiovascular causes, nonfatal MI, nonfatal stroke, revascularization, heart failure, or resuscitated cardiac arrest. The secondary outcome was the composite of death from cardiovascular causes, nonfatal MI, nonfatal stroke, revascularization, heart failure, resuscitated cardiac arrest, or angina with evidence of ischemia. Additional outcomes included death from any cause, each of the individual components comprising the co-primary and secondary outcomes, a new diagnosis of diabetes, cognitive function (among those individuals age ≥ 70 years), and erectile dysfunction (among men).

Table 4.3 Some useful NNTs (a)

Target disorder	Interventions	Primary outcome	Control event rate (CER)	Experimental event rate (EER)	Follow-up time	Number needed to treat	Number needed to harm
			Event rate				
Systolic blood pressure (SBP) (a)	Intensive blood pressure (BP) control (SBP < 120 mm Hg) vs standard BP control (SBP 135–139 mm Hg)	First acute coronary syndrome (ACS), stroke, heart failure, or cardiovascular (CV) death	6.8%	5.2%	3.26 years (trial stopped early)	63	
Acute respiratory distress syndrome (ARDS) (b)	High-frequency oscillatory ventilation vs control	In-hospital mortality	47%	35%	Until hospital discharge		8
Clostridium difficile recurrence (c)	Duodenal infusion of donor feces vs vancomycin 500 mg four times daily × 14 days	Cure without relapse at 10 weeks*	31%	94%	10 weeks	2	
HemoglobinA₁c (in patients with type 2 diabetes mellitus [DM2] and obesity) (d)	Intensive medical therapy (IMT) + Roux-en-y gastric bypass vs IMT alone	Achievement of hemoglobin (Hb) A₁c ≤ 6.0%*	12%	42%	1 year	3	

Smoking cessation (e)	Nicotine patch without behavioural support vs no intervention	30-day smoking abstinence*	3%	7.6%	6 months	22
Human immunodeficiency virus (HIV) screening test (f)	Active choice vs opt-out for HIV testing	Rates of HIV testing	51.3%	65.9%	NA	7
Symptomatic high-grade stenosis (g)	Carotid endarterectomy (compared with medical therapy)	Death or major stroke	18%	8%	2 years	10
Diastolic blood pressure 90–109 mm Hg (h)	Antihypertensive drugs	Death, stroke, or myocardial infarction (MI)	5.5%	4.7%	5.5 years	128
Diastolic blood pressure 115–129 mm Hg (i)	Antihypertensive drugs	Death, stroke, or MI	13%	1.4%	1.5 years	3

*These are outcomes that we hope to increase (rather than prevent, as with most randomized controlled trials). Therefore, the EER is higher than the CER, but this is the desired outcome distribution, and we have to account for this in computing the ARR and NNT by reversing the difference (EER − CER rather than CER − EER).

Please see www.cebm.utoronto.ca for additional NNTs.

a. N Eng J Med. 2015;373(22):2103–2116.
b. N Eng J Med. 2013;368(9):795–805.
c. N Eng J Med. 2013;368(5):407–415.
d. N Eng J Med. 2012;366(17):1567–1576.
e. JAMA. 2016;176(2):184–190.
f. BMJ. 2016;532:h6895.
g. N Eng J Med. 1991;325:445–453.
h. BMJ. 1995;291:97–104.
i. JAMA. 1967;202:116–22.

4

those receiving standard blood pressure [BP] control) to prevent one additional composite event, including first ACS event, stroke, heart failure, or cardiovascular death.

We can describe the adverse effects of therapy in an analogous fashion, as the number needed to harm (NNH) one more patient from the therapy. The NNH is calculated as 1/ARI. In the MRC trial, 0.03% of the control group experienced rhabdomyolysis compared with 0.05% of patients who experienced this in the group that received a statin. This absolute risk increase of $|0.03\% - 0.05\%| \equiv 0.02\%$ generates an NNH of 5000 over 5 years. This means that we would need to treat 5000 patients with a statin for 5 years to cause one additional patient to have rhabdomyolysis. Thus, the NNT and NNH together provide us with a nice measure of the effort that we and our patients have to expend to prevent a bad outcome balanced against the potential associated risks. The utility of these formulae as an effort/yield ratio (or "poor clinicians' cost-effectiveness analysis") is readily apparent.

In the study by Yusuf et al, the first co-primary outcome, which was the composite of death from cardiovascular causes, nonfatal MI, or nonfatal stroke, had an ARR of 1.1%, which yields an NNT of 91 over the 5.6 years of follow-up. If we look at the raw data provided in the "discussion" section, only 1 of 6361 participants that received rosuvastatin developed rhabdomyolysis, compared with 0 of 6344 participants that received placebo. This results in an ARI of 0.000157% and an NNH of 636,100 (although the CI for this estimate is large).

To understand NNTs, we need to consider some additional features. First, they always have a dimension of follow-up time associated with them. Quick reference to Table 4.3 reminds us that the NNT of 10 to prevent one more major stroke or death by performing endarterectomy on patients with symptomatic high-grade carotid stenosis refers to outcomes over a 2-year period (in this case, from an operation that is over in minutes). One consequence of this time dimension is that if we want to compare NNTs and NNHs for different follow-up times we have to make an assumption about them and a "time adjustment" to at least one of them. Say we wanted to compare the NNTs to prevent one additional stroke, MI, or death with medications among patients with mild versus severe hypertension. Another quick look at Table 4.3 gives us an NNT of 3 at 1.5 years for patients with severe hypertension (these are patients that already have end organ damage) and an NNT of 128 at 5.5 years for patients with mild hypertension (most of whom are free of end organ complications). To compare their NNTs, we need to adjust at least one of them so that they relate to the same follow-up time. The assumption that we make here is that the RRR from antihypertensive therapy is constant over time (i.e., we assume that antihypertensive therapy exerts the same relative benefit in year 1 as it does over the next 4 years). If we are comfortable with that assumption, we can then proceed to make the time adjustment. This assumption is probably reasonable for antihypertensives because most of them exert their effect within a few weeks and, if taken as prescribed, their effect is durable over time. However, it may not be valid for other treatments like analgesic agents to which patients may become desensitized over time.

Let's adjust the NNT for the group of patients with mild hypertension (128 over the "observed" 5.5 years) to an NNT corresponding to a "hypothetical" 1.5 years. We can do this by setting up a balanced equation:

$$NNT_{(Hypothetical)} \div Time_{(Hypothetical)} \equiv NNT_{(Observed)} \div Time_{(Observed)}$$

Rearranging we obtain:

$$NNT_{(Hypothetical)} \equiv NNT_{(Observed)} \times [Time_{(Hypothetical)} / Time_{(Observed)}]$$

Plugging in the values, we get:

$$NNT_{(1.5)} \equiv 128 \times (1.5/5.5) = 35$$

(By convention, we round any decimal NNT upward to the next whole number.)

Now we can appreciate the vast difference in the yield of clinical efforts to treat patients with mild versus severe hypertension: We need to treat 35 of the former, but only three of the latter for 1.5 years to prevent one additional bad outcome. The explanation lies in the huge difference in CERs, which were far higher among patients with severe hypertension followed up for just 1.5 years than among patients with mild hypertension followed up for 5.5 years—meaning that we saw a much more substantial ARR in the cohort of patients with severe hypertension.

Considering our scenario, the first co-primary outcome, which was the composite of death from cardiovascular causes, nonfatal MI, or nonfatal stroke, had an ARR of 1.1%, which yields an NNT of 91 over the 5.6 years of follow-up. Remember that this is a finding among a population at intermediate risk of cardiovascular events. The "Myocardial Ischemia Reduction with Aggressive Cholesterol Lowering" (MIRACL) trial examined the use of statins in a population of patients at high risk of cardiovascular events.[23] In this study, 3086 patients with recent unstable angina or non-ST elevation MI were randomized to receive atorvastatin 80 mg versus placebo, daily, within 4 days of hospitalization. The primary outcome, similar but not identical to the HOPE-3 (Heart Outcomes Prevention Evaluation 3) trial, was the composite of all-cause mortality, nonfatal MI, cardiac arrest requiring resuscitation, or rehospitalization for an ACS. The rate of this composite outcome was 14.8% in the intervention group versus 17.4% in the control group, yielding an ARR of 2.6% and an NNT of 39 over 16 weeks of follow-up. Already we can see that the NNT is more impressive, and that too, over a MUCH shorter period! If we want to make the NNTs comparable over the same period, we can adjust the NNT from HOPE-3 to a follow-up period of 16 weeks:

$$NNT_{(HOPE3)} \div Time_{(HOPE3)} \equiv NNT_{(MIRACL)} \div Time_{(MIRACL)}$$

After rearranging, we obtain:

$$NNT_{(HOPE3)} \equiv NNT_{(MIRACL)} \times [Time_{(HOPE3)} / Time_{(MIRACL)}]$$

By plugging in the values, we get:

$$NNT_{(HOPE3)} \equiv 39 \times (291.2/16) \equiv 710$$

As you can see, if the patients at only intermediate risk were to be prescribed statins, we would need to treat 710 patients for 16 weeks to reduce the risk of the composite endpoint (death from cardiovascular causes, nonfatal MI, or nonfatal stroke) in just one of them! In contrast, for high-risk patients, we only need to treat 39 individuals!

We can also adjust the NNT depending on the baseline risk of the patient. Returning to Table 4.2 and our MRC trial example, we calculated an NNT of 72 for that study—but patients can have a different baseline risk of the outcome (depending on the presence of comorbid illnesses, etc.), and therefore they may be at higher or lower risk of the event than the "average" patient in the study. The NNT can be adjusted for our patient's individual baseline risk of the outcome, and this will be discussed in detail on page 104.

2. How precise is this estimate of the treatment effect?

CIs are a tool that we can use to convey the precision of a study result. The CI provides the range of values that are likely to include the true risk and quantifies the uncertainty in our measurement. A commonly used parameter is the 95% CI, and this specifies the limits within which the true association lies, 95% of the time.

We can work through this concept by considering the NNT, which, as noted, is like any other clinical measure in that it is simply an *estimate* of the truth—therefore, we should specify the limits within which we can confidently state that the true NNT lies. In the PROGRESS trial, blood pressure lowering after stroke or TIA "reduced the absolute rates of ischemic stroke from 14% to 10%."[24] This amounted to an RRR = 28%; 95% confidence interval: (17% to 38%). We were provided this CI in the paper. The way to interpret this is that we have 95% confidence that the true RRR value lies between 17% and 38%, with 28% being the most likely value.

The absolute risk reduction for this result from the PROGRESS (Perindopril pROtection aGainst REcurrent Stroke Study) trial is 4% (14% − 10%), for which we can also calculate a 95% CI. We do this by recalling that RRR ≡ (|CER − EER|/CER) and ARR is simply |CER − EER|, which we can obtain from the RRR by multiplying the RRR by the CER:

$$\text{ARR} \equiv \text{RRR} \times \text{CER} \equiv (|\text{CER} - \text{EER}|/\,\cancel{\text{CER}}\,) \times \cancel{\text{CER}} \equiv |\text{CER} - \text{EER}|$$

In our example, the CER is 14% or 0.14 and the boundaries of the RRR CI, which are reported in the paper, are (17%–38%). Therefore, to get the ARR 95% CI:

$$\text{ARR 95\% CI} \equiv \text{RRR 95\% CI} \times \text{CER} \equiv (17\% - 38\%) \times 14\%$$
$$\equiv (2.38\% - 5.32\%)$$

It is important to consider whether the confidence interval contains "the null," where the "null" means that there is no benefit with a therapy. The null depends on the measure of association that is being used. For an ARR, which is |CER − EER| (meaning a risk difference), no benefit is demonstrated by a value of 0 (i.e., CER ≡ EER). This means that when the confidence interval crosses 0, it is including the possibility of no effect. This means that the result is not statistically significant—that is, the p value is greater than 0.5. We will describe the relationship between confidence intervals and p values in greater detail below. We can see that in our example, the ARR 95% CI is (2.38%–5.32%), and it does not include 0%; therefore, this is a statistically significant finding, and the possibility of no benefit is unlikely in this study.

Finally, we can calculate the confidence interval for the NNT by simply taking the inverse of the ARR confidence intervals (because NNT ≡ 1/ARR): 1/0.0238 and 1/0.0532. Thus, the 95% CI for the NNT is 43 to 19, which we rewrite as (19–43).

The smaller the number of patients in the study that generated the NNT, the wider its CI because we are "less confident" that the results

4

Box 4.3 Confidence intervals and significance tests

Confidence intervals (CIs) and significance tests are closely related. Generally, a "significant" p value of $p < 0.05$ will correspond to a 95% CI, which excludes the value indicating no difference. The "no difference" value is 0 for a difference of measures (e.g., absolute risk reduction, otherwise known as a risk difference) and is 1 for a ratio (e.g., the relative risk, odds ratio, or hazard ratio).

For example, an absolute risk difference of 5% (95% CI –5% to +15%) is not statistically significant because the 95% CI includes 0, whereas a risk difference of 5% (95% CI 2%–8%) would be statistically significant because if does not include 0. Similarly, a relative risk of 0.80 (95% CI 0.50–1.1) would not be statistically significant because it includes 1, whereas a relative risk of 0.80 (95% CI 0.70–0.90) would be statistically significant because it does not include 1 (the "no effect" value for ratio measures).

Most statisticians now agree that estimations, including CIs, are preferable for summarizing the results of a study, but CIs and p values are interchangeable and many papers present both. For more information about confidence intervals, including details about how to calculate them, refer to Appendix 1 (LINK).

---

represent a true effect if there are only a few patients in whom we performed the experiment (fewer patients mean that the result we see may have occurred through bias or chance). Nonetheless, even when the CI is wide, it can provide us with some guidance, and we should look at the limits of the CI.[25] The PROGRESS trial example above shows a positive effect, but we need to look at the upper limit of the CI for the NNT. Is the value of 43 clinically important? If we decide that it is not, the study results are unhelpful, even though it is statistically significant (i.e., even though "$p < 0.05$"). Similarly, if the study results are negative, we can look at the limits of the CI to see if a potentially important positive benefit has been excluded. A result that isn't statistically significant (that is "$p > 0.05$") can still be helpful to us! Incidentally, confidence intervals and p values are closely related (Box 4.3).

Practising evidence-based medicine in real time: calculating the measures of treatment effect—a shortcut

Rather than memorizing the formula described above, we could instead use an evidence-based medicine (EBM) calculator whenever we need to calculate the measure of the treatment effect (i.e., if the results of the study aren't presented in the article using these measures). This tool saves us time and decreases the risk of a mathematical error. You can download an EBM calculator at: http://www.cebm.utoronto.ca/practise/

Randomized Controlled Trial Calculator

Return to Calculator Index

This calculator was created for your own personal use and testing purposes. It is to be used as a guide only. Medical decisions should NOT be based solely on the results of this program. Although this program has been tested thoroughly, the accuracy of the information cannot be guaranteed.

Randomized Controlled Trial Calculator

	Outcome		No Outcome	
Experimental		A		B
Control		C		D

get results   reset

Results

Chi-squared   --   --

	Estimate	95% CI
RRR	--	--
ARR	--	--
NNT	--	--

Fig. 4.2 CEBM statistics calculator. (© CEBM, University of Toronto, reproduced with permission.)

ca/statscal/ (Fig. 4.2). Let's try to repeat the calculations that we completed in Table 4.2 by using the EBM calculator. In the dropdown box on the calculator, click on the "RCT" option. We can enter the data from the table, and at the click of a button, we can obtain the measures of effect and their CIs.

Practising EBM in real time: using preappraised evidence

When retrieving evidence to answer our clinical question, we also completed a search of the *ACP Journal Club* and identified an entry for the study by Yusuf et al. that we have been appraising.[1,26] We know that this article has passed some quality filters because it appears in this journal. Furthermore, it has been rated on clinical relevance and newsworthiness by clinicians. Contrast the more informative abstract provided by the *ACP Journal Club* with the one from the original article. Using the *ACP Journal Club*, we can quickly see that it was a randomized, placebo-controlled study in which patients, clinicians, outcomes assessors, and members of the steering committee were all blinded. The investigators used an ITT analysis, and 99% follow-up was achieved. Of note, a declarative title and the clinical question that the trial addressed (using the PICO [population, intervention, comparison, outcome] format!) are included: "Rosuvastatin reduced major cardiovascular events in patients at intermediate cardiovascular risk." Using the *ACP Journal Club* abstract, we can appraise the trial's validity and importance in less than a minute and quickly move to decide if we can apply the evidence to our patient! Moreover, there is a commentary by an expert clinician who provides a clinical bottom line and places the evidence from this article in context with other evidence.

We can also find this article in a search of Evidence Alerts https://plus.mcmaster.ca/EvidenceAlerts/QuickSearch.aspx?Page=1#Data (Fig. 4.3). Indeed, we had already seen this article in a weekly e-mail that we receive and we had saved it to our own, searchable database within "Evidence Alerts." We were able to retrieve the citation, which appears below. The citation includes comments from clinicians from primary care, internal medicine, and cardiology. Comments on study quality and clinical context may help us with our interpretation and use of the evidence.

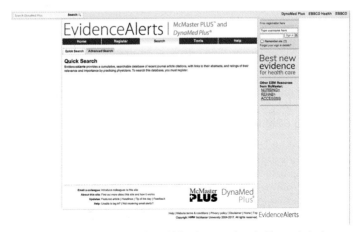

Fig. 4.3 Evidence Alerts. (© McMaster University, reproduced with permission.)

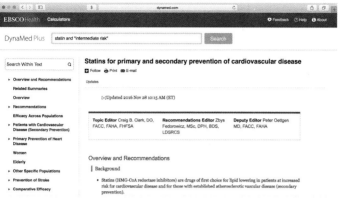

Fig. 4.4 Screenshot from DynaMed Plus showing results of statin search. (© EBSCO, reproduced with permission.)

We could also look for an answer to our question about statins in intermediate risk patients in "Clinical Evidence (CE)." As mentioned on Chapter 2, CE (www.clinicalevidence.org) uses explicit, rigorous methods to retrieve, appraise, summarize, and update relevant evidence. Another resource that can provide preappraised evidence at the bedside is DynaMed (Fig. 4.4) (http://www.dynamed.com/resultlist?q=statin+and +%22intermediate+risk%22&filter); all these resources also offer a free trial. We can search for the relevant sections in these resources that describe the evidence for statins in intermediate-risk patients. Using this preappraised evidence, we can obtain the answer to our clinical question in less than 30 seconds—making it feasible to practise EBM in real time at the bedside! Access these resources for yourself!

Are the valid, important results of this individual study applicable to our patient?

Now that we have decided that the evidence we have found is both valid and important, we need to consider if we can apply it to our own patient. To apply evidence, we need to integrate the evidence with our clinical experience and expertise and with our patient's values and preferences. The guides for doing this are in Box 4.4.

> **Box 4.4** Is this valid and important evidence (from an individual randomized trial) applicable to our patient?
>
> 1. Is our patient so different from those in the study that its results cannot apply?
> 2. Is the treatment feasible in our setting?
> 3. What are our patient's potential benefits and harms from the therapy?
> 4. What are our patient's values and expectations for both the outcome we are trying to prevent and the treatment we are offering?

1. Is our patient so different from those in the study that its results cannot apply?

We need to use our clinical expertise to decide if our patient is so different from those in the study that the study results will not apply. One approach would be to demand that our patient fit all the inclusion criteria for the study and reject the study if our patient does not fit each one. This is not a very sensible approach because most differences between our patients and those in trials tend to be quantitative, along a spectrum. For example, patients may have different ages, different degrees of risk of the outcome event, or differential responsiveness to the therapy. Differences between our patients and trial participants are less likely to be absolute—in terms of a total absence of responsiveness to treatment or risk of event. We would suggest that it is more appropriate to consider whether our patient's sociodemographic features or pathobiology are so different from those in the study that its results are useless to us and our patient; only then should we discard its results and resume our search for relevant evidence. There are only a few occasions when this might be the case: different pharmacogenetics, absent immune responses, comorbid conditions that prohibit the treatment, to name but a few. As a consequence of this clinical (as opposed to actuarial) approach, it is rare that we have to reject a study because of a lack of applicability. Note that one important difference that we do need to consider is the patient's perspectives, values, and goals and how these might influence the proposed therapeutic regimen, which we will discuss in detail later.

Sometimes treatments appear to produce qualitative differences in the responses of subgroups of patients so that they appear to benefit some subgroups but not others. Such qualitative differences in response are extremely rare. For example, some early trials of aspirin for transient ischemic attacks (TIAs) showed large benefits for men but none for

---

Box 4.5 Guides for whether to believe apparent qualitative differences in the efficacy of therapy in some subgroups of patients

---

A qualitative difference in treatment efficacy among subgroups is likely only when *all* the following questions can be answered "yes":
1. Does it really make biological and clinical sense?
2. Is the qualitative difference both clinically (beneficial for some but useless or harmful for others) and statistically significant?
3. Was it hypothesized before the study began (rather than the product of dredging the data)?
4. Was it one of just a few subgroup analyses carried out in the study?
5. Is this subgroup difference suggested by comparisons within rather than between studies?
6. Has the result been confirmed in other independent studies?

---

women; subsequent trials and SRs showed that this was a chance finding and that aspirin *is* efficacious in women. If you think that the treatment you are examining may work in a qualitatively different way among different subgroups of patients, you should refer to the guides in Box 4.5. To summarize them, unless the difference in response makes biological sense, was hypothesized before the trial, and has been confirmed in a second, independent trial, we would suggest that you accept the treatment's overall efficacy as the best starting point for estimating its efficacy in your individual patient.

4

In the study by Yusuf et al., the average age of patients was 65 years, about 45% of them were women, and a majority of the patients had an elevated waist-to-hip ratio. Prespecified hypothesis-based subgroup analyses defined across several variables, including, but not limited to, gender, racial or ethnic group, age, and baseline and cardiovascular risk, did not demonstrate heterogeneity of the results. These demographic factors are similar to those of our patient.

---

2. Is the treatment feasible in our setting?

Next, we need to consider if the treatment is feasible in our practice setting. Is the treatment available in our setting? Can our patient, or the health care system, pay for the treatment, its administration, and the required monitoring?

Cholesterol-lowering therapies are variable in cost—with some of the newer agents being quite expensive. However, with many patents now expired, several statins are available in generic formulations. Therefore, if you believe in a "class effect" (the outcomes seen with one statin are likely to be reproduced with another statin), then you can consider substitutions within a class of medication if cost is a factor. Depending on the patient's insurance status, these medications may also be covered if appropriate treatment criteria are met.

3. What are the potential benefits and harms from the therapy to our patient?

After we have decided that the study is applicable to our patients and that the treatment is feasible, we need to estimate our patient's unique benefits and risks of therapy. There are two general approaches to doing this. The first and longer approach begins by coming up with the best possible estimate of what would happen to our patient if she were not treated, her individual CER or the "patient's expected event rate" (PEER). To make this estimate we can apply the overall RRR (for the events we hope to prevent with therapy) and the RRI (for the adverse effects of therapy) and generate the corresponding NNT and NNH for our specific patient. Before demonstrating this concept, we note that the second (and much quicker) approach skips this PEER step and works directly from the NNT and NNH in the study. With either approach, we assume that the relative benefits and risks of therapy are the same for patients with high and low PEERs. Because the second method is so much quicker, you may choose to skip to page 105, but if you want to learn the long way (first), read on.

The long way, via PEER

There are four ways to estimate our patient's PEER. First, we can simply assign our patient the overall CER from the study; this is easy, but sensible only if our patient is like the "average" study patient. Second, if the study has a subgroup of patients with characteristics similar to our own patient, we can assign to our patient the CER for that subgroup. (Indeed, in the unlikely event that we could say "yes" to all of the questions posed in Box 4.5, we could even apply the ARR for that subgroup to generate an NNT for our patient.) Third, if the study report includes a valid clinical prediction guide, we could use it to assign a PEER to our patient. Fourth, we could look for another paper that described the prognosis of untreated patients like ours and use its results to assign our patient a PEER. All four of the methods that we have described generate a PEER for our patient—what we would expect to happen to them if they received the "control" or comparison intervention in the study we are using. To convert this into an NNT or NNH for patients just like ours, we have to apply the corresponding RRR and RRI to them, using the formula:

$$NNT \equiv 1/(PEER \times RRR) \text{ or}$$

$$NNH \equiv 1/(PEER \times RRI)$$

where $RRR \equiv (|CER - EER|/CER)$, and the CER and EER are obtained from the trial. The same formula applies for the RRI but the CER and EER are for the adverse events.

For example, suppose that we find a paper that suggests that our patient has a risk of MI of 10% over 10 years given her intermediate risk (so her PEER is 10%). The trial by Yusuf et al. generated an overall adjusted RRR of 23% at 5.6 years, so the NNT for patients like ours is $1/(10\% \times 23\%) \equiv 43$.

As you can see, these calculations can be cumbersome to do without a calculator, and fortunately Dr. G. Chatellier and his colleagues published the convenient nomogram, shown in Figure 4.5, to help us. Alternatively, we could use the EBM calculator from our website (www.cebm.utoronto.ca).

Now we will turn our attention to the short way of computing our patient's unique risk and benefit, sticking with NNT/NNH. This is a faster and easier method of estimating an NNT or NNH for our patient and is the one we usually use at the bedside or in the clinic. In this approach, the estimate we make for our patient's risk of the outcome event (if the patient were to receive just the "control" therapy) is specified relative to that of the average control patient, and expressed as a "decimal fraction," which we call f_t. For example, if we think that our patient (if left untreated) has twice the risk of the outcome as control patients in the trial, $f_t \equiv 2$; alternatively, if we think our patient is at only half their risk, then $f_t \equiv 0.5$. We can use our past clinical experience and expertise in coming up with a value for f_t, or we can use any of the information sources described in the previous section. Remembering our assumption that the treatment produces a constant RRR across the range of susceptibilities, the NNT for patients just like ours is simply the reported NNT divided by f_t. In our MRC trial example, we calculated an NNT of 72, meaning that we would need to treat 72 patients like those in the trial

4

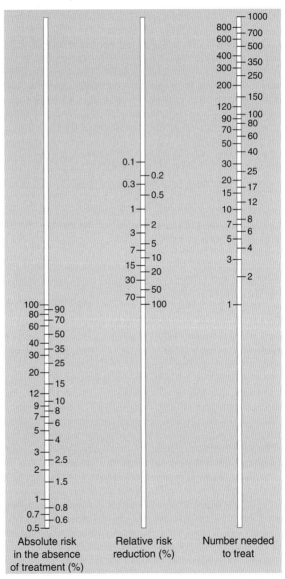

Fig. 4.5 Nomogram for determining numbers needed to treat (NNTs). (From Chatellier G, et al. The number needed to treat: a clinically useful nomogram in its proper context. *BMJ*. 1996;312:426–429, with permission).

with a statin for a mean of 5 years to prevent one more of them from experiencing a stroke. If, however, we judge that our patient is at three times the risk of stroke without treatment as the patients in the control group, $f_t \equiv 3$ and $NNT/f_t \equiv 72/3 \equiv 24$. This means that we would only need to treat 24 higher-risk patients like ours for 5 years to prevent an additional stroke.

Again, we need to consider our patient's risk of adverse events from the therapy. To do this, we can use any of the same methods that we used to individualize our patient's NNT. Using the simplest one, we may decide that our patient is at three times the risk of adverse events as patients in the control group of the study ($f_h \equiv 3$), or we may decide that our patient is at one-third the risk ($f_h \equiv 0.33$). Assuming the RRI of harm is constant over the spectrum of susceptibilities, we can adjust the study NNH of 5000 with f_h (just as we did for the NNT), and generate NNH values of 1667 and 15,152 corresponding to f_h values of 3 and 0.33, respectively.

> Returning to the study by Yusuf et al., we may believe that our patient's risk of MI/stroke/death from a cardiovascular cause was greater than those in the control group. Imagine it is 2 times that of the control group; f_h is therefore 2 and the NNT becomes 91/2 or 46. We would only need to treat 46 people like our patient to reduce one occurrence of MI/stroke/death from cardiovascular cause.

4

4. How can we present this information to the patient in a way that can support shared decision making? What are our patient's values and expectations for both the outcome we are trying to prevent and the treatment we are offering?

Thus far, we have individualized the benefits and risks of therapy for our patient but we have ignored the patient's values and preferences. How can we incorporate these into a treatment recommendation? There are several models available for providing shared decision-making support, including elaborate ("Rolls Royce") ways of doing this, such as a formal CDA, which incorporates the patient's likelihood of the outcome events with his or her own values for each health state. However, performing a CDA for each patient is not usually feasible; instead, we tend to rely on finding an existing CDA. To be able to use the existing CDA, either our patient's values (and risks) must approximate those in the analysis, or the CDA must provide information about the impact of variation in patient values (and risks) on the results of the CDA. We will discuss decision analyses in detail in a later section. For now, suffice it to say that even expert clinical decision analysts find them prohibitively slow to use in the real world! Clinicians can also use validated decision aids that present descriptive and probabilistic information about the target disorder, management options, and outcome events to facilitate shared decision making. Well-validated decision aids can be tough to find. If you're interested in finding some, there is a growing repository available at: http://decisionaid.ohri.ca/decaids.html.

Is there some quick way of incorporating patient specific risks that doesn't do too much violence to the truth? In an attempt to meet the needs of comprehensibility, applicability, and ease of use for busy clinical services, we proposed a patient-centred measure of the likelihood of being helped and harmed by an intervention based on the NNT for target events produced by the intervention (as an expression of the likelihood of being helped), the NNH for the adverse effects of therapy (to express the likelihood of being harmed), and their ratio. This result, when adjusted by an individual patient-centred conviction about the relative severities of these two events, provides an understandable, quality-adjusted, rapidly calculated measure of the likelihood of being helped or harmed (LHH) by a particular therapy.

Returning to our patient, we found that the NNT was 91 over 5.6 years. We could use this to tell our patient that she has a 1 in 91 chance of being helped by rosuvastatin in reducing the occurrence of MI/stroke/ death from a cardiovascular cause. Similarly, looking at her risk of harm, we could tell her she has a 1 in 636,100 chance of experiencing harm (rhabdomyolysis) with this therapy. Our first approximation of her likelihood of being helped versus harmed then becomes:

$$LHH \equiv (1/NNT) : (1/NNH)^{\dagger}$$
$$\equiv (1/91) : (1/636,100)$$
$$\equiv 6990$$

We could then tell our patient that rosuvastatin therapy is 6990 times more likely to help than harm her. But, again, this ignores her unique potential benefit and harm from therapy. We might think that her baseline risk of death is lower than that of patients in the control group (and as in the previous section, we have several options for determining her

---

†Note that we could also say LHH ≡ ARR : ARI.

PEER, but for now, we will stick with the f_t method). We could estimate f_t and f_h from our clinical experience, and we might decide that her risk of MI/stroke/death from a cardiovascular cause is 0.5 times that of the control group in the study ($f_t \equiv 0.5$) and similarly we might think her risk of rhabdomyolysis was higher than that of the control group (let's assume $f_h = 1000$ for convenience in doing the math). Her LHH now becomes:

$$LHH \equiv (1/NNT) \times f_t : (1/NNH) \times f_h$$
$$\equiv [(1/91) \times 0.5] : [(1/636,100) \times 1000]$$
$$\equiv 3.5$$

This now means that our patient is 3.5 times as likely to be helped as harmed by the therapy.

Observe that in our calculation above, we multiplied rather than divided by f_t in this case because we are adjusting $1/NNT$, so we are essentially inverting our previous modification.

We now tell our patient that based on her unique benefits and harms, she is 3.5 times more likely to be helped than harmed by the therapy.

But, this doesn't incorporate our patient's unique values and preferences. How can we convert these into a form that permits our patient to make a personalized treatment decision? We begin this in the time-honored way of describing both options and any other alternatives in a way that respects the patient's cultural and linguistic needs, making use of visual aids to address literacy constraints, creating a safe space for patients and their loved ones to ask questions, and repeating the options as needed. When the treatment option is a common one (e.g., whether to take long-term aspirin after an MI), we might conclude our discussion with a written description of what outcomes might be expected if the patient either accepts or forgoes treatment. This leads us to the most critical step in calculating the LHH—the process of eliciting our patient's preferences.

Practising EBM in real time: preappraised literature for patients

Medline Plus is a website that provides high quality information to patients (https://vsearch.nlm.nih.gov/vivisimo/cgi-bin/query-meta?v%3 Aproject=medlineplus&v%3Asources=medlineplus-bundle&query =%22statins%22&_ga=2.243421964.865596624.1495023798-563915735 .1495023798) (Fig. 4.6). In our search on statins, we retrieve a synopsis

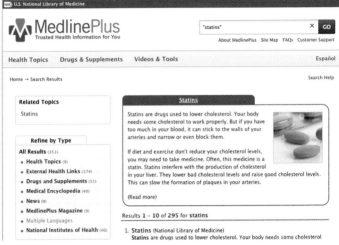

Fig. 4.6 Screenshot from Medline search. (© NIH, reproduced with permission.)

of the evidence that highlights how statins work and provides references that our patient may want to review. This material is generated by the U.S. National Library of Medicine. It is freely available and a resource that we can provide to our patients.

We ask our patient to make value judgements about the relative severity of the bad outcome we hope to prevent with therapy and the adverse event we might cause with it. We work with the patient to help her express how severe she considers one of them to be relative to the other—is MI/stroke/death 20 times as severe as rhabdomyolysis? Five times as severe? This can be accomplished in a quick and simple way by asking our patient to tell us which outcome is worse, and by how much. If the patient has difficulty making this comparison in a direct fashion, we present her with a rating scale (Fig. 4.7), the ends of which are anchored at 0 (≡ death or stroke or ??[8]) and 1 (≡ full health); this describes the "utility" that the patient experiences with each outcome. So, for instance, we ask our patient to place a mark where she would consider the value of the target event we hope to prevent with treatment; in our case, suppose the patients assigns this a value of 0.025. Similarly,

---

[9]Yes, our patients sometimes identify fates worse than death, in which case we extend the line below zero.

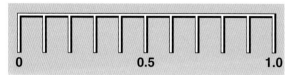

Fig. 4.7 Rating scale for assessing values.

we ask her to place a second mark to correspond with the value for rhabdomyolysis, the adverse event that we are trying to prevent; our patient assigned the adverse event a value of 0.45, which constitutes a moderate "disutility." Comparing these two ratings, we can say that our patient believes that MI/stroke/death is 18 (0.45/0.025) times worse than the rhabdomyolysis that may occur as an adverse drug effect. We call this relative value the severity or "s" factor. We then ask her whether this comparison makes sense, and usually repeat this process on a second visit to see whether this relative severity is stable over time and reflective of consistent values and wishes.

Integrating this with our risk-adjusted LHH, the LHH becomes:

$$LHH \equiv [(1/NNT) \times f_t] : [(1/NNH) \times f_h] \times s$$
$$\equiv [(1/91) \times 0.5] : [(1/636,100) \times 1000] \times 18$$
$$\equiv 3.5 \times 18$$
$$\equiv 63$$

Thus, in the final analysis, our patient is 63 times as likely to be helped versus harmed by rosuvastatin therapy based on her values and preferences.

If we are unsure of our patient's "f" for benefit or harm, or if our patient is uncertain about her "severity" factor, we can do a sensitivity analysis by inserting other clinically sensible values for "f" and "s" and see how they affect the size and direction of the LHH.

The foregoing discussion demonstrates a quick and easy model for arriving at the LHH, but it is a far cry from the "Rolls Royce" of CDA. We could add a few features to the basic LHH, making it a more robust means of comparing two active treatments (instead of just a placebo versus experimental treatment as in our example). And, if there were several serious adverse events that could result from the treatment(s), we could add each of them to generate the fully adjusted LHH. Finally, as we will describe later in this chapter, we can also discount future events as in a CDA.

However, we have found that the method we have just described to arrive at an LHH can be used in the busy clinical setting (median time to complete it is 6.5 minutes). Furthermore, it is intelligible to both clinicians and patients and it is patient centred. Here is the link to the video that explains tailoring of evidence to patients (https://goanimate .com/videos/0WfftaXs-K78?utm_source=linkshare&utm_medium =linkshare&utm_campaign=usercontent.) As other approaches in this rapidly developing field are validated in clinical settings, they will appear in future editions of this book.

Now that we have completed a critical appraisal of the paper that we retrieved, we may want to keep a permanent record of this. We find that critically appraised topics (CATs) are useful as teaching tools. CAT banks are great practice tools if we can find sites that describe and use rigorous methodology for the creation, peer review, and updating of CATs. However, these tasks require tremendous resources and few CAT banks that we have found meet these needs.

Further reading about individual randomized trials

Guyatt G, Rennie D, Meade M, Cook DJ, editors. Users' guides to the medical literature. A manual for evidence-based clinical practice. 3rd ed. Chicago, IL: McGraw-Hill Education; 2015.

Haynes RB, Sackett DL, Guyatt GH, Tugwell P. Clinical epidemiology: how to do clinical practice research. Philadelphia, PA: Lippincott Williams & Wilkins; 2006.

Straus SE. Individualizing treatment decisions. The likelihood of being helped versus harmed. Eval Health Prof 2002;25:210–24.

Reports of systematic reviews

It might appear that this section is out of order—the first target of any search about therapy should be an SR because SRs are the most powerful and useful evidence available. However, because the critical appraisal of an SR requires the skill to appraise the individual trials that comprise it, we have switched the order in this book.

An SR is a summary of the clinical literature that uses explicit methods to systematically search, critically appraise, and synthesize the evidence base on a specific issue. Its goal is to minimize bias (usually by not only restricting itself to randomized trials but also seeking published and unpublished reports in every language) and random error (by amassing very large numbers of individual study participants). SRs may, but need not, include some statistical method for combining the results of individual studies, generating a type of study called a *meta-analysis*. In contrast, traditional literature reviews usually do not include an exhaustive literature search or synthesis of studies and do not utilize this kind of rigorous methodology. The guides that we consider when appraising an SR follow. Not surprisingly, many of them (especially around importance and applicability) are the same as those for individual reports, but those for validity are different. We will start with assessing validity using the guides in Box 4.6; the guides for considering the importance of the results are outlined in Box 4.7.

We see a patient in the emergency department. He is a 65-year-old, previously healthy man presenting with cough productive of yellow sputum, shortness of breath, and fever. He is hypoxic with an oxygen saturation of 86% on room air, has bronchial breath sounds over the right base, has an elevated white blood cell count, and has consolidation on chest radiography. He is admitted to General Internal Medicine with a diagnosis of community-acquired pneumonia, and relevant investigations are ordered. The resident on call starts antibiotics, and she wonders whether this patient should receive concomitant corticosteroids. Together, we formulate the question: In a patient with community-acquired pneumonia, does treatment with corticosteroids along with antibiotics decrease his risk of death, intensive care unit (ICU) admission, or need for intubation? We search PubMed Clinical Queries using the terms "corticosteroids," "pneumonia," and "adults," and we retrieve a SR by Siemieniuk et al., published in 2015.[27]

4

Box 4.6 Is the evidence from this systematic review valid?

1. Is this a systematic review of randomized trials?
2. Does it describe a comprehensive and detailed search for relevant trials?
3. Were the individual studies assessed for validity?
   A less frequent point:
1. Were individual patient data (or aggregate data) used in the analysis?

Box 4.7 Is the valid evidence from this systematic review important?

1. Are the results consistent across studies?
2. What is the magnitude of the treatment effect?
3. How precise is the treatment effect?

Are the results of this systematic review valid?

1. Is this a systematic review of randomized trials?

Initially, we need to determine whether the SR combines randomized or nonrandomized trials. SRs, by combining all relevant randomized trials, reduce both bias and random error and thus provide the highest level of evidence currently achievable about the effects of health care.[h] In contrast, SRs of nonrandomized trials can compound the problems of individually misleading trials and produce a lower quality of evidence. For this reason, if the SR we find includes both randomized and non-randomized trials, we avoid it unless it separates these types of trials in its analyses. As mentioned previously, individual trials may not have sufficient follow-up to provide estimates of adverse events, and this is an advantage of SRs because they pool results from multiple studies. However, if these adverse events are not reported in the trials, we may need to look for SRs that include observational studies.

> Our review includes randomized trials investigating the use of antibiotics with corticosteroids or placebo in patients admitted to hospital with community-acquired pneumonia.

2. Does it describe a comprehensive and detailed search for relevant trials?

We need to scrutinize the methods section to determine whether it describes how the investigators found all the relevant trials. If not, we drop it and continue looking. If they did carry out a search, we seek reassurance that it went beyond standard bibliographic databases because these have been shown to fail to correctly label up to half of the published trials in their files.[29] A more rigorous SR would include hand-searching of journals, conference proceedings, theses, and the databanks of pharmaceutical firms, as well as contacting authors of published articles. Negative trials are less likely to be submitted and selected for publication (which could result in a false-positive conclusion in an SR restricted to published trials). And if the SR's authors restricted their search to reports

---

[h]This is why the Cochrane Collaboration has been compared with the Human Genome Project; however, we think that the Cochrane Collaboration faces an even greater challenge given the infinite number of trials versus the finite number of genes! Clarke and Mallett have suggested that at least 10,000 SRs are needed to cover studies relevant to health care as identified by the Cochrane Collaboration in 2003.[28]

in just one language, this, too, could bias the conclusions. It has been observed, for example, that bilingual German investigators were more likely to submit trials with positive results to English language journals and those with negative results to German language journals.[i] More journals are now requiring authors to identify and describe the impact of excluding studies because of language restrictions on their findings and conclusions. As with the reporting of individual trials, journals are asking for a flow diagram outlining the search strategy and the path to article selection. This process is governed by the "Preferred Reporting Items for Systematic Reviews and Meta-Analyses" (PRISMA) statement,[30] aimed at enhancing the accuracy of reporting of reviews. Figure 4.8 provides the flow diagram for the study we found.

The authors of our review replicated the search strategy used in a review previously published by the Cochrane Collaboration in December 2010. (Ideally, we should see that the search has been appraised by an information scientist using the PRESS checklist.[31]) They then searched PubMed, EMBASE, and the Cochrane Central Register of Controlled Trials from January 1, 2010, to May 24, 2015. They also manually searched the references of included articles as well as any other articles citing the included publications (called *forward citation searching*). They selected studies in any language. This yielded 13 RCTs, nine of which were not included in the original 2010 review.

4

---

3. Were the individual studies assessed for validity?

The methods section of the report should also include a statement describing how the investigators assessed the validity of the individual studies (using criteria such as those listed in Box 4.1). We would feel most confident in an SR in which multiple independent reviewers assessed the individual studies and demonstrated good agreement in their findings. These independent assessments help reduce bias. The independent assessments should occur at each stage of the review process. For example, the titles and abstracts of the retrieved articles should be reviewed independently by two investigators to determine whether they meet inclusion criteria, the full text articles should be reviewed independently by two individuals, and data abstraction and risk of bias should be assessed by two independent reviewers.

---

[i]This observation applies to allopathic interventions; the situation is reversed for trials assessing complementary medical therapies!

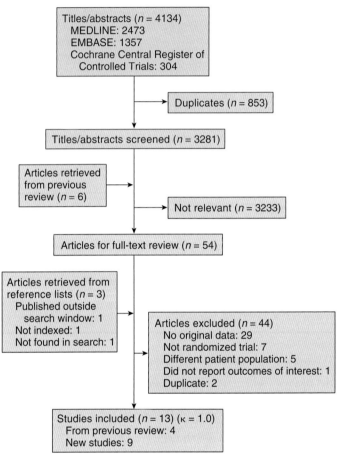

Fig. 4.8 PRISMA flow diagram for systematic review. (From Siemieniuk RAC, et al. Corticosteroid therapy for patients hospitalized with community-acquired pneumonia: systematic review and meta-analysis. *Ann Intern Med.* 2015;163(7):519–528, with permission.)

In the SR we found, two independent reviewers extracted data and used the Grading of Recommendations Assessment, Development, and Evaluation (GRADE) system to make recommendations about the strength of the evidence. Factors that were included in their consideration were "study design (in this case, randomized controlled trials); risk of bias, precision, consistency, and directness of the evidence; and the possibility of publication bias." They employed a modified version of the Cochrane Risk of Bias tool to evaluate the risk of bias of the individual studies.

4. Were individual patient data (or aggregate data) used for the analysis?

A less frequent point to consider is whether the authors used individual patient data (rather than summary tables or published reports) for their analysis. We would feel more confident about the conclusions of the study, especially as it related to subgroups, if individual patient data were used, because they provide the opportunity to test promising subgroups from one trial against an identical subgroup from other trials (you might want to refer to Box 4.5). Individual patient data allow us to ensure appropriate follow-up and to perform more reliable analyses of patients' time to specific clinical events. Individual patient data analysis also allows us to conduct more accurate subgroup analyses. Analysis of published, aggregate data can give different answers to an individual patient data MA because of exclusion of trials, or of individual patients, or as a result of differences in key study factors, such as the length of follow-up.

Once we are satisfied with the validity of the SR, we can turn to its results. Box 4.7 outlines the guides that we can use.

Are the valid results of this systematic review important?

1. Are the results consistent across studies?

Were the effects of treatment consistent from study to study? We are more likely to believe the results of an SR if the results of every trial included show a treatment effect that is going in the same direction (what we call "qualitatively" similar results). We shouldn't expect the results to show exactly the same degree of efficacy (or "quantitatively" identical results), but we should be concerned if some trials confidently conclude a beneficial effect of treatment and others in the same review clearly exclude benefit or even demonstrate harm. More generally, we can look at the degree to which the CIs overlap from the various trials.

Ideally, we would like to find that the investigators tested their results using statistical methods to see whether any lack of consistency (otherwise known as "heterogeneity") was caused by differences between the trials or by the effects of chance. One way to do this is to compute the I^2 statistic. The term "I^2 statistic" refers to the proportion of total variation observed between the trials that can be attributed to differences between the trials themselves rather than sampling error. If the authors did find statistically significant heterogeneity, did the authors satisfactorily explain why it was observed?[j] They might invoke factors that are clinical differences, such as the baseline characteristics of the study patients, dosage, or duration of therapy, or methodological differences, such as the study design, which includes the outcome measurements, or the risk of bias.

If the study results are consistent with each other—in other words, the findings are homogeneous—the authors may choose to summarize the results using statistical methods, thereby performing a quantitative review or MA. Note that even if statistical heterogeneity occurs, investigators can complete an MA; however, in that case it is important for the investigators to explore the impact of the heterogeneity in the studies on the MA.

Twelve of the 13 trials looked at the all-cause mortality. Pooled results demonstrated that 7.9% of patients in the control group died, compared with 5.3% of patients in the corticosteroids group, risk ratio (RR) 0.67 (95% CI 0.45–1.01; $I^2 \cong 6\%$; interaction $p \cong 0.010$). However, upon more careful inspection, the results varied depending on the severity of pneumonia. Turning our attention to Figure 4.9, we can see that among patients with severe pneumonia, all the trials show a trend toward benefit, even though only two out of six of the trials showed statistically significant results (the CIs do not cross the null, which in this case is 1 because we are using a ratio as our measure of association—recall Box 4.3 on CIs). For the subgroup of patients with severe pneumonia, the authors obtained RR 0.39 (95% CI 0.20–0.77; $I^2 \cong 0\%$). Therefore, we conclude that among the subgroup of patients with severe pneumonia, there appears to be a significant benefit. However, all-cause mortality among patients with less severe pneumonia did not show improved outcomes:

---

[j]According to the Cochrane Handbook, substantial heterogeneity is suggested by an I^2 greater than 75%, and in that case, the authors should explore the potential causes.

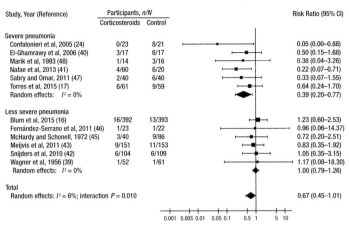

Fig. 4.9 A Forest plot. (From Siemieniuk RA, et al. Corticosteroid therapy for patients hospitalized with community-acquired pneumonia: a systematic review and meta-analysis. *Ann Intern Med.* 2015;163(7):519–528, with permission.)

4

Three out of six studies showed no benefit, and none of the six studies had statistically significant results for this outcome. For this subgroup, RR 1.00 (95% CI 0.79–1.26; $I^2 \equiv 0\%$). We conclude that the benefit on all-cause mortality was being driven in great part by the subgroup of patients with more severe pneumonia.

Note that in this study, heterogeneity was assessed using "visual inspection, a test for heterogeneity, and the I^2 statistic." Clinical heterogeneity was present across trials with differences in patient characteristics, the choice of steroid used including dose, timing, and duration of drug use. Sensitivity analyses were completed to determine the impact of heterogeneity, and there was no meaningful impact on the results.

2. What is the magnitude of the treatment effect?

Just as we examined the results of single therapeutic trials, we need to find a clinically useful expression for the results of SRs, and here we become victims of history and some high-level statistics (the toughest in this book). Although growing numbers of SRs present their results as NNTs, most of them still use ORs or RRs.[k] Note that RRs are also sometimes referred to as *risk ratios.* Earlier in this chapter, we showed that the RRR doesn't preserve the CER or the patient's expected event rate (PEER), and this disadvantage extends to ORs and RRs.

SRs often present results as a Forest plot (Fig. 4.9). In this study, the forest plot we are examining represents the effect of steroids on all-cause mortality in hospitalized patients with community-acquired pneumonia. The findings are grouped by the severity of pneumonia. As we can see, a Forest plot is a graphical representation of the estimate of the treatment effect and its CI. It is particularly helpful in SRs because the authors can include the measure of association—e.g., the RR—along with CI for each individual study, as well as the pooled result (which is the result of the MA). On the left side of this figure, each citation is presented. Moving horizontally, each citation is followed by its results from both the intervention and the control arms. The RR for each study is presented as a square, and the CI is represented by two lines emanating from either side of the RR and equidistant from the RR. The key things to focus on in these figures are the line of no difference and the lengths of the CI.

The line of no difference is drawn for an RR of 1. This makes sense because we are dealing with a measure of association that is a ratio, so if there is no difference between the two groups, the numerator and denominator will be identical, yielding an RR of 1. Next, we scan to see if the estimate of the RR (for each individual study and for the summary estimate) falls to the left or right of this line and whether the CI for this estimate crosses this line (of no association). In Figure 4.9, when the RR and its CI lie to the left of the line of no difference, this means that mortality is decreased with steroids. If the RR and its CI fall to the right of the line of no difference, this means that mortality is increased with steroids, and this would favour not treating patients with pneumonia with adjunctive steroids.

---

[k]An OR is the odds of an event in a patient in the experimental group relative to that of a patient in the control group (using a 2×2 table to demonstrate the interventions and outcomes, this amounts to OR $\equiv$ ad/bc). An RR (or risk ratio) is the risk of an event in a patient in the experimental group relative to that of a patient in the control group (in a 2×2 table of interventions and outcomes, the RR $\equiv$ [a/a+b]/[c/c+d]). Without getting into too much detail, we can see that if we are dealing with rare events, then a is small, so a/a+b is approximated by a/b. Likewise if c is small, c/c+d can be approximated by c/d. Therefore, when dealing with rare events the RR $\equiv$ ad/bc $\equiv$ OR. In other words, for rare events, the RR approximates the OR.

If we look at the all-cause mortality results of the trials with severe pneumonia in the Figure 4.9, we can first see that four trials are not statistically significant (the CIs overlap with 1—recall Box 4.3 above), but that two trials are statistically significant (the CIs of the studies by Confalonieri et al. and Nafae et al. do not include 1). We can be reassured by the consistency in these findings—that all of them trend in the same direction. Furthermore, the pooled RR (0.39 [CI 0.20–0.77]) also lies to the left of the line of no difference, and its CI is contained entirely on the left side, not crossing the line of no difference, indicating it is statistically significant.

For patients with less severe pneumonia, the results are equivocal—the results of three of the studies are to the left of the line of no difference, and the results of the other three are to its right. All the individual trial results cluster close to the line of no difference, and all their CIs cross the line of no difference. The pooled RR for these studies of patients with less severe pneumonia is 1.00 (CI 0.79–1.26)!

With all this useful information, we can look at the results from all of the included studies, (the impact of steroids on all-comers, irrespective of pneumonia severity), and we see that the pooled RR is 0.67 (CI 0.45–1.01). If we had looked at this pooled estimate in isolation, we would not have recognized that the benefit was driven by the subgroup of patients with more severe pneumonia!

4

Although ORs and RRs are of very limited use in the clinical setting, they can be converted to NNTs (or NNHs) using the formulae in Box 4.8. Better yet, we've provided the results of some typical conversions in Tables 4.4 and 4.5. And finally, we can take a shortcut and use the EBM calculator (https://ebm-tools.knowledgetranslation.net/calculator) that we have developed that allows us to convert an OR to an NNT at the click of a button (https://ebm-tools.knowledgetranslation.net/calculator/converter/). We interpret the NNTs and NNHs derived from SRs in the same way as we would for individual trials. In this case, although an RR is reported, we need to calculate the event rate in each of the arms ourselves, because NNT $\equiv$ 1/ARR, where the ARR $\equiv$ CER − EER.

Are the valid, important results of this systematic review applicable to our patient?

An SR provides an overall, average effect of therapy, which may be derived from a quite heterogeneous population. How do we apply this

---

Box 4.8 Formulae to convert odds ratios (ORs) and relative risks (RRs) to numbers needed to treat (NNTs)

For RR < 1:

$$NNT \equiv 1/(1-RR) \times PEER$$

For RR > 1:

$$NNT \equiv 1/(RR-1) \times PEER$$

For OR < 1:

$$NNT \equiv 1-[PEER \times (1-OR)]/(1-PEER) \times (PEER) \times (1-OR)$$

For OR > 1:

$$NNT \equiv 1+[PEER \times (OR-1)]/(1-PEER) \times (PEER) \times (OR-1)$$

PEER, Patient expected event rate.

Table 4.4 Translating odds ratios (ORs) to NNTs when OR < 1

Patient expected event rate (PEER)	For odds ratio < 1						
	0.9	0.9	0.7	0.6	0.5	0.4	0.3
0.05	209 (a)	104	69	52	41	34	29 (b)
0.10	110	54	36	27	21	18	15
0.20	61	30	20	14	11	10	8
0.30	46	22	14	10	8	7	5
0.40	40	19	12	9	7	6	4
0.50	38	18	11	8	6	5	4
0.70	44	20	13	9	6	5	4
0.90	101 (c)	46	27	18	12	9	4 (d)

(a) The relative risk reduction (RRR) here is 10%.
(b) The RRR here is 49%.
(c) The RRR here is 1%.
(d) The RRR here is 9%.

evidence to our individual patient? The same way we did for individual trials—by applying the guides for applicability listed in Box 4.4. One advantage that SRs have over most randomized trials is that SRs may provide precise information on subgroups, which can help us to individualize the evidence to our own patients. To do this, we need to remind ourselves of the cautions about subgroups that we have summarized in

Table 4.5 Translating odds ratios (ORs) to NNTs when OR > 1

Patient expected event rate (PEER)	For odds ratio > 1						
	1.1	1.25	1.5	1.75	2	2.25	2.5
0.05	212	86	44	30	23	18	16
0.10	113	46	24	16	13	10	9
0.20	64	27	14	10	8	7	6
0.30	50	21	11	8	7	6	5
0.40	44	19	10	8	6	5	5
0.50	42	18	10	8	6	6	5
0.70	51	23	13	10	9	8	7
0.90	121	55	33	25	22	19	18

The numbers in the body of the table are the NNTs for the corresponding ORs at that particular PEER. This table applies both when a good outcome is increased by therapy and when a side effect is caused by therapy.

(Adapted from John Geddes, personal communication, 1999.)

Box 4.9 Is this valid and important evidence from a systematic review applicable to our patient?

1. Is our patient so different from those in the study that its results cannot apply?
2. Is the treatment feasible in our setting?
3. What are our patient's potential benefits and harms from the therapy?
4. What are our patient's values and expectations for both the outcome we are trying to prevent and the adverse effects we may cause?

Box 4.5. As noted above, SRs can provide information on risks and benefits of therapy by pooling the findings from individual studies, which can be helpful for us as we are weighing the risks and benefits of therapy with our patients (Box 4.9).

Methods for conducting SRs are constantly evolving, particularly with regard to strategies that can be used to integrate qualitative and quantitative data. Some of the novel methods include critical interpretive synthesis, integrative review, meta-narrative review, meta-summary, mixed studies review, narrative synthesis, and realist review.[32] These methods vary in their strengths and limitations. One additional methodology that is garnering increasing attention is network MA. Network MA is a strategy that allows researchers to make inferences about how different interventions might compare to each other, in the absence of a head-to-head RCT, by setting up a network of RCTs that permit indirect comparisons.[33] For example, if patient populations and outcomes are similar in several studies, a trial of drug A versus placebo might be nested in the same network as a second trial comparing drug B versus placebo. Using a transitive relation, we might use the data in these studies to compare drug A versus drug B. The advantages of network MA include the ability to evaluate all possible interventions against each other—including ranking their relative effectiveness and safety—and making use of both direct and indirect evidence.

Further reading about systematic reviews

Egger M, Davey SG, Altman DG. Systematic reviews in health care: meta-analysis in context. London, UK: BMJ Books; 2008.

Guyatt G, Rennie D, Meade M, Cook DJ, editors. Users' guides to the medical literature. A manual for evidence-based clinical practice. 3rd ed. Chicago, IL: AMA Press; 2015.

Haynes RB, Sackett DL, Guyatt G, Tugwell P. Clinical epidemiology: how to do clinical practice research. Philadelphia, PA: Lippincott Williams & Wilkins; 2006.

A few words on qualitative literature

In this book, we have focused primarily on searching for and appraising quantitative literature. Qualitative research can help us to understand clinical phenomena with an emphasis on understanding the experiences and values of our patients. The field of qualitative research has an extensive history in the social sciences but its exploration and development are newer to clinical medicine. We do not consider ourselves experts in this area, and we suggest that you take a look at the references we have included at the end of this section. We have included some guides in Box 4.10, which might be useful for evaluating the validity, importance, and applicability of a qualitative study.

Let's consider an example. Patients who are suffering from chronic diseases may have to take long-term medications, as in our example of a woman who was at intermediate risk of cardiovascular disease and was contemplating statin therapy. We might want to explore the literature describing how patients arrive at a decision to take lifelong medications and to better understand how to incorporate patient values and perspectives into clinical decision making. A search of the literature

Box 4.10 Is the evidence from this qualitative study valid, important, and applicable?

Are the results of this qualitative study valid?
1. Was the selection of participants explicit and appropriate?
2. Were the methods for data collection and analysis explicit and appropriate?

Are the results of this valid qualitative study important?
1. Are the results impressive?

Are the valid and important results of this qualitative study applicable to my patient?
1. Do these same phenomena apply to my patient?

led us to a qualitative study by Sale et al., which explored factors contributing to patients' decisions to take medications for osteoporosis, published in the journal *BMC Musculoskeletal Disorders* in 2011.[34]

Are the results of this qualitative study valid?

4

1. Was the selection of participants explicit and appropriate?

We would like to find that the authors included an appropriate spectrum of patients. By "appropriate," we mean that they represent the population that we are interested in and that are relevant to the study question. In qualitative studies, purposive sampling of participants may be used instead of random sampling. Purposive sampling is a strategy in which investigators explicitly select individuals who meet their specific criteria to reflect the experience that they are trying to assess.

In this study, rather than randomly sampling a group of patients, the investigators sampled purposively—identifying patients that had been prescribed medications for osteoporosis—to learn what shaped their experiences. Identified patients were either men or women, age 65 years and older, at a fracture clinic at a single urban teaching hospital. They had to have sustained a fragility fracture within the last 5 years, they were at "high risk" for future fractures, and they were prescribed a medication for osteoporosis. They had to be English speakers and cognitively intact to participate.

2. Were the methods used for data collection and analysis explicit and appropriate?

There are many different methods for collecting and analyzing data in a qualitative study, and we need to ensure that the methods are explicitly outlined. We would suggest that you refer to some of the works mentioned at the end of this section to learn more about these methods. Nonetheless, we offer a few starting points for your consideration. Did the investigators use direct observation (or audiotapes)? Did they conduct individual face-to-face interviews or focus groups? Was a text analysis used? Did the authors develop a conceptual framework and use the collected data to challenge and refine this framework in an iterative fashion?

> In this patient perspective study, the investigators used semi-structured, face-to-face interviews (with the use of an interview guide); the interviews lasted 1 to 2 hours and were audiotaped. Transcriptions of the interviews were uploaded to the software NVivo, which facilitates analysis of qualitative data. Two of the authors independently coded the data and met after reviewing each transcript to revise the interview guide in an iterative fashion as new and important themes emerged. They also developed and refined a coding template following analysis of several transcripts and looked for interrelationships between the codes. Multiple themes were reviewed within the larger research team.

Unlike quantitative research, where we try to find articles that describe blinded outcome assessors, blinding may not always be appropriate in qualitative research because it can limit the investigator's ability to interpret the data. Here, we are reassured that the investigators initially reviewed the data independently so that they arrived at an interpretation without bias from within the research team. Qualitative researchers may also use journals or memos as a reflective exercise to consider their own biases that might influence the analysis. Triangulation of source material can also occur; for example, interviews could be completed alongside field observations or document analysis.

Are the valid results of this qualitative study important?

1. Are the results impressive?

Does the report provide sufficient detail for us to obtain a clear picture of the phenomena described? Usually, the results are presented narratively with relevant examples and quotes included to highlight themes. Sometimes, authors include a quantitative component to outline dominant themes and demographic details. We include a sample from the patient perspective study below.

Experience with initiating medications for osteoporosis[34]

There were 21 participants, of which 15 were female. For 12 of the patients, minimal contemplation about taking the medication was required, whereas for the other nine patients, there was considerable consideration in advance of taking therapy for osteoporosis. Those who made the decision easily had strong physician–patient alliances and voiced trust in their physicians over trust necessarily in the medication; they did not consider the risks of taking these medications in their consideration of whether to initiate therapy. Those that had a more difficult time arriving at a decision were also influenced by care providers, but in this case, they required more information to be convinced of the need for medications. One patient stated: "*He [specialist] didn't say anything that convinced me that I needed to take the medication*." Another patient in this group took issue with the attitude of her physician: "*I got the impression from her [the GP] that she automatically put women on bone density medication once they were 50 or over … so I was not convinced to take it because … I wasn't convinced that I needed it. Not at all.*"

4

Are the valid, important results of this qualitative study applicable to our situation?

1. Do we think these same phenomena apply to our patient/participant?

Does this report describe participants like our own, and do the phenomena described seem relevant to our participant? Ideally, the paper should provide sufficient information to allow us to determine whether our participant or the situation is sufficiently similar to those included in the study. In our case, although our patient would be taking a statin for primary prevention of cardiovascular events, it is nonetheless useful to recognize the importance of the physician–patient therapeutic alliance and the role for counselling regarding the indication, risks, and benefits of the medication.

Further reading about individual randomized trials and qualitative studies

Creswell JW. Qualitative inquiry and research design. London, UK: Sage Publications; 1998.

Guyatt G, Rennie D, Meade M, Cook DJ, editors. Users' guides to the medical literature. A manual for evidence-based clinical practice. 3rd ed. Chicago, IL: AMA Press; 2015.

Reports of clinical decision analyses

Occasionally, when we are attempting to answer a question about therapy, the results of our search will yield a CDA. A CDA applies explicit, quantitative methods to compare the likely consequences of pursuing different treatment strategies, integrates the risks and benefits associated with the various treatment options, and incorporates values associated with potential outcomes. A CDA starts with a diagram called a *decision tree*, which begins with the disorder of interest and branches out based on the alternative treatment strategies, revealing the possible outcomes that may occur with each strategy. A simple example is shown in Figure 4.10, which looks at the possible strategies for the management of atrial fibrillation, including anticoagulation—which can be further divided into the use of warfarin or direct oral anticoagulants (DOACs), antiplatelet therapy, and no antithrombotic prophylaxis, as well as electrical and chemical cardioversion. The point at which a treatment decision is made is marked with a box called a *decision node*. The possible outcomes that arise from each of the treatment strategies follow this decision node. These outcomes are preceded by circles, called *chance nodes*. They are so named because after a treatment is administered there is an element of chance as to whether the individual has a positive, negative, or neutral outcome. The probabilities for each of the outcomes that might occur with each of the treatments are estimated from the literature (hopefully with a modicum of accuracy!) or occasionally from the clinician's expertise. A triangle is used to denote a terminal outcome. The patient's utility for each outcome is placed after the triangle. A utility is the measure of a person's preference for a particular health state and is usually expressed as a decimal from 0 to 1. Typically, perfect health is assigned a value of 1, and death is assigned a value of 0, although there are some outcomes that patients may think are worse than death, and the scale may need to be extended below zero. Formal methods should be used to elicit

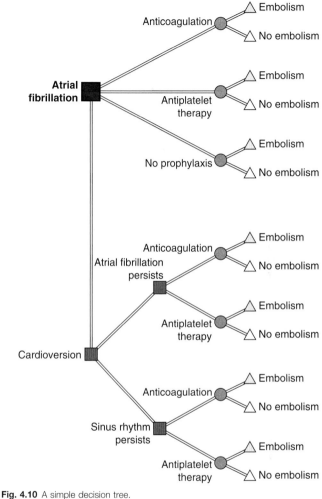

Fig. 4.10 A simple decision tree.

utilities. Among these methods are the "standard gamble" and "time trade-off" techniques, among others. These are methods that ask patients to quantify the value they place on a particular health state. They strive to make empiric something that is otherwise rather subjective. With the standard gamble method, patients must articulate the percentage risk of death they might be willing to accept with a therapy, if that therapy could assure perfect health if it works. With the time trade-off method, patients indicate how much of their life they would be willing to trade in exchange for perfect health. There are also other methods, including validated questionnaires that generate a utility score. In the end, all of these methods are used to generate a number represented as life-years, or quality-adjusted life-years (QALYs), where a year in a higher-quality health state contributes more to the outcome than a year in a poor-quality health state; another number that might be used to approximate utility is the number of cases of disease or complications that are prevented.

After a decision tree is constructed, a process that you can see is built in a forward direction from a disease, through the possible treatments, culminating in the possible outcomes and their associated utilities, we then analyze the decision tree by moving in the reverse direction. We must take the utility of each outcome and multiply it by the probability that this particular outcome will occur. Then, we must sum each possible outcome across each chance node in the treatment branch to generate an average utility for that branch of the tree. The "winning" strategy, and preferred course of clinical action, is the one that leads to the highest absolute utility. Note that we could make the decision tree very complex and include the possibility of patients experiencing more than one outcome or health state at any given time (including short-term and long-term outcomes).

As you can see, CDAs are exquisitely labour intensive to use while on a busy clinical service, and very few skilled clinicians are able to readily implement them in real time. To be used correctly, CDAs have to accurately identify and integrate probabilities and patient utilities for all pertinent outcomes. The result is elegant, and we sometimes wish we could do it for all our patients, but the process of creating even a simple tree will take longer than the time available to many of us at the bedside. Creation of more complex decision trees often requires special software and training. We have opted to use the more rough-and-ready but humanly feasible approaches for integrating evidence and patients' values, such as the LHH. We don't consider ourselves experts in CDAs, and if you are interested in reading more about how to do them, check out the references at the end of this section. Typically, CDAs are most useful in policy decisions, for instance, in making decisions about whether to pay for specific treatments.

But even if we do not generate our own CDAs, we sometimes read reports that incorporate them, and the rest of this section will briefly describe how we decide whether they are valid, important, and applicable to a patient.

Are the results of this CDA valid?

Box 4.11 outlines the questions we need to consider here. The CDA should include all the known treatment strategies (including the option of "no treatment") and the full range of outcomes for each strategy (good, bad, and no change) that we (and our patients) think are important. For example, if we are interested in looking at a CDA that might help us determine the best management of patients with non-valvular atrial fibrillation and the CDA we find does not include aspirin as an alternative treatment to oral anticoagulants, we should be skeptical about its usefulness (because the use of aspirin is a viable, albeit less effective, treatment for atrial fibrillation). A CDA should explicitly describe a comprehensive, systematic process that was used to identify, select, and combine the best external evidence into probabilities for all the potential important clinical outcomes. There may be some uncertainty around a probability estimate, and the authors should specify a range; this may come from the range of values from different studies or from a 95% CI from a single study or systematic review. The methods that were used to assess the evidence for validity (see pages 73 and 113) should also be included in the study. If a systematic review was not found to provide an estimate of the probability, were the results of the studies that were found combined in some sensible way? Finally, some investigators may use expert opinion to generate probability estimates, if the estimates are not readily available in the literature, and these estimates will not be as valid as those obtained from evidence-based sources. In this case it would be particularly important to do a sensitivity

---

Box 4.11 Is this evidence from a clinical decision analysis (CDA) valid?

1. Were all important therapeutic alternatives (including no treatment) and outcomes included?
2. Are the probabilities of the outcomes valid and credible?
3. Are the utilities of the outcomes valid and credible?

---

analysis to determine how our estimates might change if the probabilities are different from what was assumed.

Were the utilities obtained in an explicit and sensible way from valid sources? Ideally, utilities are measured in patients using valid, standardized methods, such as the standard gamble or time trade-off techniques described earlier. Occasionally, investigators will use values already present in the clinical literature or values obtained by "consensus opinion" from experts. These latter two methods are not nearly as credible as measuring utilities directly in appropriate patients.

Ideally, in a high-quality CDA, the investigators should "discount" future events. For example, most people would not trade a year of perfect health now for one 20 years in the future—we usually value the present greater than the future. Discounting the utility will take this into account.

If we think the CDA has satisfied all the above criteria, we move on to considering whether the results of this CDA are important. If it does not satisfy the criteria, we will have to go back to our search.

Are the valid results of this CDA important? (Box 4.12)

Was there a clear "winner" in this CDA so that one course of action clearly led to a higher average utility? Surprisingly, experts in this area often conclude that average gains in QALYs of as little as 2 months are worth pursuing (especially when their confidence intervals are big so that some patients enjoy really big gains in QALYs). However, gains of a few days to a few weeks are usually considered "toss-ups" in which both courses of action lead to, relatively speaking, identical outcomes and the choice between them is inconsequential.

Before accepting the results of a positive CDA we need to make sure it determined whether clinically sensible changes in probabilities or utilities altered its conclusion. If such a "sensitivity analysis" generated no switch in the designation of the preferred treatment, it is a robust analysis—meaning that the "winning" course is durable regardless of a change in the inputs, a change that might reflect individual patient variability in probabilities of outcomes and utilities from outcomes. If, however, the designation of the preferred treatment is sensitive to small

---

Box 4.12 Is this valid evidence from a clinical decision analysis (CDA) important?

1. Did one course of action lead to clinically important gains?
2. Was the same course of action preferred despite clinically sensible changes in probabilities and utilities?

Box 4.13 Is this valid and important evidence from a clinical decision analysis (CDA) applicable to our patient?

---

1. Do the probabilities in this CDA apply to our patient?
2. Can our patient state his or her utilities in a stable, useable form?

---

changes in one or more probabilities or utilities, the results of the CDA are uncertain, and it may not provide any substantive guidance in our shared clinical decision making with patients.

Are the valid, important results of this CDA applicable to our patient? (Box 4.13)

Once we've decided that the conclusions of a CDA are both valid and important, we still need to decide whether we can apply it to our specific patient. Are our patient's probabilities of the various outcomes included in the sensitivity analysis? If they lie outside the range tested, we will need to either recalculate the components of the decision tree or at least be very cautious in following its overall recommendations. Similarly, we might want to generate utilities for our patient to see if they fall within the range tested in the CDA. A crude technique that we use on our clinical service begins by drawing a line on a sheet of paper with two anchor points on it: one at the top labelled "perfect health," which is given a score of 1, and one near the bottom labelled "death," which is given a score of 0 (making it precisely 10 cm long helps by creating a visual analogue that can assist patients in empiricizing their values). After explaining it, we ask the patient to mark the places on the scale that correspond to her current state of health and to all the other outcomes that might result from the choice of interventions. The locations that the patient selects are used to represent the utilities (if time permits, we leave the scale with the patient so that she can reflect on, and perhaps revise, the utilities). We can then see whether our patient's utilities (both initially and on reflection) lie within the boundaries of the study's sensitivity analysis.

Further reading about clinical decision analysis

Guyatt G, Rennie D, Meade M, Cook DJ, editors. Users' guides to the medical literature. A manual for evidence-based clinical practice. 3rd ed. Chicago, IL: AMA Press; 2015.

Hunink M, Glasziou P, Siegel J, et al. Decision making in health and medicine: integrating evidence and values. Cambridge, UK: Cambridge University Press; 2001.

Reports of economic analyses

Sometimes our search for an answer to a therapeutic or other clinical question will yield an economic analysis that compares the costs and consequences of different management decisions. We warn you at the outset that economic analyses are difficult to interpret and often controversial (even among health economists), and we won't claim to have described all of their nuances here (if you are interested in understanding them, we have suggested some additional resources at the end of this section). They are very demanding to conduct for their investigators and hard to decipher for us as readers as well. They are most useful in making policy decisions. These analyses teach us to stop thinking linearly only about the costs of a new treatment in terms of dollars and cents but, instead, to start thinking laterally about the other things we cannot do if we use scarce resources to fund a new treatment. This "cost as sacrifice" is better known as "opportunity cost" and is a useful way of thinking in everyday practice—for example, when internists "borrow" a bed from surgical colleagues to admit a medical emergency tonight, the opportunity cost of this decision includes cancelling tomorrow's elective surgery on a patient for whom the bed was initially reserved.

These papers are pretty tough to read and you might want to confine your initial searches to curators of evidence-based medicine (e.g., *ACP Journal Club*), which not only provide a standard, clear format for reporting economic analyses but also provide expert commentaries. The following guides (outlined in Boxes 4.14, 4.15, and 4.16) should help you decide whether an economic analysis is valid, important, and useful.

Box 4.14 Is this evidence from an economic analysis valid?

1. Are all well-defined courses of action compared?
2. Does it provide a specified view from which the costs and consequences are being viewed?
3. Does it cite comprehensive evidence on the efficacy of alternatives?
4. Does it identify all the costs and consequences we think it should and select credible and accurate measures of them?
5. Was the type of analysis appropriate for the question posed?

Box 4.15 Is this valid evidence from an economic analysis important?

1. Are the resulting costs or cost/unit of health gained clinically significant?
2. Did the results of this economic analysis change with sensible changes to costs and effectiveness?

Box 4.16 Is this valid and important evidence from an economic analysis applicable to our patient?

1. Do the costs in the economic analysis apply in our setting?
2. Are the treatments likely to be effective in our setting?

Are the results of this economic analysis valid?

We need to begin by remembering that economic analyses are about choices and that we must therefore ensure that the study we are evaluating included all the possible, sensible, alternative courses of action (e.g., various oral anticoagulants, antiplatelet therapy, and cardioversion for patients with nonvalvular atrial fibrillation [NVAF]). If, for example, we found a report that only described the costs of antiplatelet therapy for patients with NVAF, that's an exercise in accounting, not economic analysis, and it wouldn't help us. A valid economic analysis also has to specify the point of view from which the costs and outcomes are being viewed. Did the authors specify if costs and consequences are evaluated from the perspective of the patient, hospital, local government, or the public? For example, a hospital might shy away from in patient cardioversion in favour of discharging a patient with NVAF on oral anticoagulants that would be paid for by the patient or from the family physician's drug budget, whereas society as a whole may want the most cost-effective approach from an overall point of view.

Because economic analyses assume (rather than prove) that the alternative courses of action have highly predictable effects, we need to determine whether they cite and summarize solid evidence on the efficacy of alternatives (the same caution we must remember when reading a CDA). Was an explicit and sensible process used to identify and appraise the evidence that would satisfy the criteria for validity listed in Box 4.1?

All the costs and effects of the treatment should be identified, and credible measures should have been made of all of them. The cost side here can be tricky because investigators and readers may have different standards about what comprises cost. Do we need to consider only direct costs (e.g., cost of medication, hospitalization) or also indirect costs (e.g., time lost from work)? As noted above, the individual(s) bearing each of these costs may be different. Moreover, a high-quality economic analysis should also include (and explain!) discounting future costs and outcomes.

We need to consider if the type of analysis was appropriate for the question the investigators posed, and this is not as hard as it sounds. If the question was "Is there a cheaper way to care for this patient without substantially changing the quality of care?" the paper should ignore the outcomes and simply compare costs (a "cost minimization" analysis). If the question was "Which way of treating this patient gives the greatest health 'bang for the buck'?" the method of analysis is determined by the sorts of outcomes being compared. If outcomes are identical for all the treatment alternatives ("Is it cheaper to prevent embolic stroke in NVAF patients with warfarin or a direct oral anticoagulant [DOAC]?"), the appropriate analysis is a "cost-effectiveness" analysis. If, however, the outcomes as well as the interventions differ ("Do we get a bigger bang for our buck treating kids for leukemia or older adults for Alzheimer disease?"), the authors will have had to come up with some way of measuring these disparate outcomes with the same yardstick. There are two accepted ways to do this. First, they could convert all outcomes into monetary values—a "cost–benefit" analysis. The challenge with a cost–benefit analysis is the process of setting monetary values—how can we put a value on life itself (how would we place a monetary value on treating children versus older adults)? No wonder that a cost–benefit methodology lacks popularity. An alternative is to undertake a "cost–utility analysis." Rather than considering monetary value, in this type of analysis, we use another common yardstick to measure disparate outcomes in terms of their social value—utility. With this framework, we consider how patients view the desirability of a particular outcome compared with other outcomes (e.g., perfect health, imperfect health, death, and fates worse than death). Utilities can be combined with time to generate QALYs, a concept referenced earlier in the discussion on CDAs. A QALY articulates not just time lived but also the quality of the time lived. For example, 1 year in perfect health is judged equivalent to 3 years in a poststroke state, a state with a diminished utility of, say, 0.3. In this way, it becomes possible to compare otherwise widely disparate outcomes (treating children for leukemia or older adults for Alzheimer disease).

If the economic analysis fails the above tests for validity, we go back to searching. If it passes, we can proceed to considering whether its valid results are important.

Are the valid results of this economic analysis important?

Specifically, are the resulting costs or cost/unit of health gained clinically significant? We need to consider whether the intervention will provide a benefit at an acceptable cost. If it is a cost-minimization analysis, we should consider if the difference in cost is big enough to warrant switching to the cheaper alternative. For a cost-effectiveness analysis, we consider whether the difference in effectiveness is great enough for us to justify spending the difference between the two costs. In a cost–utility analysis, we determined how the QALYs generated from spending resources on this treatment compare with the QALYs that might result if different decisions about resource allocation were made. This comparison is made easier by cost–utility "league tables."[1]

Are the valid, important results of this economic analysis applicable to our patient/practice?

As usual, we begin by considering whether our patient is so different from those included in the study that its results are not applicable to our situation. We can do this by estimating our patient's probabilities of the various outcomes, and by asking the patient to generate the utilities for these outcomes, using the strategies outlined previously. If the values that we obtain fall within the ranges used in the analysis, we can be satisfied that the "effectiveness" results can be applied to our patient. Next, we can consider whether the intervention would be used in the same way in our practice. We compare the costs of applying this intervention in the study to the costs that would apply in our own setting. Costs may be different because of different practice patterns or different local prices for resources. If we think that they are different, we need to determine whether our personal cost estimates are contained within the range of possible costs tested in the sensitivity analysis. If the report satisfies these tests, we can apply it to our context! But if it fails any of them, we go back to searching!

---

[1]If you want to learn more about league tables, we recommend this resource: Mason J, Drummond M, Torrance G. Some guidelines on the use of cost-effectiveness league tables. *BMJ*. 1993;306:570–572. There are also some useful tutorials on the topic that are freely available; one can be found at https://www.nlm.nih.gov/nichsr/hta101/ta10107 .html.

Further reading about economic analysis

Guyatt G, Rennie D, Meade M, Cook DJ, editors. Users' guides to the medical literature. A manual for evidence-based clinical practice. 3rd ed. Chicago, IL: AMA Press; 2015.

Reports of clinical practice guidelines

It seems that we cannot scan a journal without finding information about a new CPG. CPGs are systematically developed statements to help clinicians and patients with decisions about appropriate health care for specific clinical circumstances.[35] In addition, they may inform decisions made by policymakers and managers. Huge amounts of time and money are being invested in their production, application, and dissemination. Unfortunately, this often occurs with unnecessary duplication. Moreover, not all guidelines are created equal. In a review of the quality of 11 guidelines published between 2006 and 2011 on the diagnosis, assessment, and management of hypertension, Al-Ansary et al. found that less than 20% of them met sufficient criteria for assessing rigour in the development of these guidelines.[36] Another challenge that we encounter as clinicians related to the overlap of guidelines is the lack of collaboration across their developers. For example, in our practice, we have guidelines on the assessment and management of hypertension, dyslipidemia, diabetes, stroke, and cardiovascular disease, but what we really need is a single guideline that informs how to optimize vascular risk factors. This is a model that has been applied by the New Zealand Guidelines Group, an organization that is leading the world in trying to achieve this kind of cohesive approach to guideline generation.[37] The National Institute for Health and Care Excellence (NICE) in the United Kingdom is likewise paving the way, with its recent guidelines on the clinical assessment and management of multimorbidity—a review that supports health care providers in caring for patients in a more holistic and patient-centred way.[38] It is this type of approach that will enhance our ability to actually use the evidence from guidelines. The goal of this next section is to help busy clinicians evaluate whether a guideline is worth using.

In a nutshell, if we are considering using a guideline, we need to evaluate two distinct components, as depicted in Table 4.6—first, the evidence summary ("Here is the average effect of this intervention on the typical patient who accepts it"), and second, the detailed instructions for applying that evidence to our patient. We apply our eye and nose

Table 4.6 The two components of practice guidelines

	Evidence component	Detailed instructional component
Bottom line	"Here's the typical effect of this diagnostic/ therapeutic/preventive intervention on the typical patient."	"Here is exactly what to do to/with this patient."
Underlying requirements	Validity, importance, up-to-datedness	Local relevance
Expertise required by those executing this component	Human biology, consumerism, clinical epidemiology, biostatistics, database searching	Clinical practice, patient values, current practice, local geography, local economics, local sociology, local politics, local traditions
Site where this component should be performed	National or international	Local
Form of output	Levels/Grade of evidence	Grades/Strength of recommendations, detailed instructions, flow charts, protocols

4

Box 4.17 The killer Bs

1. Is the *burden* of illness (frequency in our community, or our patient's pretest probability or expected event rate [PEER]) too low to warrant implementation?
2. Are the *beliefs* of individual patients or communities about the value of the interventions or their consequences incompatible with the guideline?
3. Would the opportunity cost of implementing this guideline constitute a bad *bargain* in the use of our energy or our community's resources?
4. Are the *barriers* (geographic, organizational, traditional, authoritarian, legal, or behavioural) so high that it is not worth trying to overcome them?

to the first component, the evidence summary—our eye to see if all of the relevant evidence has been tracked down and graded for its validity and our nose to smell whether it has updated its review recently enough to still be fresh. Then, we apply our ear to the second component to listen for any "killer Bs" (Box 4.17) in our local context that would make the detailed instructions impossible to implement.

Valid guidelines create their evidence components from systematic reviews of all of the relevant worldwide literature. The reviews that provide the evidence components for guidelines are "necessity driven" and synthesize the best evidence (even if it is of dubious quality) that can be found to guide an urgent decision that has to be made. It necessarily follows that some recommendations in the second component of a guideline may be derived from evidence of high validity and others from evidence that is much more prone to error.

Are the results of this practice guideline valid? (Box 4.18)

Detailed guides for assessing the validity of practice guidelines have been developed using rigorous methodology, and we would suggest that you turn to these if you are particularly interested in this topic.[39] For example, the Appraisal of Guidelines for Research and Evaluation (AGREE) Collaboration[39] has developed an instrument for assessing the validity of guidelines that includes items targeting six domains—scope and purpose, stakeholder involvement, rigour of development, clarity of presentation, applicability, and editorial independence. Recently AGREE has been refined and validated. Similarly, the Institute of Medicine has created standards for creating trustworthy guidelines.[40] In this section, we present a more basic version that you can use when appraising the validity of guidelines (see Box 4.18).

Similar to high-quality CDAs and economic analyses, valid practice guidelines should include all relevant strategies (e.g., for diagnosis, screening, prognosis, and/or treatment) and the full range of outcomes (including the good and the bad) that are important. For example, a guideline by the Canadian Task Force for Preventive Health Care (available at: http://canadiantaskforce.ca) found that there was moderate-quality evidence of no benefit and potential harm with routine mammography in women aged 40 to 49 years.[41] It was crucial for this guideline to include data not only on the impact of this screening intervention on mortality but also on the potential harm, including the emotional distress associated with unnecessary breast biopsies. Similarly, a guideline on

---

Box 4.18 Guides for deciding whether a guideline is valid

1. Did its developers carry out a comprehensive, reproducible literature review within the past 12 months?
2. Is each of its recommendations both tagged by the level of evidence upon which it is based and linked to a specific citation?

---

prostate cancer assessment and management should include the evidence around impact of screening with prostate-specific antigen (PSA), including overdiagnosis and overtreatment. This highlights the need for relevant stakeholder engagement to ensure that all important outcomes are considered.

A valid practice guideline should include a comprehensive, reproducible literature review; indeed, a systematic review should be the base unit of guidelines. A comprehensive review needs to include all relevant articles in all relevant languages. For example, some of the most important evidence for guidelines about family supports for patients with schizophrenia was published in Mandarin, and this would have been missed had the world literature on this topic not been included. Ideally, the guideline should explicitly describe the methods used to retrieve, appraise, and synthesize the evidence.

We have previously described the reasons that we would like to see therapy recommendations supported by evidence from systematic reviews of randomized trials. However, such evidence might not always be available. It follows that some guideline recommendations may be derived from high-quality evidence and others from evidence that is more prone to error. Because the strength of the evidence supporting guideline recommendations may vary, it is useful to have the recommendations graded based on the quality of the evidence that was found. In other words, the different "levels" of evidence should be explicitly noted alongside any clinical recommendations. Only in this way can we separate the solid recommendations from the tenuous ones and (if we want to appraise the evidence for ourselves) track them back to their original sources. This need was recognized back in the 1970s by the Canadian Task Force on the Periodic Health Exam.[42] Since that time, even more sophisticated ways of describing and categorizing levels of evidence have been developed.[43] In an attempt to standardize the methods by which evidence is graded and the strength of recommendations are communicated, an international collaboration has developed the GRADE system.[44] GRADE classifies the overall certainty in the evidence into one of four levels—high, moderate, low, and very low. For example, we might think that a randomized trial is of a high quality based on the methods that have been described, but on assessing it further, we find that it did not adhere strictly to the study protocol or the results have wide CIs, so it is downgraded to a lower quality. The strength of recommendations is graded as "strong" or "weak." When desirable effects of an intervention outweigh undesirable effects, a strong recommendation is made. Other factors that influence the strength of a recommendation are uncertainty,

4

variability in values and preferences, or ill-defined cost implications. There are pros and cons to the GRADE approach (as with all approaches), and training is required for using GRADE in guideline development.[45] A nonprofit program to help bring GRADE to the bedside is working to create practice guidelines, evidence summaries, and decision aids that are dynamically updated, user-friendly, and available online.[46] We await evidence that demonstrates that these tools enhance decision making by clinicians and patients.

As you can see, satisfying these validity guides is a formidable task, and successful development of guidelines requires a combination of clinical, informational, and methodological skills, not to mention protected time and funding. For this reason, the first component of guideline development is best satisfied by a national or international collaboration of sufficient scope and size to not only carry out the systematic review but also update it as often as is required to include important new evidence that might appear on the scene.

Is this valid guideline applicable to my patient/practice/ hospital/community?

The first (and most important) advice here is that if a guideline was developed in another setting, we should be wary about its applicability in advising us how to treat patients in our local context. The ADAPTE and Can-IMPLEMENT groups[47,48] have provided approaches for adapting guidelines to local contexts. They describe multistep process that can be used by decision makers when considering how to modify a guideline—while trying to preserve the validity of the recommendations.

Although advances have been made in the science of guideline development, less work has been done to improve the actual implementation of guidelines. Recommendations often lack sufficient information or clarity to allow clinicians, patients, or other decision makers to implement them. Guidelines are often complex and contain a large number of recommendations with varying evidentiary support, health impact, and feasibility of use in clinical practice. Various groups are attempting to help guideline developers and clinicians who use guidelines to enhance the implementability of guidelines. For example, GUIDE-M is one such tool that was based on a realist review of the literature.[49]

Good guideline development clearly separates the evidence component ("Here is what you can expect to achieve in the typical patient who accepts this intervention.") from the detailed recommendations component ("Admit to an ICU, carry out this enzyme-linked immunosorbent assay [ELISA] test, order that treatment, monitor it minute by minute, and have your neurosurgeon examine the patient twice a day."). What if local factors mean that there is no ICU, you cannot afford ELISA tests, you must get special permission from the Ministry of Health to use the treatment, you are caring for a patient whose next of kin does not like this sort of treatment, you are chronically short-staffed, or your nearest neurosurgeon is 3 hours away? We can see that the local context matters a great deal.

The applicability of a guideline depends on the extent to which it is in harmony or conflict with four local (sometimes patient-specific) factors, and these are summarized as the potential "killer Bs" of Box 4.17. Although we list four potential barriers, there are of course many more. Indeed, a systematic review of barriers faced by physicians in guideline implementation has identified more than 250 of them, and this doesn't even consider barriers at the level of the patient or health system![50] Here, we describe common ones. If you hear any of these four Bs buzzing in your ear when you consider the applicability of a guideline, be cautious. We should also bear in mind that barriers can become facilitators, and we should also determine what facilitators to implementation might exist in our local setting.

First, is the *burden* of illness too low to warrant implementation? Is the target disorder rare in our area (e.g., malaria in northern Canada)? Or is the outcome we hope to detect or prevent unlikely in our patient (e.g., the pretest probability for significant coronary stenosis in a young woman with nonanginal chest pain)? If so, implementing the guideline may not only be a waste of time and money, but it might also do more harm than good. Reflecting on this "B" requires that we consider our patient's unique circumstances and risk of the event as we do when assessing the applicability of any piece of evidence.

Second, are our patients' or community's *beliefs* about the values or utilities of the interventions themselves, or the benefits and harms that they produce, compatible with the guideline's recommendations? Ideally, guidelines should include some mention of values, who assigned these values (patients or authors), and whether they came from one or many sources. The values assumed in a guideline, either explicitly or implicitly, may not match those in our patient or in our community. Even if the values seem, on average, to be reasonable, we must avoid forcing them on individual patients because patients with identical risks may not hold the same beliefs, values, and preferences as those included in the generation of the guideline. In fact, some may be quite averse to

143

undergoing the recommended procedures. For example, patients with early breast cancer with identical risks, given the same information about chemotherapy, might make fundamentally different treatment decisions based on how they weigh the long-term benefit of reducing the risk of recurrence against the short-term harm of adverse drug effects.[51] Similarly, patients with severe angina at identical risk of coronary events, given the same information about treatment options, exhibit sharply contrasting treatment preferences because of the different values they place on the risks and benefits of surgery.[52] Although the average beliefs in a community are appropriate for deciding, for example, whether chemotherapy or surgery should be paid for with public funds, decisions for individual patients must reflect their own personal beliefs and preferences.

Third, would the opportunity cost of implementing this guideline (rather than some other one(s)) constitute a *bargain* in the use of our energy or our community's resources? We need to remember that the cost of shortening the wait list for orthopedic surgery might be lengthening the wait time for psychotherapy in the treatment of depression. As decision making of this sort gets decentralized, different communities are bound to make different economic decisions, and "health care by postal code" will and ought to occur, especially under democratic governments.

And finally, are there insurmountable *barriers* to implementing the guideline in our patient (whose preferences indicate that they would be more likely to be harmed than helped by the intervention/investigation, or who would flatly refuse the investigations or intervention) or in our community? Barriers can be geographic (if the required interventions are not available locally), organizational (if there is no stroke unit available in a hospital that admits patients with acute stroke), traditional (if there is a predilection for following the status quo), authoritarian (if decision making occurs top-down, with little input from the frontlines), legal (if there is fear of litigation when a conventional but useless practice is abandoned), or behavioural (if clinicians fail to apply the guideline or patients fail to take their medicine). Another way to categorize barriers is to assess them at each stakeholder level—patients/public, health care providers, managers, and policymakers. Yet another is to classify barriers (and facilitators) on the basis of whether they pertain to knowledge, attitudes, or behaviours.[53] Whatever classification is used, it is important to consider the local factors that might serve as an impediment to implementation. If there are major barriers, the potential benefits of implementing a guideline may not be worth the effort and resources (or opportunity costs) required to overcome them.

Changing our own, our colleagues', and our patients' behaviours often requires much more than simply knowing what needs to be done. If implementing a guideline requires changing behaviour, we need to identify which barriers are operating and what we can do about them. Significant attention is now being paid to evaluate methods of overcoming these barriers, including changing physician behaviour. Providing evidence from clinical research to physicians is a necessary but insufficient condition for the provision of optimal care. This finding has created interest in knowledge translation, the scientific study of the methods for closing the knowledge-to-practice gap and the analysis of barriers and facilitators inherent in the process.[54]

So, in deciding whether a valid guideline is applicable to our patient/practice/hospital/community, we need to identify the four Bs that pertain to the guideline and our local context and decide whether they can be reconciled. The only people who are "experts" in the Bs are the patients and providers at the sharp edge of implementing the application component. Note that none of these Bs has any effect on the validity of the evidence component of the guideline, and it is clear that validity of the evidence is not all that matters.

4

n-of-1 trials

You may not always be able to find a randomized trial or systematic review relevant to your patient. Traditionally, when faced with this dilemma, clinicians have conducted a "trial of therapy" during which we start our patient on a treatment and follow him or her to determine whether the symptoms improve or worsen while on treatment. Performing this standard trial of therapy may be misleading (and is prone to bias) for several reasons:

1. Some target disorders are self-limiting, and patients may get better on their own.

2. Both extreme laboratory values and clinical signs, if left untreated and reassessed later, often return to normal.

3. A placebo can lead to substantial improvement in symptoms.

4. Both our own and our patient's expectations about the success or failure of a treatment can bias conclusions about whether a treatment actually works.

5. Polite patients may exaggerate the effects of therapy.

If a treatment were used during any of the above situations, it would tend to appear efficacious when, in fact, it was useless.

The *n-of-1 trial* applies the principles of rigorous clinical trial methodology to overcome these problems when trying to determine the best treatment for an individual patient. It randomizes time and assigns the patient (using concealed randomization and hopefully blinding of the patient and clinician) to active therapy or placebo at different times so that the patient undergoes cycles of experimental and control treatment resulting in multiple crossovers (within the same patient) to help us decide on the best therapy. It is employed when there is significant doubt about whether a treatment might be helpful in a particular patient and is most successful when directed toward the control of symptoms or prevention of relapses resulting from a chronic disease. It is also helpful in determining whether symptoms may be caused be a medication. For example, a group of investigators in Australia evaluated a series of n-of-1 trials among patients with one of three clinical diseases in which the optimal treatment option remained uncertain—osteoarthritis, chronic neuropathic pain, and attention-deficit hyperactivity disorder (ADHD).[55] They found a successful strategy for supporting patients requiring expensive medications for the treatment of chronic diseases.

Guides that we use for deciding whether to execute an n-of-1 trial are listed in Box 4.19. The crucial first step in this process is to have a discussion with the involved patients to determine their interest, willingness to participate, expectations of the treatment, and desired outcomes. Next, we need to determine whether formal ethics approval is required.[m] If, after reviewing these guides, you decide to proceed with an n-of-1 trial, we recommend the following strategies (they are described in detail elsewhere[n]):

1. Come to agreement with the patient on the symptoms, signs, or other manifestations of the target disorder that we want to improve and set up a data collection method so that the findings can be recorded regularly.

---

[m]At our institutions, this is variable—in some places ethics and written consent is required and at others it isn't necessary because the objective is improved care for an individual patient who is our co-investigator.

[n]Kravitz RL, Duan N, eds, and the DEcIDE Methods Center N-of-1 Guidance Panel (Duan N, Eslick I, Gabler NB, Kaplan HC, Kravitz RL, Larson EB, Pace WD, Schmid CH, Sim I, Vohra S). *Design and Implementation of N-of-1 Trials: A User's Guide.* AHRQ Publication No. 13(14)-EHC122-EF. Rockville, MD: Agency for Healthcare Research and Quality; February 2014. Available at: www.effectivehealthcare.ahrq.gov/N-1-Trials .cfm.

Box 4.19 Guides for n-of-1 randomized trials

---

1. Is an n-of-1 trial indicated for our patient?
   - Is the effectiveness of the treatment really in doubt for our patient?
   - Will the treatment, if effective, be continued long-term?
   - Is our patient willing and eager to collaborate in designing and carrying out an n-of-1 trial?
2. Is an n-of-1 trial feasible in our patient?
   - Does the treatment have a rapid onset?
   - Does the treatment cease to act soon after it is discontinued?
   - Is the optimal treatment duration feasible?
   - Can outcomes that are relevant and important to our patient be measured?
   - Can we establish sensible criteria for stopping the trial?
   - Can an unblinded run-in period be conducted?
3. Is an n-of-1 trial feasible in our practice setting?
   - Is there a pharmacist available to help?
   - Are strategies for interpreting the trial data in place?
4. Is the n-of-1 study ethical?
   - Is approval by our medical research ethics committee necessary?

---

2. Determine (in collaboration with a pharmacist and our patient) the active and comparison (usually placebo) treatments, treatment durations, and rules for stopping a treatment period.

3. Set up pairs of treatment periods, in which our patient receives the experimental therapy during one period and the placebo during the other (with the order of treatment randomized).

4. If possible, both we and our patient remain blind to the treatment being given during any period, even when we examine the results at the end of the pair of periods. This means having a pharmacist independently prepare medications.

5. Pairs of treatment periods are continued and analyzed until we decide to unblind the results and decide whether to continue the active therapy or abandon it.

6. Monitor treatment targets regularly—using relevant outcomes decided upon by the patient and clinician.

Further reading about n-of-1 trials

Guyatt G, Rennie D, Meade M, Cook DJ, editors. Users' guides to the medical literature. A manual for evidence-based clinical practice. 3rd ed. Chicago, IL: AMA Press; 2015.

Kravitz RL, Duan N; the DEcIDE Methods Center N-of-1 Guidance Panel (Duan N, Eslick I, Gabler NB, et al.), editors. Design and implementation of N-of-1 trials: a user's guide. AHRQ Publication No. 13(14)-EHC122-EF. Rockville, MD: Agency for Healthcare Research and Quality; 2014. Available at: www.effectivehealthcare.ahrq.gov/N-1-Trials.cfm.

References

1. Yusuf S, Bosch J, Dagenais G, Zhu J, Xavier D, Liu L, et al. Cholesterol Lowering in Intermediate-Risk Persons without Cardiovascular Disease. N Engl J Med 2016;374(21):2021–31.

2. Schulz KF, Altman DG, Moher D. CONSORT 2010 statement: updated guidelines for reporting parallel group randomized trials. Ann Intern Med 2010;152(11):726–32.

3. Stampfer MJ, Colditz GA. Estrogen replacement therapy and coronary heart disease: a quantitative assessment of the epidemiologic evidence. Prev Med 1991;20:47–63.

4. Hulley S, Grady D, Bush T, et al. Randomized trial of estrogen plus progestin for secondary prevention of coronary heart disease in postmenopausal women. JAMA 1998;280:605–13.

5. Rossouw JE, Anderson G, Prentice RL, et al. Risks and benefits of estrogen and progestin in healthy postmenopausal women: principal results from the Women's Health Initiative randomized controlled trial. JAMA 2002;288:321–3.

6. The EC/IC Bypass Study Group. Failure of extracranial - intracranial arterial bypass to reduce the risk of ischemic stroke. Results of an international randomized trial. N Engl J Med 1985;313:1191–200.

7. Echt DS, Liebson PR, Mitchell LB, et al. Mortality and morbidity in patients receiving encainide, flecainide, or placebo. The Cardiac Arrhythmia Suppression Trial. N Engl J Med 1991;324:781–8.

8. Moore T. Deadly medicine: Why tens of thousands of heart patients died in America's worst drug disaster. New York: Simon & Schuster; 1995.

9. Ronksley PE, Brien SE, Turner BJ, Mukamal KJ, Ghali WA. Association of alcohol consumption with selected cardiovascular disease outcomes: a systematic review and meta-analysis. BMJ 2011;342.

10. Schultz KF, Grimes DA. Allocation concealment in randomized trials. Lancet 2002;359:614–18.

11. Consolidated Standards of Reporting Trials [December 2016]. Available from: http://www.consort-statement.org/.

12. Deshauer D, Moher D, Fergusson D, et al. Selective serotonin reuptake inhibitors for unipolar depression: a systematic review of classic long-term randomized controlled trials. CMAJ 2008;178:1293–301.

13. Bassler D, Montori VM, Briel M, et al. Early stopping of randomized clinical trials for overt efficacy is problematic. J Clin Epidemiol 2008; 61:241–6.

14. Stegert M, Kasenda B, von Elm E, You JJ, Blumle A, Tomonaga Y, et al. An analysis of protocols and publications suggested that most discontinuations of clinical trials were not based on preplanned interim analyses or stopping rules. J Clin Epidemiol 2016;69:152–60.

15. Porta N, Bonet C, Cobo E. Discordance between reported intention-to-treat and per protocol analyses. J Clin Epidemiol 2007; 60(7):663–9.

16. Barnett HJ, Taylor DW, Eliaszew M, et al. Benefits of carotid endarterectomy in patients with symptomatic moderate or severe stenosis. N Engl J Med 1998;339:1415–25.

17. Devereaux PJ, Manns B, Ghali WH, et al. Physician interpretations and textbook definitions of blinding terminology in randomized control trials. JAMA 2001;285:2000–3.

18. Lewis HD Jr, Davis JW, Archibald DG, Steinke WE, Smitherman TC, Doherty JE 3rd, et al. Protective effects of aspirin against acute myocardial infarction and death in men with unstable angina. Results of a Veterans Administration Cooperative Study. N Engl J Med 1983; 309(7):396–403.

19. Ferreira-Gonzalez I, Permanyer-Miralda G, Busse JW, et al. Methodologic discussions for using and interpreting composite endpoints are limited but still identify major concerns. J Clin Epidemiol 2007;60:651–7.

20. The ADVANCE Collaborative Group. Intensive blood glucose control and vascular outcomes in patients with type 2 diabetes. N Engl J Med 2008;358:2560–72.

21. Intensive glucose control did not prevent important complications in type 2 diabetes. ACP J Club 2008;149(3).

22. Wilson MC. Top Strategies to Weave EBM into Your Clinical Teaching. Lecture presented at Association of Program Directors in Internal

4

Medicine (APDIM): Chief Residents Workshop; 2013; Lake Buena Vista, Florida.

23. Schwartz GG, Olsson AG, Ezekowitz MD, Ganz P, Oliver MF, Waters D, et al. Effects of atorvastatin on early recurrent ischemic events in acute coronary syndromes: the MIRACL study: a randomized controlled trial. JAMA 2001;285(13):1711–18.

24. Randomised trial of a perindopril-based blood-pressure-lowering regimen among 6,105 individuals with previous stroke or transient ischaemic attack. Lancet 2001;358(9287):1033–41.

25. Glasziou P, Doll H. Was the study big enough? Two cafe rules. Evid Based Med 2006;11(3):69–70.

26. Eaton CB. Rosuvastatin reduced major cardiovascular events in patients at intermediate cardiovascular risk. Ann Intern Med 2016; 165(2):JC6.

27. Siemieniuk RA, Alonso-Coello P, et al. Corticosteroid therapy for patients hospitalized with community acquired pneumonia. Ann Intern Med 2015;163(7):519–28. doi:10.7326/M15-0715.

28. Mallett S, Clarke M. How many Cochrane reviews are needed to cover existing evidence on the effects of health care interventions? ACP J Club 2003;139(1):A11.

29. Health Information Research Unit. Hedges. 2016 [Accessed 3 December 2016]. Available from: http://hiru.mcmaster.ca/hiru/HIRU_Hedges_home.aspx.

30. Liberati A, Altman DG, Tetzlaff J, et al. The PRISMA statement for reporting systematic reviews and meta-analyses of studies that evaluate health care interventions. Ann Intern Med 2009;151:4.

31. McGowan J, Sampson M, Salzwedel DM, Cogo E, Foerster V, Lefebvre C. PRESS Peer Review of Electronic Search Strategies: 2015 Guideline Statement. J Clin Epidemiol 2016;75:40–6.

32. Tricco AC, Antony J, Soobiah C, Kastner M, MacDonald H, Cogo E, et al. Knowledge synthesis methods for integrating qualitative and quantitative data: a scoping review reveals poor operationalization of the methodological steps. J Clin Epidemiol 2016;73:29–35.

33. Mills EJ, Thorlund K, Ioannidis JP. Demystifying trial networks and network meta-analysis. BMJ 2013;346:f2914.

34. Sale JE, Gignac MA, Hawker G, Frankel L, Beaton D, Bogoch E, et al. Decision to take osteoporosis medication in patients who have had a fracture and are 'high' risk for future fracture: a qualitative study. BMC Musculoskelet Disord 2011;12:92.

35. Institute of Medicine. Clinical practice guidelines: directions for a new program. Washington DC: National Academy Press; 1990.

36. Al-Ansary LA, Tricco AC, Adi Y, Bawazeer G, Perrier L, Al-Ghonaim M, et al. A Systematic Review of Recent Clinical Practice Guidelines on the Diagnosis, Assessment and Management of Hypertension. PLoS ONE 2013;8(1):e53744.

37. Sheerin I, Hamilton G, Humphrey A, Scragg A. Issues in the assessment of cardiovascular risk in selected general practices in Canterbury, New Zealand. N Z Med J 2007;120(1261).

38. National Institute for Health and Care Excellence. Multimorbidity: clinical assessment and management. London: NICE Guideline; 2016.

39. Canadian Institute of Health Research. AGREE: Advancing the science of practice guidelines [internet]. 2014 [cited 4 December 2016]. Available from: http://www.agreetrust.org/about-the-agree-enterprise/agree-research-teams/agree-collaboration/.

40. The National Academies of Sciences. Standards for Developing Trustworthy Clinical Practice Guidelines [internet]. 2016 [cited 11 December 2016]. Available at: http://www.nationalacademies.org/hmd/Reports/2011/Clinical-Practice-Guidelines-We-Can-Trust/Standards.aspx.

41. Canadian Task Force on Preventive Health Care. Screening for Breast Cancer [internet]. 2011 [cited 3 December 2016]. Available at: http://canadiantaskforce.ca/ctfphc-guidelines/2011-breast-cancer/.

42. The Canadian Task Force on the Periodic Health Examination. The periodic health examination. Can Med Assoc J 1979;121:1093–254.

43. Guyatt G, Rennie D, Meade M, Cook DJ, editors. Users' guides to the medical literature. A manual for evidence-based clinical practice. 3rd ed. Chicago: AMA Press; 2015.

44. Guyatt G, Oxman A, Vist G, Kunz R, Falck-Ytter Y, Alonso-Coello P, et al. for the GRADE working group. GRADE: an emerging consensus on rating quality of evidence and strength of recommendations. BMJ 2008;336:924–6.

45. Brouwers MC, Somerfield MR, Browman GP. A for Effort: Learning from the application of the GRADE approach to cancer guideline development. J Clin Oncol 2008;26(7):1025–6.

46. Making Grade the Irresistible Choice [internet]. 2016 [cited 3 December 2016]. Available at: http://magicproject.org.

47. ADAPTE Group. ADAPTE manual for guideline adaptation. 2007. Available from: http://www.adapte.org. Accessed 27 May 2008.

4

48. Lippincott's Nursing Center.com. CAN-IMPLEMENT [internet]. 2016 [cited 3 December 2016]. Available at: http://www.nursingcenter.com/evidencebasedpracticenetwork/canimplement.aspx?id=1917711.

49. Brouwers MC, Makarski J, Kastner M, Hayden L, Bhattacharyya O. The Guideline Implementability Decision Excellence Model (GUIDE-M): a mixed methods approach to create an international resource to advance the practice guideline field. Implement Sci 2015;10:36.

50. Cabana M, Rand C, Powe N, Wu A, Wilson M, Abboud P, et al. Why don't physicians follow clinical practice guidelines? A framework for improvement. JAMA 1999;282:1458–65.

51. Levine MN, Gafni A, Markham B, MacFarlane D. A bedside decision instrument to elicit a patient's preference concerning adjuvant chemotherapy for breast cancer. Ann Intern Med 1992;117:53–8.

52. Nease RF, Kneeland T, O'Connor GT, et al. Variation in patient utilities for outcomes of the management of chronic stable angina: implications for clinical practice guidelines. JAMA 1995;273:1185–90.

53. Legare F, O'Connor AM, Graham ID, Saucier D, Cote L, Blais J, et al. Primary health care professionals' views on barriers and facilitators to the implementation of the Ottawa Decision Support Framework in practice. Patient Educ Couns 2006;63:380–90.

54. Straus SE, Tetroe J, Graham ID. Knowledge translation in health care: moving from evidence to practice. 2nd ed. Oxford: Wiley/Blackwell/BMJ Books; 2013.

55. Scuffham PA, Nikles J, Mitchell GK, Yelland MJ, Vine N, Poulos CJ, et al. Using N-of-1 trials to improve patient management and save costs. J Gen Intern Med 2010;25(9):906–13.

5 Diagnosis and screening

Clinical diagnosis is a complex and uncertain process, which is part intuition and part rational. Before we look in detail at the rational "evidence-based medicine (EBM)" part of the process, we should look briefly at the wider process of diagnosis.

Experienced clinicians appear to combine two modes of thinking when engaged in clinical diagnosis.[1,2] In one mode, the clinician rapidly recognizes the patient's illness as a case of a familiar disorder; this is described as pattern recognition or nonanalytic reasoning. In the second mode, the clinician relates features of the patient's illness to knowledge from memory and uses it to induce the diagnostic possibilities and to deduce the best diagnostic explanation for the illness; this is termed "analytic reasoning." Excellent clinicians employ both modes, using the faster, nonanalytic method when it suffices, but slowing down to use the analytic approach when it is needed.[2] Within the analytic mode of reasoning, clinicians use several different approaches to analyzing patients' illness. In this chapter. we'll focus on the probabilistic approach.[3] Consider how we might approach the following clinical scenario.

5

A 40-year-old woman with fatigue

We can think of diagnosis as occurring in three stages:[3] initiation of diagnostic hypotheses ("I wonder if the patient has ... ."); refinement of the diagnosis by ruling out or narrowing possibilities ("It is not X or Y; what type of infection could it be?"); and finally some confirmation of the final, most likely diagnosis ("We should do a biopsy to confirm this before treating."). These processes and some examples are illustrated in Figure 5.1.[4] Initiation of the diagnosis includes gathering clinical findings and selecting patient-specific differential diagnoses for each potential diagnosis. For our patient with fatigue, we would look for other features that might narrow the diagnostic range—which, for fatigue, is unfortunately vast; otherwise we are left with checking of common causes, such as depression, stress/anxiety, medication side effects, or anemia. Refining the diagnosis includes hypothesis-driven use of additional clinical findings or tests used to raise or lower our estimates of the likelihood of each potential disorder and arriving at the final diagnosis when we are able to verify a diagnosis or cross a test/treat threshold, which is discussed later in this chapter.

Stage | Strategy

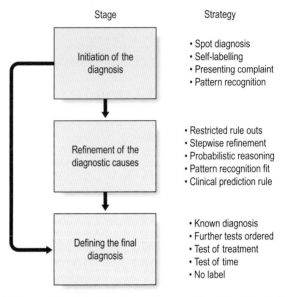

Initiation of the diagnosis
- Spot diagnosis
- Self-labelling
- Presenting complaint
- Pattern recognition

Refinement of the diagnostic causes
- Restricted rule outs
- Stepwise refinement
- Probabilistic reasoning
- Pattern recognition fit
- Clinical prediction rule

Defining the final diagnosis
- Known diagnosis
- Further tests ordered
- Test of treatment
- Test of time
- No label

Fig. 5.1 Stages and strategies in the diagnostic process. From Heneghan C, Glasziou P, Thompson M et al. Diagnostic strategies used in primary care. BMJ 2009;338, with permission.

In learning to be better diagnosticians, we need to learn the many possible patterns that we may encounter, whether visual or nonvisual. With many thousands of possible diagnoses, that is a big task and essential to the initiation phase—if we don't know of a diagnostic possibility, we cannot consider it. Each phase of the diagnostic process can be informed by relevant evidence. For example, evidence on the accuracy of the clinical examination can help us with the initiation of diagnosis. Additionally, research articles on disease probability can inform our attempts to define the pretest probability of various diagnoses. However, in the next phases, we will need to refine the diagnostic possibilities by using various diagnostic "tests" (including analysis of symptoms and signs, laboratory tests, and imaging) to refine and finally confirm the diagnosis. In this chapter, we will focus on three questions about these diagnostic "tests":

A. Is this evidence about the accuracy of a diagnostic test valid?

B. Does this (valid) evidence show that the test is useful?

C. How can I apply this valid, accurate diagnostic test to a specific patient?

After retrieving evidence about a test's accuracy, questions 1 and 2 suggest that we need to decide if it's valid and important before we can apply the evidence to our individual patients. As with therapy, the order in which we consider validity and importance may not be crucial and depends on individual preference. But both should be done before applying the study results. Because the screening and early diagnosis of cases without symptoms have some similarities to, but also some crucial differences from, cases with diseases, we'll close with a special section devoted to these acts at the interface of clinical medicine and public health. Tests may also be used for refining prognosis or for monitoring a disease, but we will not cover those in this chapter.

A central theme of this chapter is making sense of the uncertainties and inaccuracies in the process of diagnosis. Figure 5.2 shows the interpretation of the highly sensitive D-dimer for diagnosing deep vein thrombosis (DVT). The figure shows the posttest probabilities after positive (upper curve) and negative (lower curve) D-dimer results for the range of possible pretest probabilities of DVT. The graph is based on the highly sensitive D-dimer having a *sensitivity* of 97.7% (i.e., of those with DVT, 97.7% will have a positive result) and 46% specificity (i.e., of those without DVT, 46% will have a negative result). The first question, on validity, asks if we can believe the information in the graph. The second question, on importance, asks if the results show clinically worthwhile shifts in uncertainty (the further apart the posttest curves, the larger is this shift) and, specifically, whether the test helps to rule in or rule out the target disorder. The figure suggests that the highly sensitive D-dimer is helpful in ruling out most of the conditions in the pretest range but does not help to rule in a specific condition. For example, for patients with a moderate (17%) chance of DVT based on the Well score, the chance after a negative D-dimer is about 1%, but after a positive D-dimer, it is still only about 28%. The third question implies that we need to understand how the test results might change our diagnostic uncertainty on application, not only for the patients in the study but, more importantly, for a particular individual patient as well.

So let's return to the opening scenario, and pick up after some initial tests have been done, and we need to consider how to interpret whether the ferritin is "abnormal."

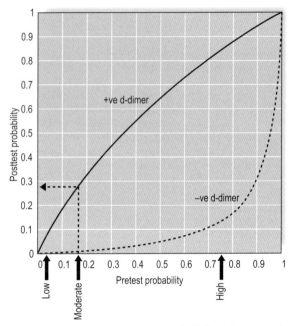

Fig. 5.2 Probability revision graph showing a test's (D-dimer) impact on diagnostic uncertainty by how it changes the pretest probability to the posttest probability (of deep vein thrombosis [DVT]).

A 40-year-old woman with fatigue and anemia

Suppose that in performing the workup for a patient with fatigue, we find that she has anemia and think that the probability that she has iron-deficiency anemia is 50% (i.e., the odds that the anemia is caused by iron deficiency are about 50:50). When we present the patient to our supervisor, she asks for an Educational Prescription to determine the usefulness of performing a serum ferritin test as a means to detecting iron-deficiency anemia.[5] By the time we've tracked down and studied the external evidence, the result of our patient's serum ferritin test comes back at 60 mmol/L. How should we put all this together?

Before looking at the scenario and our three questions, we should take a short detour through the land of "abnormality" so that we understand what could be meant by "normal" or "abnormal" ferritin.

What is normal or abnormal?

Most test reports will end up calling some results "normal" and others "abnormal." There are at least six definitions of "normal" in common use (listed in Box 5.1). This chapter will focus on definition #5 ("diagnostic" normal) because we think that the first four have important flaws, which can lead to misdiagnosis and overdiagnosis (i.e., giving a patient a diagnostic label that will not help during his or her lifetime). The first two (the Gaussian and percentile definitions) focus just on the diagnostic test results in either a normal (the left-hand cluster in Fig. 5.3) or an undifferentiated group of people (an unknown mix of the left and right clusters in Fig. 5.3), with no reference standard or clear consequences for being "abnormal." They not only imply that all "abnormalities" occur at the same frequency (5%) but suggest that if we perform more and more diagnostic tests on our patient, we are increasingly likely to find something "abnormal," which would lead to all sorts of inappropriate further testing.

The third definition of "normal" (culturally desirable) represents the sort of value judgement seen in fashion advertisements and can confuse medicine with social norms, for example, homosexuality being included in the early versions of the *Diagnostic and Statistical Manual of Mental Disorders* (DSM). The fourth (risk factor) definition has the drawback that it "labels" or stigmatizes patients above an arbitrary cut-off whether or not we can intervene to lower their risk—a big problem with much genetic testing and other screening maneuvers, as you'll learn in the concluding section of this chapter. The fifth (diagnostic) definition is

---

Box 5.1 Six definitions of normal

1. Gaussian—the mean ±2 standard deviations—this one assumes a normal distribution for all tests and results in all "abnormalities" having the same frequency.
2. Percentile—within the range, say of 5–95%—has the same basic defect as the Gaussian definition. Implies a specificity of 95% but with unknown sensitivity.
3. Culturally desirable—when "normal" is that which is preferred by society, the role of medicine gets confused.
4. Risk factor—carrying no additional risk of disease—nicely labels the outliers, but does changing a risk factor necessarily change risk?
5. Diagnostic—range of results beyond which target disorders become highly probable; the focus of this discussion.
6. Therapeutic—range of results beyond which treatment does more good than harm; means we have to keep up with advances in therapy!

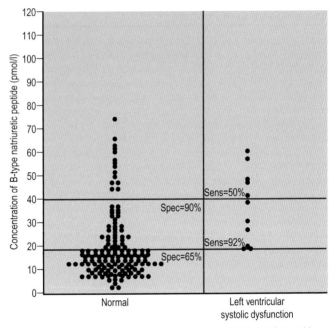

Fig. 5.3 Distribution of B-type natriuretic peptide (BNP) results in nondiseased (normal left ventricular ejection fraction [LVEF]) and diseased (reduced LVEF) groups; two cut-offs are shown for 20 and 40 pmol/L.

the one that we will focus on here, and we will show you how to work with it in the next section of this chapter. The final (therapeutic) definition (Does treating at and beyond this level do more good than harm?) is, in part, an extension of the fourth (risk factor) definition but has the great clinical advantage that it changes with our knowledge of efficacy. Thus, the definition of "normal" blood pressure has changed radically over the past several decades because we have developed better anti-hypertensives and learned that treatment of progressively less pronounced elevations of blood pressure does more good than harm.

Is this evidence about the accuracy of a diagnostic test valid?

Having found a possibly useful article about a diagnostic test, how can we quickly critically appraise it for its proximity to the truth? The patients

---

Box 5.2 Is this evidence about a diagnostic test valid?

---

1. **Representativeness**: Was the diagnostic test evaluated in an appropriate spectrum of patients (like those in whom we would use it in practice)?
2. **Ascertainment**: Was the reference standard ascertained regardless of the diagnostic test result?
3. **Measurement**: Was there an independent, blind comparison with a reference standard?
   Fourth question to be considered for clusters of tests or clinical prediction rules:
4. **Validity**: Was the cluster of tests validated in a second, independent group of patients?

---

in the study should have undergone both the diagnostic test in question (say, an item of the history or physical examination, a blood test, etc.) and the reference (or "gold") standard (an autopsy or biopsy or other confirmatory "proof" that they do or do not have the target disorder, or long enough follow-up so that the disease should have declared itself). We can check that this was done well by asking some simple questions, and often we'll find their answers in the article's abstract. Box 5.2 lists these questions for individual reports, but we can also apply them to the interpretation of a systematic review of several different studies of the same diagnostic test for the same target disorder.[a]

1. Representative: Was the diagnostic test evaluated in an appropriate spectrum of patients (e.g., those in whom we would use it in practice)?

Did the report include patients with all the common presentations of the target disorder (including those with its early manifestations) and patients with other, commonly confused conditions? Studies that confine themselves to florid cases versus asymptomatic volunteers (a diagnostic "case-control" study) are useful only as a first crude check of the test because when the diagnosis is obvious to the eye we don't need any

---

[a]We'll stress throughout this book that systematic reviews provide us with the most valid and useful external evidence on just about any clinical question we can pose. They are still quite rare for diagnostic tests, and for this reason, we'll describe them in their usual, therapeutic habitat, in chapter 4. When applying Box 4.6 and Box 4.7 (on p. 113) to diagnostic tests, simply substitute "diagnostic test" for "treatment" as you read. We look for the same things when considering the validity of diagnostic systematic reviews; specifically, was a comprehensive search completed, was a quality assessment of retrieved articles performed, and was there heterogeneity?

diagnostic test. (Note that these study designs tend to overestimate test accuracy.) The really useful articles will describe the diagnostic dilemmas we face and include patients with mild as well as severe conditions; early as well as late cases of the target disorder; and both treated and untreated individuals.

2. Ascertainment: Was the reference standard ascertained regardless of the diagnostic test's result?

When patients have a negative diagnostic test result, investigators are tempted to forgo the reference standard, and when the latter is invasive or risky (e.g., angiography), it may be wrong to carry it out on patients with negative test results. To overcome this, many investigators now employ a reference standard for proving that a patient does not have the target disorder, and this standard requires that the patient doesn't suffer any adverse health outcome during a long follow-up despite the absence of any definitive treatment (e.g., convincing evidence that a patient with clinically suspected DVT did not have this disorder would include no ill-effects during a prolonged follow-up despite the absence of antithrombotic therapy).

3. Measurement: Was there an independent, blind comparison with a reference ("gold") standard?[b]

In a study of test accuracy, we must determine whether the test we're interested in was compared with an appropriate reference standard. Sometimes investigators have a difficult time coming up with clear-cut reference standards (e.g., for psychiatric disorders), and we'll want to

---

[b]Note that to approximate the sequence of steps in the critical appraisal of therapy articles, we could consider the appraisal questions using the following order: **r**epresentativeness, **a**scertainment, and **m**easurement. You'll notice that the first letters of these words produce the acronym "RAM," which some learners might find useful for remembering the appraisal questions. Alternatively, when considering the validity of reports of diagnostic test accuracy, others might find it easier to consider the most crucial question first: Was there a comparison with an appropriate reference standard? If an appropriate reference standard was not used, we can toss the article without reading further, thus becoming more efficient knowledge managers. If the report we're reading fails one or more of these three tests, we'll need to consider whether it has a fatal flaw that renders its conclusions invalid. If so, it's back to more searching (either now or later; if we've already used up our time for this week, perhaps we can interest a colleague or trainee in taking this on as an "Educational Prescription"—see page 30 if this term is new to you). However, if the report passes this initial scrutiny and we decide that we can believe its results, and we haven't already carried out the second critical appraisal step of deciding whether these results are important, then we can proceed to the next section.

give careful consideration to their arguments justifying the selection of their reference standard. Moreover, we caution you against the uncritical acceptance of reference standards, even when they are based on "expert" interpretations of biopsies; in a note in the *Evidence-Based Medicine Journal,* Kenneth Fleming[6] reported that the degree of agreement over and above chance in pathologists' reading of breast, skin, and liver biopsies is less than 50%! The results of one test should not be known to those who are applying and interpreting the other (e.g., the pathologist interpreting the biopsy that comprises the reference standard for the target disorder should be "blind" to the result of the blood test that comprises the diagnostic test under study). In this way, investigators avoid the conscious and unconscious bias that might otherwise cause the reference standard to be "overinterpreted" when the diagnostic test is positive and "underinterpreted" when it is negative. By "independent," we mean that the completion and interpretation of the reference test (or the test we're interested in) is not dependent on, and does not incorporate, the results of the other test(s).

Does this (valid) evidence demonstrate an important ability of this test to accurately distinguish patients who do and don't have a specific disorder?

5

In deciding whether the evidence about a diagnostic test is important, we will focus on the accuracy of the test in distinguishing patients with and without the target disorder. We'll consider the ability of a valid test to change our minds, going from what we thought before the test (we'll call that the "pretest" probability of some target disorder) to what we think afterward (we'll call that the "posttest" probability of the target disorder). Diagnostic tests that produce big changes from pretest to posttest probabilities are important and likely to be useful to us in our practice.

The study's main results will be the proportion of patients with the target disease in (1) those classified as positive by the test and (2) those classified as negative. These are known as the "posttest" probability of disease given a positive test result (also called the "positive predictive value" [PPV]) and the "posttest" probability of non-disease given a negative test result (or the "negative predictive value" [NPV], which refers to chances of *not* having disease if the test is negative). Returning to our clinical scenario, suppose further that in filling our prescription, we find a systematic review[7] of several studies of this diagnostic test

Table 5.1 Results of a systematic review of serum ferritin as a diagnostic test for iron-deficiency anemia*

		Target disorder (iron-deficiency anemia)		
		Present	Absent	Totals
Diagnostic test	Positive	731	270	1001
result (serum	(<65 mmol/L)	a	b	a + b
ferritin)	Negative	78	1500	1578
	(≥65 mmol/L)	c	d	c + d
		809	1770	2579
Totals		a + c	b + d	a + b + c + d

*These data come from: Guyatt GH, Oxman AD, Ali M, Willan A, Malloy W, Patterson C. Laboratory diagnosis of iron-deficiency anaemia: an overview. *J Gen Intern Med.* 1992;7:145–153.
Prevalence = (a + c)/(a + b + c + d) ≡ 809/2579 ≡ 31%.
Positive predictive value ≡ a/(a + b) ≡ 731/1001 ≡ 73%.
Negative predictive value ≡ d/(c + d) ≡ 1500/1578 ≡ 95%.
Sensitivity ≡ a/(a + c) ≡ 731/809 ≡ 90%.
Specificity ≡ d/(b + d) ≡ 1500/1770 ≡ 85%.
LR+ ≡ sens/(1 − spec) ≡ 90%/15% ≡ 6.
LR− ≡ (1 − sens)/spec ≡ 10%/85% ≡ 0.12.
Study pretest odds ≡ prevalence/(1 − prevalence) ≡ 31%/69% ≡ 0.45.
Posttest odds ≡ pretest odds × likelihood ratio.
Posttest probability ≡ posttest odds/(posttest odds + 1).

(evaluated against the reference standard of bone marrow staining for iron), decide that it is valid (based on the guides in Box 5.2), and find the results as shown in Table 5.1. The prevalence (or study pretest probability) overall is 809/2579 ≡ 31%. For low ferritin (<65 mmol/L— note this cut-off varies by guideline, but we'll return to level-specific interpretation in a later section), the posttest probability of iron-deficiency anemia among patients in the studies is a/(a + b) ≡ 731/1001 ≡ 73%. This study posttest probability is known as the PPV. For high ferritin (>65 mmol/L), the posttest probability of iron-deficiency anemia among patients in the studies is c/(c + d) ≡ 78/1578 ≡ 5%. This study posttest probability of 5% means that the study probability of not having iron-deficiency anemia after a negative result is 95%, which is known as the NPV. So, within the study, the uncertainty regarding iron deficiency has been shifted from the initial 31% to probabilities of either 73% or 5%—both appear to be clinically important shifts.

Sensitivity, specificity, and likelihood ratios

The study's posttest probabilities would apply directly to our patient if they had the same pretest chances of diseases. However, that is rarely the case, so instead, we will usually use an indirect process that involves a little math, which will we try to simplify for you.

Recall that we thought our patient's pretest probability of iron-deficiency anemia was greater than that in the study; in fact, we estimated it to be 50%, rather than the study's 31%. We could do a direct adjustment of the predictive values for the patient's different pretest probability by using the following equation:

patient posttest odds ≡ study posttest odds
× (patient pretest odds/study pretest odds)

which is analogous to the adjustment of a treatment trial's number needed to treat (NNT) for the patient's expected event rate (PEER). This is fine if you have the study in hand, but generally it is easier to derive some test accuracy measures—sensitivity and specificity, or the likelihood ratios—and apply these directly to the patient's individual pretest probability. So, let's look at these measures.

As you can see from Table 5.1, our patient's result (60 mmol/L) places her in the top row of the table, either in cell a or cell b. You might note from this table that 90% of patients with iron deficiency have serum ferritins in the same range as does our patient $[a/(a + c)]$; that property, the proportion of patients with the target disorder who have positive test results, is called *sensitivity*.

sensitivity ≡ probability of a positive test given disease

The complement of this proportion describes the proportion of patients who do not have the target disorder who have negative or normal test results, $d/(c + d)$, and is called *specificity*, that is:

specificity ≡ probability of a negative test given non-disease

(Note that "non-disease" here doesn't mean "no disease" but, rather, that it is not the target disease of the test).

You might also note that only 15% of patients with other causes of their anemia have results in the same range as does our patient, which means that our patient's result would be about six times as likely (90%/15%) to be seen in someone with iron-deficiency anemia as in someone without the condition; that ratio is called the *likelihood ratio* for a positive test result (LR+). The likelihood ratio positive is:

LR+ ≡ probability of positive test result given disease/
probability of positive test result given non-disease

We thought ahead of time (before we had the result of the serum ferritin) that our patient's odds of iron deficiency were 50 : 50; this is called *pretest odds* of 1 : 1. As you can see from the formulae toward the bottom of Table 5.1, we can multiply that pretest odds of 1 by the likelihood ratio of 6 to get the posttest odds of iron-deficiency anemia after the test ($1 \times 6 \equiv 6$); that's a posttest odds of 6 : 1 in favour of iron-deficiency anemia. Since, like most clinicians, you may be more comfortable thinking in terms of probabilities than odds, this posttest odds of 6 : 1 converts (as you can see at the bottom of Table 5.1) to a posttest probability of $6/(6 + 1) = 6/7 \equiv 86\%$. (To confirm the results of your calculations, try calculating the posttest probability for the same ferritin result for a patient who, as in Table 5.1, has a pretest odds of 0.45;[c] you'll know you did it right if you end up with an answer for posttest probability that is identical to its equivalent, the PPV.) Note that we could use the graph in Figure 5.4 that allows us to determine the posttest probability by drawing a line from the 50% pretest probability to the posttest positive line and across to the 86% posttest probability.

Once we know the sensitivity and specificity from a valid study, we can consider whether the test is useful and whether it can "rule out" or "rule in" the target disorder of interest. Can this test discriminate better compared with chance classification?

Is my test better than a coin toss? If we toss a coin and call "heads" positive and "tails" negative, what is the sensitivity and specificity? Since one-half the diseased cases will be detected, the sensitivity must be 50%. And since one-half the non-diseased cases will be negative, the specificity must be 50%. Can you work out what the sensitivity and specificity of two coin tosses is if we call any pair with a head "positive"?

As you might have guessed from our coin "test," if the sensitivity% and specificity% only add to 100%, then the test is useless. It leaves the probabilities unchanged (and the posttest lines both lie on the diagonal of the pretest/posttest graph). So, for a test to be useful, the sensitivity%

---

[c]The posttest odds are $0.45 \times 6 \equiv 2.7$ and the posttest probability is $2.7/3.7 \equiv 73\%$. Note that this is identical to the PPV.

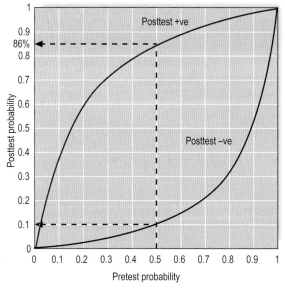

Fig. 5.4 Probability revision graph. A test's impact on uncertainty: from pretest to posttest probabilities.

5

+ specificity% – 100% (known as the *Youden Index*) must be greater than zero and preferably be at least 50% (and ideally 100%!).

Can the test rule in or rule out?

Extremely high values (approaching 100%) of sensitivity and specificity with only modest specificity or sensitivity respectively can be useful. When a test has a very high sensitivity (e.g., the loss of retinal vein pulsation in increased intracranial pressure), a negative result (the presence of pulsation) effectively rules out the diagnosis (of raised intracranial pressure), and one of our clinical clerks suggested that we apply the mnemonic "SnNout" to such findings (when a sign has a high Sensitivity, a Negative result rules out the diagnosis) (Fig. 5.5). Similarly, when a sign has a very high Specificity (e.g., the face of a child with Down syndrome), a Positive result effectively rules in the diagnosis (of Down syndrome); not surprisingly, our clinical clerks call such a finding a "SpPin" (when a sign has high Specificity, a Positive result rules in the

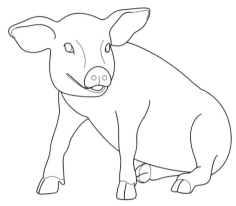

Fig. 5.5 SnNout. When a sign has a high Sensitivity, a Negative result rules out the diagnosis.

diagnosis). Keep in mind that tests with extremely high sensitivity or specificity are rare! If you can find a perfect test that has 100% sensitivity and specificity, do let us know!

We can generate likelihood ratios directly or by reference to the sensitivity and specificity by using the formulae provided in Table 5.1. The formula for the likelihood ratio for a positive test result is:

$$LR+ \equiv \text{sensitivity}/(1 - \text{specificity})$$

and the formula for the likelihood ratio for a negative test result is:

$$LR- \equiv (1 - \text{sensitivity})/\text{specificity}$$

Finally, you might sometimes come across the "diagnostic odds ratio," which is simply the LR+/LR−. If the diagnostic odds ratio is 1, then the Youden Index will be 0. Table 5.2 illustrates the sensitivity, specificity, Youden Index, and likelihood ratios for some "tests" from the clinical examination. The first three are SnNouts, and the next two are SpPins, but the last two rows are the most common—tests that are neither SpPins nor SnNouts, but they do give some information.

How can I apply this valid, important diagnostic test to a specific patient?

Having found a valid systematic review or individual report about a diagnostic test, and having decided that its accuracy is sufficiently high

Table 5.2 Accuracy of selected tests from the physical examination

Test*; condition	Sensitivity	Specificity	Youden Index	LR+ / LR−
Postural pulse increase >30/minute; large blood loss	98	99	97	98 / 50
Brachioradial delay; severe aortic stenosis	97	62	59	2.5 / 0.04
Dullness >10.5 cm from midsternal line; CTR >0.5	97	61	58	2.5 / 0.05
Diastolic BP <50 mm Hg; moderate-to-severe aortic stenosis	30–50	98	38	20 / 0.6
Lachman sign; anterior cruciate ligament tear	48–96	90–99	66	17 / 0.2
Pulse >90 beats/min; hyperthyroidism	80	82	62	4.4 / 0.24
Eyelid retraction; hyperthyroidism	34	99	33	33.2 / 0.7

*All tests taken from McGhee S. *Evidence-Based Physical Diagnosis*. 3rd ed. St. Louis, MO: Saunders; 2012.
BP, Blood pressure; CTR, Cardiothoracic ratio; LR, likelihood ratio.

5

to be useful, how do we apply it to our patient? To transfer the study results, adapt them to our patient's unique pretest probability, and decide this would be clinically useful, we should ask three questions, which are summarized in Box 5.3.

1. Is the diagnostic test available, affordable, accurate, and precise in our setting?

We obviously can't order a test that is not available. Even if it is available, we may want to confirm that it is performed in a similar manner as in the study; that it is interpreted in a competent, reproducible fashion; and that its potential consequences (see below) justify its cost. For example, some of us work on medical units at more than one hospital and have found that the labs at these different hospitals use different assays for assessing B-type natriuretic peptide (BNP)—making the interpretation for the clinician more challenging! Moreover, diagnostic tests often have different outcomes among different subsets of patients,

---

Box 5.3 Are the results of this diagnostic study applicable to my patient?

---

1. Is the diagnostic test available, affordable, accurate, and precise in our setting?
2. Can we generate a clinically sensible estimate of our patient's pretest probability?
   a. Is it based on personal experience, prevalence statistics, practice databases, or primary studies?
   b. Are the study patients similar to our own?
   c. Is it unlikely that the disease possibilities or probabilities have changed since this evidence was gathered?
3. Will the resulting posttest probabilities affect our management and help our patient?
   a. Could it move us across a test-treatment threshold?
   b. Would our patient be a willing partner in carrying it out?
   c. Would the consequences of the test help our patient reach his or her goals in all this?

---

generating higher likelihood ratios in later stages of florid disease and lower likelihood ratios in early, mild stages.

At least some diagnostic tests based on symptoms or signs lose power as patients move from primary care to secondary and tertiary care. Refer back to Table 5.1 and you will understand the reason for this. When patients are given referrals, in part because of symptoms, their primary care clinicians will be giving these referrals to patients in both cell *a* and cell *b*, and subsequent evaluations of the accuracy of their symptoms will tend to show falling specificity as a result of the referral of patients with false-positive findings. If we think that any of these factors may be operating, we can try out what we judge to be clinically sensible variations in the likelihood ratios for the test result and see whether the results alter our posttest probabilities in a way that changes our diagnosis (the short-hand term for this sort of exploration is "sensitivity analysis").

2. Can we generate a clinically sensible estimate of our patient's pretest probability?

This is a key topic, and it deserves its own "section-within-a-section." As we said above, unless our patient is a close match to the study population, we'll need to "adjust" the study posttest probability to account for the pretest probability in our patient. How can we estimate our patient's pretest probability? We've used five different sources for this vital information—clinical experience, regional or national prevalence statistics, practice databases, the original report we used for deciding on the accuracy and importance of the test, and studies devoted specifically to determining pretest probabilities. Although the last is ideal, we'll consider each in turn.

First, we can recall our clinical experience with prior patients who presented with the same clinical problem, and backtrack from their final diagnoses to their pretest probabilities. While easily and quickly accessed, our memories are often distorted by our last patient, our most dramatic (or embarrassing) patient, our fear of missing a rare but treatable cause, and the like, so we use this source with caution.[d] And if we're early in our careers, we may not have enough clinical experience to draw upon. Thus, although we tend to use our remembered cases, we need to learn to supplement them with other sources, unless we have the time and energy to document all of our diagnoses and generate our own database.

Second, we could turn to regional or national prevalence statistics on the frequencies of the target disorders in the general population or some subset of it. Estimates from these sources are only as good as the accuracy of their diagnoses, and although they can provide some guidance for "baseline" pretest probabilities before taking symptoms into account (useful, say, for patients walking into a general practice), we may be more interested in pretest probabilities in just those persons with a particular symptom.

Third, we could overcome the foregoing problems by tracking down local, regional, or national practice databases that collect information on patients with the same clinical problem and report the frequency of disorders diagnosed in these patients. Although some examples exist, such databases are mostly things of the future. As before, their usefulness will depend on the extent to which they use sensible diagnostic criteria and clear definitions of presenting symptoms.

Fourth, we could simply use the pretest probabilities observed in the study we critically appraised for the accuracy and importance of the diagnostic test. If the full spectrum of patients with the symptom or clinical problem (the second of our accuracy guides) was sampled, we can extrapolate the pretest probability from their study patients (or some subgroup of it) to our patient.

---

[d]If you want to read more about how our minds and memories can distort our clinical reasoning, start with Kassirer JP, Kopelman RI. Cognitive errors in diagnosis: instantiation, classification and consequences. *Am J Med*. 1989;86:433–441.

Box 5.4 Guides for critically appraising a report about pretest probabilities of disease

---

1. Is this evidence about pretest probability valid?
   a. Did the study patients represent the full spectrum of those who present with this clinical problem?
   b. Were the criteria for each final diagnosis explicit and credible?
   c. Was the diagnostic workup comprehensive and consistently applied?
   d. For initially undiagnosed patients, was follow-up sufficiently long and complete?
2. Is this evidence about pretest probability important?
   a. What were the diagnoses and their probabilities?
   b. How precise were these estimates of disease probability?

Fifth and finally, we could track down a research report of a study expressly devoted to documenting pretest probabilities for the array of diagnoses that present with a specific set of symptoms and signs similar to those of our patient. Well-done studies performed on patients closely similar to our patient provide the least biased source of pretest probabilities for our use. Although such studies are challenging to carry out (one of us led a group that generated guides for the critical appraisal of such studies),[8] they may be more readily available than widely believed. We've summarized these guides in Box 5.4. We've provided examples of pretest probabilities on our website (www.cebm.utoronto.ca).

3. Will the resulting posttest probabilities affect our management and help our patient?

There are three elements in the answer to this final question, and we begin with the bottom line: Could its results move us across some threshold that would cause us to stop all further testing? Two thresholds should be borne in mind, as shown in Figure 5.6. First, if the diagnostic test was negative or generated a likelihood ratio near 0.1, the posttest probability might become so low that we would abandon the diagnosis we were pursuing and turn to other diagnostic possibilities. Put in terms of thresholds, this negative test result has moved us from above to below the "test threshold" in Figure 5.6, and we won't do any more tests for that diagnostic possibility. However, if the diagnostic test came back with a positive result or generated a high likelihood ratio, the posttest probability might become so high that we would also abandon further

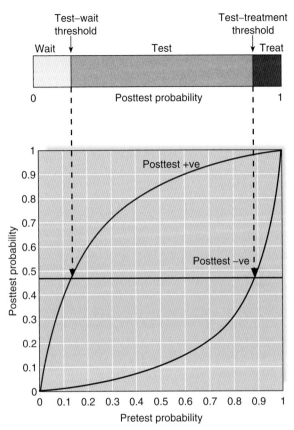

Fig. 5.6 Test–treatment thresholds.

testing because we've made our diagnosis and would now move to choosing the most appropriate therapy; in these terms, we've now crossed from below to above the "treatment threshold" in Figure 5.6.

Only when our diagnostic test result leaves us stranded between the test and treatment thresholds would we continue to pursue that initial diagnosis by performing other tests. Although there are some very fancy ways of calculating test–treatment thresholds from test accuracy and the

171

risks and benefits of correct and incorrect diagnostic conclusions,[e] intuitive test–treatment thresholds are commonly used by experienced clinicians and are another example of individual clinical expertise. We suggest you look at several pretest scenarios using a posttest probability graph (see Fig. 5.4) to get a feel of when the test results in clinically useful shifts in decisions.

We may not cross a test–treatment threshold until we've performed several different diagnostic tests, and here is where another nice property of the likelihood ratio comes into play: Provided the tests are independent we can "chain" the likelihood ratios. The posttest odds resulting from the first diagnostic test we apply becomes the pretest odds for our second diagnostic test. Hence we can simply keep multiplying the running product by the likelihood ratio generated from the next test. For example, when a 45-year-old man walks into our office, his pretest probability of greater than 75% stenosis of one or more of his coronary arteries is about 6%. Suppose that he gives us a history of atypical chest pain (only two of the three symptoms of substernal chest discomfort, brought on by exertion, and relieved in less than 10 minutes by rest are present, generating a likelihood ratio of about 13) and that his exercise electro-cardiography (ECG) reveals 2.2 mm of nonsloping ST-segment depression (generating a likelihood ratio of about 11). Then his posttest probability for coronary stenosis is his pretest probability (converted into odds) times the product of the likelihood ratios generated from his history and exercise ECG, with the resulting posttest odds converted back to probabilities (through dividing by its value + 1), that is:

$$(0.06/0.94) \times 13 \times 11 \equiv 9.13, \text{ and then } 9.13/10.13 \equiv 90\%$$

The final result of these calculations is strictly accurate as long as the diagnostic tests being combined are "independent" (i.e., given the "true" condition, the accuracy of one test does not depend on further testing). However, some dependence is common, and it means that we tend to overestimate the informativeness of the multiple tests. Accordingly, we would want the calculated posttest probability at the end of this sequence to be comfortably above our treatment threshold before we would act upon it. This additional example of how likelihood ratios make lots of implicit diagnostic reasoning explicit is another argument in favour of seeking reports of overall likelihood ratios for sequences or clusters of diagnostic tests (see section on Multiple Tests).

---

[e]See the recommendations for additional reading, or Pauker SG, Kassirer JP. The threshold approach to clinical decision making. *N Eng J Med.* 1980;302:1109.

We should have kept our patient informed as we worked our way through all the foregoing considerations, especially if we've concluded that the diagnostic test is worth considering. If we haven't yet done so, we certainly need to do so now. Every diagnostic test involves some invasion of privacy, and some are embarrassing, painful, or dangerous. We'll have to be sure that the patient is an informed, willing partner in the undertaking. In particular, the patient should be aware of the possibility of false-positive or false-negative outcomes so that this is not a surprise when the patient returns for the discussion of results. The ultimate question to ask about using any diagnostic test is whether its consequences (reassurance obtained by a negative result; labeling and unpleasant diagnostic and prognostic news when the result is positive, need for further diagnostic tests and treatments, etc.) will help our patient achieve his or her goals of therapy. Included here are considerations of how subsequent interventions match clinical guidelines or restrictions on access to therapy designed to optimize the use of finite resources for all members of our society.

More extreme results are more persuasive

The more extreme a test result is, the more persuasive it is. Although the dichotomized serum ferritin's sensitivity (90%) and specificity (85%) look impressive, expressing its accuracy with *level-specific* likelihood ratios reveals its even greater power and, in this particular example, shows how we can be misled by the restriction to just two levels (positive and negative) of the test result. Many test results, like that of serum ferritin, can be divided into several levels, and in Figure 5.6, we show you an approach called *critically appraised topic* (CAT), which is a particularly useful way of dividing test results into five levels.

When we use level-specific likelihood ratios, we see how much more informative extreme ferritin results are. The likelihood ratio for the "very positive" result is huge (52) so that one extreme level of the test result can be shown to rule in the diagnosis, and in this case we can SpPin 59% (474/809) of the patients with iron-deficiency anemia despite the unimpressive sensitivity (59%) that would have been achieved if the ferritin results had been split just below this level. Likelihood ratios of 10 or more, when applied to pretest probabilities of 33% or more $(0.33/0.67 \equiv$ pretest odds of 0.5), will generate posttest probabilities of $5/6 \equiv 83\%$ or more.

Similarly, the other extreme level (>95) is a SnNout 75% (1332/1770) for those who do not have iron-deficiency anemia (again despite a not-very-impressive specificity of 75%). Likelihood ratios of 0.1 or less, when applied to pretest probabilities of 33% or less ($0.33/0.67 \equiv$ pretest odds of 0.5), will generate posttest probabilities of $0.05/1.05 \equiv 5\%$ or less. The two intermediate levels (moderately positive and moderately negative) can move a 50% prior probability (pretest odds of $1:1$) to the useful but not necessarily diagnostic posttest probabilities of $4.8/5.8 \equiv 83\%$ and $0.39/1.39 \equiv 28\%$. And the indeterminate level ("neutral") in the middle (containing about 10% of both sorts of patients) can be seen to be uninformative, with a likelihood ratio of 1. When diagnostic test accuracy results are around 1, we've learned nothing by ordering them. To give you a better "feel" for this, the impacts of different likelihood ratios on different pretest probabilities are shown in Figure 5.7. We've provided additional examples of likelihood ratios on this book's website (www.cebm.utoronto.ca). To learn more about this, you can watch a 30-minute video about how to work out and use likelihood ratios using the ferritin example at: http://www.edge-cdn.net/video_919158?playerskin = 37016.

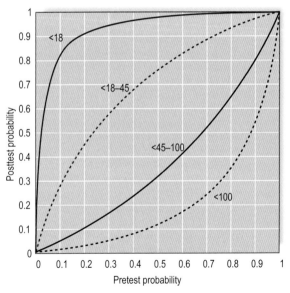

Fig. 5.7 Different posttest probabilities for four ferritin results.

An easier way of manipulating all these calculations is the nomogram of Figure 5.8. You can check out your understanding of this nomogram by using it to replicate the results of Table 5.1.

Now, return to our patient with a pretest probability for iron deficiency of 50% and a ferritin result of 60 mmol/L. To your surprise (we reckon!), our patient's test result generates an indeterminate likelihood ratio of only 1, and the test which we thought might be very useful, based on the old sensitivity and specificity way of looking at things, really hasn't been helpful in moving us toward the diagnosis. We'll have to think about other tests (including perhaps the reference standard of a bone marrow examination) to sort out her diagnosis.

More and more reports of diagnostic tests are providing multilevel likelihood ratios as measures of their accuracy. When their abstracts report only sensitivity and specificity, we can sometimes find a table with more levels and generate our own set of likelihood ratios; at other times we can find a scatterplot (of test results vs diagnoses) that is good enough for us to be able to split them into levels.

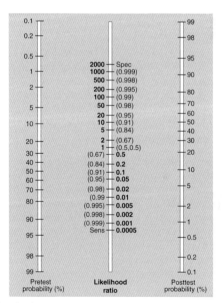

Fig. 5.8 Likelihood ratio nomogram.

Table 5.3 Examples of clinical prediction rules

Prediction rule	Sensitivity	Specificity
Ottawa ankle rule[8]	99.6%	48%
ABCD rule for melanoma[9]	84%	56%
Well's DVT rule[10]	Multilevel test	
ABCD rule for stroke prediction after TIA[11]	Multilevel test	

ABCD, Asymmetry, irregular Borders, more than one or uneven distribution of Color, or a large (greater than 6 mm) Diameter; DVT, deep vein thrombosis; TIA, transient ischemic attack.

Multiple tests

Some reports of diagnostic tests go beyond even likelihood ratios, and one of their extensions deserves mention here. This extension considers multiple diagnostic tests as a cluster or sequence of tests for a given target disorder. These multiple results can be presented in different ways, either as clusters of positive/negative results or as multivariate scores, and in either case they can be ranked and handled just like other multilevel likelihood ratios. Some examples of common clinical prediction rules are given in Table 5.3.[9-12]

When they perform (nearly) as well in a second, independent ("test") set of patients, we often refer to them as "clinical prediction guides" (CPGs). In appraising the validity of a study of a CPG, we need to consider a fourth question in addition to those above.

4. Was the cluster of tests validated in a second, independent group of patients?

Diagnostic tests are predictors, not explainers, of diagnoses. As a result, their initial evaluation cannot distinguish between real diagnostic accuracy for the target disorder and chance associations resulting from idiosyncrasies in the initial ("training" or "derivation") set of patients. This problem is compounded for clusters of diagnostic features (the CPGs), where the large numbers of possible tests considered mean we may overestimate the value of the few chosen in the CPG. The best indicator of accuracy in these situations is the demonstration of similar levels of accuracy when the test or cluster is evaluated in a second, independent (or "test") set of patients. If it performs well in this "test" set, we are reassured about its accuracy. If it performs poorly, we should look elsewhere. And if no "test set" study has been carried out, we'd be wise to reserve judgement. Clinical prediction guides are also used to help establish a prognosis. Detailed appraisal guides for clinical prediction guides are available, and we refer you to the textbooks mentioned at the end of this chapter for more information.

Practising evidence-based medicine in real time

CPGs often include several variables, which we have to keep in mind when trying to apply these guides to our patients. Several colleagues have attempted to make this easier and have provided interactive versions of CPGs that are available on websites (e.g., http://www.mdcalc.com/).

Learning and teaching with CATs (see also p. 256)

Now that we have invested precious time and energy into finding and critically appraising an article, it would be a shame not to summarize and keep track of it so that we (and others) can use it again in the future. The means to accomplish this was invented by Stephane Sauve, Hui Lee, and Mike Farkouh, who were residents on Dave Sackett's clinical service several years ago—a standardized one-page summary of the evidence that is organized as a "CAT." A CAT begins with a declarative title and quickly states a clinical "bottom line" describing the clinical action that follows from the paper. To assist later updating of the CAT, the three- or four-part clinical question that started the process, and the search terms that were used to locate the paper are included in it. Next is a summary of the study methods and a table summarizing the key results. Any issues important to bear in mind when applying the CAT (e.g., rare adverse effects, costs, or unusual elements of the critical appraisal) are inserted beneath the results table. Now take a look at the CAT we generated for ferritin.

5

Screening and case finding—proceed with caution!

So far, this chapter has focused on making a diagnosis for sick patients who have come to us for help. They are asking us to diagnose their diseases and to help them to the best of our ability; however, only charlatans would guarantee them longer life at the very first encounter. This final section of the chapter focuses on making early diagnosis of presymptomatic disease among well individuals in the general public (we'll call that "screening") or among patients who have come to us for some other unrelated disorder (we'll call that "case finding"). Individuals whom we might consider for screening and case finding are not ill because of the target disorders, so we are soliciting them with the promise (overt or covert) that they will live longer, or at least better, if they let us test them. Accordingly, the evidence we need about the validity of screening and case finding goes beyond the accuracy of the test for early diagnosis; we need hard evidence that patients are better off, in the long run, when such early diagnosis is achieved.

All screening and case finding, at least in the short run, harms some people. Early diagnosis is just that: People are "labelled" as having, or as being at a high risk for developing, some pretty awful diseases (cancer of the breast, stroke, heart attack, and the like). And this labelling takes place months, years, or even decades before the awful diseases will become manifest as symptomatic illness—and sometimes the symptomatic illness will never occur, which results in so-called overdiagnosis. Labelling hurts. For example, a cohort of working men, who were studied both before and after they were labelled "hypertensive," displayed increased absenteeism, decreased psychological well-being, and progressive loss of income compared with their normotensive workmates (and the side effects of drugs could not be blamed because these bad effects occurred even among men who were never treated!).[13] What's even worse is that those with false-positive results of screening tests will experience only harm (regardless of the efficacy of early treatment). Recently, many countries have seen substantial rises in thyroid cancer detection and incidence, but with no change in the mortality rate—this overdiagnosis resulted from incidentally detected but harmless thyroid abnormalities. But even individuals with true-positive test results who receive efficacious treatment have had "healthy time" taken away from them; early diagnosis may not make folks live longer, but it surely makes all of them "sick" longer!

We've placed this discussion at the end of the chapter on diagnosis on purpose. To decide whether screening and case finding do more good than harm, we'll have to consider the validity of claims about both the accuracy of the early diagnostic test and the efficacy of the therapy that follows it. We've summarized the guides for doing this in Box 5.5. Its elements are discussed in greater detail elsewhere.[14]

1. Is there RCT evidence that early diagnosis really leads to improved survival, quality of life, or both?

Earlier detection will always appear to improve survival. The "lead time"—between screen detection and usual detection (Figure 5.9)—is

---

Box 5.5 Guides for deciding whether a screening or early diagnostic manoeuvre does more good than harm

---

1. Is there randomized controlled trial (RCT) evidence that early diagnosis really leads to improved survival, quality of life, or both?
2. Are the early diagnosed patients willing partners in the treatment strategy?
3. How do benefits and harms compare in different people and with different screening strategies?
4. Do the frequency and severity of the target disorder warrant the degree of effort and expenditure?

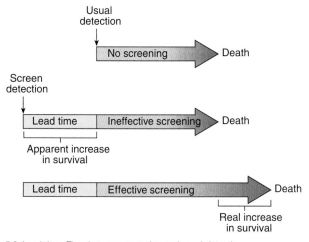

Fig. 5.9 Lead time. Time between screening and usual detection.

---

always added to apparent survival, whether or not there is any real change. This is the first of several problems in evaluating early detection. Follow-up studies of placebo groups in randomized controlled trials (RCTs) have also taught us that patients who faithfully follow health advice (by volunteering for screening or by taking their medicine) are different—and usually destined for better outcomes before they begin. Finally, early diagnostic manoeuvres preferentially identify patients with slower-progressing, more benign diseases. As a result, the only evidence we can trust in determining whether early diagnosis does more good

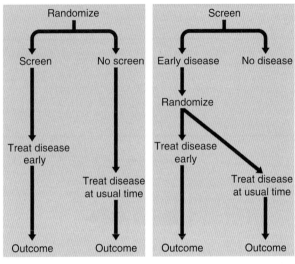

Fig. 5.10 Two structures for randomized trials of the effectiveness of screening.

than harm is a true experiment in which individuals were randomly assigned.

As shown in Figure 5.10, this may be randomization to either (1) undergo the early detection test (and, if truly positive, be treated for the target disorder) or be left alone (and only be treated if and when they developed symptomatic disease) or (2) be screened and then those with positive results be randomized to early treatment or usual care. The latter sort of evidence has been used for showing the benefits (and harms) of detecting raised blood pressure and cholesterol. The former sort of evidence showed the benefit of mammography in women 50 years of age and older for reducing deaths from breast cancer[f] and showed the uselessness (indeed, harm) of chest radiography in lung cancer. Ideally, their follow-up will consider functional and quality-of-life outcomes as well as mortality and discrete clinical events, and we should not be satisfied when the only favourable changes are confined to "risk factors."

---

[f]Because only about a third of women whose breast cancers are diagnosed early go on to prolonged survival, and even in this case, the majority of screenees with positive results are harmed, not helped, by early detection.

2. Are the early diagnosed patients willing partners in the treatment strategy?

Even when therapy is efficacious, patients who refuse or forget to take it cannot benefit from it and are left with only the damage produced by labelling. Early diagnosis will do more harm than good to these patients, and we forget the magnitude of this problem at their peril (even by self-report, only half of patients describe themselves as "compliant"). There are quick ways of diagnosing low compliance (by looking for nonattendance and nonresponsiveness and by nonconfrontational questioning), but this is a diagnosis that you need to establish before, not after, you carry out any screening or case finding.

3. How do benefits and harms compare in different people and with different screening strategies?

4. Do the frequency and severity of the target disorder warrant the degree of effort and expenditure?

These questions raise, at the levels of both our individual practice and our community, the unavoidable issue of rationing. Is going after the early diagnosis of this condition worth sacrificing the other good we could accomplish by devoting our own or our town's resources to some other purpose?

We don't want to sound too gloomy here, and we won't leave this topic without pointing you to places where you can find some of the triumphs of screening and case finding. A good place to start is the Canadian Task Force on the Periodic Health Examination (which has recently been reactivated), where there are some rigorously evaluated screening recommendations.[15]

5

Tips for teaching around diagnostic tests

We usually begin by asking learners why we perform diagnostic tests, and they often respond: "To find out what's wrong with the patient [dummy!]." This approach provides an opening for helping them to recognize that diagnosis is not about finding the absolute truth but about limiting uncertainty, and it establishes both the necessity and the logical base for introducing probabilities, pragmatic test–treatment thresholds, and the like. It's also a time to get them to start thinking about what

Continued

Tips for teaching around diagnostic tests—continued

they're going to do with the results of the diagnostic test and about whether doing the test will really help their patient (maybe they'll conclude that the test isn't necessary!). A useful sequence is to elicit some disagreement between students, for example, about a measurement or sign (but don't step in and suggest the "right" answer). The elicited disagreement can be used as an opening to unreliability and uncertainty. Comparison with a "gold standard" can introduce issues of validity. Although the formal calculations can be difficult, the qualitative ideas of SpPin and SnNout then can be introduced to get students thinking about the accuracy and utility of a test.

When teaching about early diagnosis, we often challenge our learners with the statement: "Even when therapy is worthless, early diagnosis always improves survival!" and then help them recognize the distortions that arise from drawing conclusions about volunteers, from initiating survival measurements unfairly early in screened patients, and from failing to recognize that early detection tests preferentially identify slowly—rather than rapidly—progressive disease. Once they've grasped those ideas, we think they're safe from the evangelists of early diagnosis.

References

1. Croskerry P. A universal model of diagnostic reasoning. Acad Med 2009;84:1022–8.

2. Moulton C, Regehr G, Mylopoulos M, MacRae MH. Slowing down when you should: A new model of expert judgement. Acad Med 2007;82(10 Suppl.):S109–16.

3. Richardson WS. We should overcome the barriers to evidence-based clinical diagnosis. J Clin Epidemiol 2007;60(3):217–27.

4. Heneghan C, Glasziou P, Thompson M, et al. Diagnostic strategies used in primary care. BMJ 2009;338:b946. doi:10.1136/bmj.b946.

5. Patterson C, Guyatt GH, Singer J, Ali M, Turpie I. Iron deficiency in the elderly: the diagnostic process. Can Med Assoc J 1991;144:435–40.

6. Fleming KA. Evidence-based pathology. Evid Based Med 1997;2:132.

7. Guyatt GH, Oxman AD, Ali M, et al. Laboratory diagnosis of iron deficiency anemia: an overview. J Gen Intern Med 1992;7:45–53.

8. Richardson WS, Wilson M, McGinn T. Differential diagnosis. In: Guyatt G, Rennie D, Meade M, Cook DJ, editors. Users' guides to the

medical literature. A manual for evidence-based clinical practice, 3rd ed. New York: JAMA Evidence/McGraw Hill; 2015.

9. Bachmann LM, Kolb E, Koller MT, Steurer J, ter Riet G. Accuracy of Ottawa ankle rules to exclude fractures of the ankle and mid-foot: systematic review. BMJ 2003;326:417.

10. Whited JD, Grichnik JM. The rational clinical examination. Does this patient have a mole or a melanoma? JAMA 1998;279:696–701.

11. Goodacre S, Sutton AJ, Sampson FC. Meta-analysis: the value of clinical assessment in the diagnosis of deep venous thrombosis. Ann Intern Med 2005;143:129–39.

12. Shah KH, Metz HA, Edlow JA. Clinical prediction rules to stratify short-term risk of stroke among patients diagnosed in the emergency department with a transient ischemic attack. Ann Emerg Med 2009; 53:662–73.

13. Macdonald LA, Sackett DL, Haynes RB, Taylor DW. Labelling in hypertension: a review of the behavioural and psychological consequences. J Chronic Dis 1984;37(12):933–42.

14. Barratt A, Irwig L, Glasziou P, Cumming RG, Raffle A, Hicks N, et al. Users' guides to the medical literature: XVII. How to use guidelines and recommendations about screening. Evidence-Based Medicine Working Group. JAMA 1999;281(21):2029–34.

15. Canadian Task Force on the Periodic Health Examination. The periodic health examination. Can Med Assn J 1979;121:1193–254.

5

Further reading

Guyatt G, Rennie D, Meade M, Cook DJ, editors. Users' guides to the medical literature. A manual for evidence-based clinical practice. 3rd ed. Chicago, IL: AMA Press; 2015.

Haynes RB, Sackett DL, Guyatt GH, Tugwell P. Clinical epidemiology: how to do clinical practice research. Philadelphia, PA: Lippincott Williams & Wilkins; 2006.

McGee S. Evidence-based physical diagnosis. 4th ed. St. Louis, MO: Elsevier Saunders; 2017.

McGinn T, Randolph A, Richardson S, Sackett D. Clinical prediction guides. Evid Based Med 1998;3:5–6.

6 Prognosis

Whether posed by our patients, their families, colleagues, or ourselves, we frequently need to consider questions about prognosis. For example, a patient newly diagnosed with Alzheimer dementia might ask, "What's going to happen to me?" Or a patient with a left-sided stroke might ask, "Will I regain function of my arm?" As clinicians, we might consider, "What is the prognosis in this patient with metastatic lung cancer?" or "What is the risk of stroke in a patient with nonvalvular atrial fibrillation?" Prognosis refers to determining the possible outcomes from a target disorder and the probability that they occur over a period.

To answer these questions and to make judgements about when to start and stop treatment, we need to evaluate evidence about prognosis for its validity, importance, and relevance to our patients. The guides in Box 6.1 will help us tackle these issues. We'll consider the following clinical scenario to illustrate our discussion.

> We see a 78-year-old woman recently diagnosed with dementia, most likely Alzheimer dementia; she has no neuropsychiatric symptoms currently. She comes to this appointment with her daughter who wants information on the progression of the disease and whether it will increase her mother's risk of death. Her mother has named her as her decision maker for personal care and finances. Her daughter wants to start planning for her mother's future care as she has been living alone.

6

In response to this scenario, we posed the question, "In a 78-year-old woman with newly diagnosed dementia, what is the risk of death and what prognostic factors influence progression of the disease?" We did a quick search of OVID EBM Reviews (see Fig. 7.1) using the search terms "prognosis" and "dementia" but didn't identify any systematic reviews relevant to this question. We did identify an article from the *ACP Journal Club* that was published in 2009; this article also has a companion report with additional methods details.[1-3] In an attempt to find a more recent article, we searched Evidence Updates (https://plus .mcmaster.ca/evidenceupdates/QuickSearch.aspx?Page=1#Data) using the same search terms and found an article from 2015 that might address

---

Box 6.1 Is this evidence about prognosis valid?

---

1. Was a defined, representative sample of patients assembled at a common point in the course of their disease?
2. Was follow-up of study patients sufficiently long and complete?
3. Were objective outcome criteria applied in a "blind" fashion?
4. If subgroups with different prognoses are identified:
   - Was there adjustment for important prognostic factors?
   - Was there validation in an independent group of "test-set" patients?

---

our question.[4] The article is freely accessible from PubMed Central (http://www.ncbi.nlm.nih.gov/pmc/articles/PMC4416978/). We also identified a companion article that reported the study's methods in detail;[5] this article is also freely available via PubMed Central (http://www.ncbi.nlm.nih.gov/pmc/articles/PMC3101372/).

Types of reports on prognosis

Several types of studies can provide information on the prognosis of a group of individuals with a defined problem or risk factor. The best evidence with which to answer our clinical question would come from a systematic review of prognosis studies. A systematic review that searches for and combines all relevant prognosis studies would be particularly useful for retrieving information about relevant patient subgroups. When assessing the validity of a systematic review, we'd need to consider the guides in Box 6.1 as well as those in Box 4.6. For details on appraising systematic reviews, please refer to the etiology chapter; in this current chapter, we'll focus the discussion on individual studies of prognosis.

Cohort studies (in which investigators follow one or more groups of individuals with the target disorder over time and monitor for occurrence of the outcome of interest) represent the best study design for answering prognosis questions. Randomized trials can also serve as a source of prognostic information (particularly because they usually include detailed documentation of baseline data), although trial participants may not be representative of the population with a disorder. The patients in the intervention arm can provide us with prognosis information for patients who receive treatment, whereas patients in the control arm can provide an estimate of prognosis for patients who don't receive the intervention. Case-control studies (in which investigators retrospectively determine prognostic factors by defining the exposures of cases who have already suffered the outcome of interest and controls that have not) are particularly useful when the outcome is rare or the required follow-up is long. However, the strength of inference that can be drawn from these studies is limited because of the potential for selection and measurement bias as discussed on the etiology chapter.

Determining prognosis rarely relies on a single sign, symptom, or laboratory test. Occasionally, when completing our literature search, we find articles describing tools that quantify the contributions that the clinical examination and the laboratory and radiologic investigations make in establishing a diagnosis or a prognosis for a patient. These tools that combine diagnostic and prognostic information are called clinical prediction guides and are discussed on page 176.

Are the results of this prognosis study valid?

1. Was a defined, representative sample of patients assembled at a common point in the course of their disease?

Ideally, the prognosis study we find would include the entire population of patients who ever lived who developed the disease, studied from the instant the disorder developed. Unfortunately, this is impossible and we'll have to determine how close the report we've found is to the ideal with respect to how the target disorder was defined and how participants were assembled. If the study sample fully reflects the spectrum of illness we find in our own practice (or reflecting the spectrum that is relevant to our PICO [population/intervention/comparison/outcome), we are reassured. However, considering our clinical scenario, if the study that we found included only patients from a behavioural neurology unit that specialized in care for patients with dementia and agitation, we might not be satisfied that the sample is representative of the patients that we're interested in. These patients would have passed through a filter or referral process (and likely have more severe disease) and thus don't reflect patients similar to our clinical scenario. The study should also describe standardized criteria that were used to diagnose the target disorder. In particular, we want to make sure that all patients in the cohort were diagnosed using the same, validated approach.

But from what point in the disease should patients be followed up? Consider the prognosis of an acute infectious illness; if investigators begin tracking outcomes in patients only after the course of the disease has been finished, then the outcomes for these patients might never be counted. Some patients would have recovered quickly, whereas others might have died quickly. So, to avoid missing outcomes by "starting the clock" too late, we look to see that study patients were included at a uniformly early point in the disease, ideally when it first becomes clinically manifest; this is called an "inception cohort." A study that assembled patients at any defined, common point in their disease may provide useful information if we want information only about that stage of the disease. For example, we may want to understand the prognosis of patients with metastatic lung cancer, or we may want information on the prognosis of patients with severe dementia. However, if observations were made at different points in the course of disease for various people in the cohort, the relative timing of outcome events would be difficult to interpret. For example, it would be difficult to interpret the results from a study designed to determine the prognosis of patients with rheumatoid arthritis that included patients with newly diagnosed disease as well as those who had the disease for 10 years or more. Similarly, it would be difficult to determine the prognosis of dementia in patients followed at a dementia clinic because these patients would likely be at different points in their illness. We need to look for and find a study in which participants are all at a similar stage in the course of the same disease.

We will appraise both the more recent article we identified[4,5] and the one from the *ACP Journal Club*[1-3] to compare and contrast them. Information about the study type and sampling method is usually found in the "abstract" and "methods" sections of the article.

From the more recent article, we can see that this is a cohort study of people diagnosed with possible/probable Alzheimer dementia. We need to review the methods of the 2011 and 2015 articles to identify that this is an inception cohort; note that this is a growing challenge in the clinical literature whereby readers have to find companion articles (often published in different journals) to identify all of the methods (and results), details that are needed for assessing validity and clinical decision making.

All permanent residents of Cache County, Utah, who were 65 years and older were invited to participate in the study. Participants were assessed in three incidence waves that were 3 years apart. Some patients may have been missed if they died rapidly after dementia onset because they were assessed in 3-year waves. Those patients who were lost to follow-up had a higher mortality rate. A multistage case identification process was used to diagnose dementia starting with screening using the Modified Mini-Mental State Exam. Those who had positive results in the screening were assessed via a telephone interview, and then those who had possible dementia underwent a structured examination, including neuropsychological tests administered by a trained research nurse and psychometric technician. A geriatric psychiatrist and neuropsychologist reviewed the data and made a diagnosis using the *Diagnostic and Statistical Manual of Mental Disorders*, revised 3rd edition (DSM-III-R) criteria. A geriatric psychiatrist also assessed the patient. A panel of experts reviewed all data and made a diagnosis using NINCDS-ADRDA (Neurological and Communicative Disorders and Stroke and the Alzheimer's Disease and Related Disorders Association) criteria.

From the *ACP Journal Club* abstract, we can quickly see that this study is an inception cohort, including patients with dementia diagnosed by a geriatric mental state examination algorithm. Patients from a population cohort that included those from home and inpatient settings were interviewed every 2 years to diagnose dementia. Similar to the above study, some patients may have been missed if they died rapidly after dementia onset because they were interviewed every 2 years. Those patients who were lost to follow-up or dropped out from the population cohort had higher mortality, and these would have been missed from the inception cohort.

2. Was the follow-up of the study patients sufficiently long and complete?

Ideally, every patient in the cohort would be followed until they fully recover or develop one of the other disease outcomes. If follow-up is short, it may be that too few patients develop the outcome of interest, and, therefore, we wouldn't have enough information to help us when advising our patients; in this case we'd better look for other evidence. For example, in our studies of the prognosis for patients with dementia, follow-up for only 1 month in patients who are newly diagnosed would not be helpful, given the chronic, insidious nature of the disease. In contrast, if after years of follow-up, only a few adverse events (e.g., progression to severe dementia or admission to long-term care) have occurred, this good prognostic result is very useful in reassuring our patients about their future.

The more patients who are unavailable for follow-up, the less accurate the estimate of the risk of the outcome will be. The reasons for their loss are crucial. Some losses to follow-up are both unavoidable and mostly unrelated to prognosis (e.g., moving away to a different job), and these are not a cause for worry, especially if their numbers are small. But other losses might arise because patients die or are too ill to continue follow-up (or lose their independence and move in with family), and

6

the failure to document and report their outcomes will reduce the validity of any conclusion the report draws about their prognosis.

Short of finding a report that kept track of every patient, how can we judge whether follow-up is "sufficiently complete"? There is no single answer for all studies, but we offer some suggestions that may help. An analysis showing that the baseline demographics of these patients who were lost to follow-up are similar to those followed up provides some reassurance that certain types of participants were not selectively lost, but such an analysis is limited by those characteristics that were measured at baseline. Investigators cannot control for unmeasured traits that may be important prognostically and that may have been more or less prevalent in the lost participants than in the participants who were followed.

We suggest considering the simple "5 and 20" rule: Fewer than 5% loss probably leads to little bias, greater than 20% loss seriously threatens validity, and in-between amounts cause intermediate amounts of trouble. Although this may be easy to remember, it may oversimplify clinical situations in which the outcomes are infrequent. Alternatively, we could consider the "best" and "worst" case scenarios in an approach that we'll call a *sensitivity analysis* (with apologies to statisticians for using this term here!). Imagine a study of prognosis in which 100 patients enter the study, four die, and 16 are lost to follow-up. A "crude" case-fatality rate would count the four deaths among the 84 with full follow-up, calculated as $4/84 \equiv 4.8\%$. But what about the 16 who are lost? Some or all of them might have died, too. In a "worst case" scenario, all would have died, giving a case-fatality rate of (4 known + 16 lost) $\equiv$ 20 out of (84 followed + 16 lost) $\equiv$ 100, or 20/100, that is, 20%—four times the original rate that we calculated! Note that for the "worst case" scenario, we've added the lost patients to both the numerator and the denominator of the outcome rate. However, in the "best case" scenario, none of the lost 16 would have died, yielding a case-fatality rate of 4 out of (84 followed + 16 lost), or 4/100, that is, 4%. Note that for the "best case" scenario, we've added the missing cases to just the denominator. Although this "best case" of 4% may not differ much from the observed 4.8%, the "worst case" of 20% does differ meaningfully, and we'd probably judge that this study's follow-up was not sufficiently complete and that it threatens the validity of the study. By using this simple sensitivity analysis, we can see what effect losses to follow-up might have on study results, which can help us judge whether the follow-up was sufficient to yield valid results. The larger the number of patients whose fate is unknown relative to the number who have the outcome, the more substantial the threat to validity.

In the more recent cohort study that we found, of 328 patients, 112 patients lacked follow-up data, and the reason for most of the missing data was death (n = 88). These individuals who died were older and scored lower on the initial Mini-Mental State Exam (MMSE) compared with those who were followed up, indicating they may have had more severe disease. Of the patients who survived, 93% had follow-up data on cognition and function. Given that our primary outcome of interest was risk of death, this article will still be informative; however, the information on progression of the disease will be more limited.

In the *ACP Journal Club* study that we found, all patients in the inception cohort were followed up to study completion.

3. Were objective outcome criteria applied in a blind fashion?

Diseases affect patients in many important ways; some are easy to spot, and some are more subtle. In general, outcomes at both extremes—death or full recovery—are relatively easy to detect with validity, but assigning a cause of death is often subjective (as anyone who has completed a death certificate knows!). Review of death certificates often finds cardiac arrest recorded as the cause of death—but is the death caused by pneumonia, pulmonary embolism, or something else? In-between these extremes is a wide range of outcomes that can be more difficult to detect or confirm, and where investigators will have to use judgement in deciding how to count them (e.g., readiness for return to work, or the intensity of residual pain). To minimize the effects of bias in measuring these outcomes, investigators should have established specific, standardized criteria to define each important outcome and then used them throughout patient follow-up. We'd also want to satisfy ourselves that they are sufficiently objective for confirming the outcomes we're interested in. The occurrence of death is objective, but judging the underlying cause of death is prone to error (especially as noted above when it's based on death certificates) and can be biased unless objective criteria are applied to carefully gathered clinical information. But even with objective criteria, some bias might creep in if the investigators judging the outcomes also know about the patients' prior characteristics. Blinding is crucial if any judgement is required to assess the outcome because unblinded investigators may search more aggressively for outcomes in people with the characteristic(s) felt to be of prognostic importance than in other individuals. In valid studies, investigators making judgements about clinical outcomes are kept "blind" to these patients' clinical characteristics and prognostic factors.

6

In the more recent dementia study, there are no details provided on how death was identified in the cohort. When looking at dementia severity (i.e., disease progression), the Clinical Dementia Rating was used; health status was assessed using the General Medical Health Rating. Both of these were scored by a trained research nurse at each visit; the nurse was trained by a geriatric psychiatrist. Blinding of the research nurse wasn't possible.

In the older dementia study, the authors looked at death but details of how death was determined need to be obtained from another study.[3] Participants were flagged on the Office of National Statistics NHS Central Register resulting in automatic notification of death. The need to track down this other paper highlights the challenge mentioned above for the readers of clinical literature. With encouragement of authors to publish study protocols (often separately from the results) additional study details can be obtained. However, for the busy clinician this may mean reading two or three articles to find all of the relevant information that is needed for validity assessment. The *ACP Journal Club* abstract provides some of these details, but it doesn't provide details on how mortality was determined in the current study.

4. If subgroups with different prognoses are identified, was there adjustment for important prognostic factors and validation in an independent group of "test set" patients?

Prognostic factors are demographic (e.g., age, gender), disease specific (e.g., severity of dementia at diagnosis, presence of neuropsychiatric symptoms at diagnosis), or comorbid (e.g., cardiovascular disease) variables that are associated with the outcome of interest. Prognostic factors need not be causal—and they are often not—but they must be strongly associated with the development of an outcome to predict its occurrence. For example, although mild hyponatremia does not cause death, serum sodium is an important prognostic marker in congestive heart failure (individuals with congestive heart failure and hyponatremia have higher mortality rates compared with patients who have heart failure but have normal serum sodium).[6]

Risk factors are often considered distinct from prognostic factors and include lifestyle behaviours and environmental exposures that are associated with the development of a target disorder. For example, smoking is an important risk factor for developing lung cancer, but tumour stage is the most important prognostic factor in individuals who have lung cancer.

Often, we want to know whether subgroups of patients have different prognoses (e.g., among patients with Alzheimer dementia, are older women at increased risk of faster progression or death compared with older men?). If a study reports that one group of patients had a different prognosis than another, first, we need to see if there was any adjustment for known prognostic factors. By this we mean, did the authors make sure that these subgroup predictions are not being distorted by the unequal occurrence of another, powerful prognostic factor (e.g., would it occur if women had more severe disease or had more serious cardio-vascular disease compared with men). There are both simple (e.g., stratified analyses displaying the prognoses of patients with dementia separately for men and women and for those with and without a prior cardiac event) and fancy ways (e.g., multiple regression analyses that can take into account not only prior cardiac event but also severity of disease) of adjusting for these other important prognostic factors. We can examine the methods and results sections to reassure ourselves that one of these methods has been applied before we tentatively accept the conclusion about a different prognosis for the subgroup of interest. In the dementia studies that we found, presence of comorbid disease could influence mortality. Similarly, comorbid diseases could influence functional status. Are functional status and the presence of comorbid diseases both factors that increase the risk of death in patients with dementia?

We must remember that the statistics of determining subgroup prognoses are about prediction, not explanation. They are indifferent to whether the prognostic factor is physiologically logical or a biologically nonsensical and random, noncausal quirk in the data (whether the patient lives on the north side or the south side of the street or was born under a certain astrological sign). For this reason, the first time a prognostic factor is identified, there is no guarantee that it really does predict subgroups of patients with different prognoses—it could be the result of a chance difference in its distribution between patients with different prognoses. Indeed, if investigators were to search for multiple potential prognostic factors in the same data set, a few would emerge on the basis of chance alone. The initial patient group in which prognostic factors are found is termed a "training set" or "derivation set." Because of the risk of spurious, chance identification of prognostic factors, we should look to see whether the predictive power of such factors has been confirmed in subsequent, independent groups of patients, termed "test sets" or "validation sets." To see if this was done, we'd look for a statement in the study's "methods" section describing a prestudy intention to examine this specific group of prognostic factors, based

6

on their appearance in a training set or previous study. If a second, independent study validates the predictive power of prognostic factors, we have a very useful "clinical prediction guide" (CPG) of the sort that we met earlier in this section and were discussed fully on page 176, but this time predicting our patient's outcome after he or she is diagnosed.

Blinding is also important when considering prognostic factors. If the person assessing the prognostic factor is aware that the patient had the outcome of interest, would he or she look harder for the potential prognostic factor?

In the more recent dementia study that we identified, the Global Medical Health Rating was associated with time to death; those patients with poor/fair scores had 1.6 times the risk of death compared with those with good/excellent scores. Unadjusted analyses showed that patients with some neuropsychiatric symptoms (e.g., psychosis) and those with clinically significant neuropsychiatric symptoms had an increased risk of death compared with those with milder or no symptoms. The investigators adjusted for age of disease onset, and gender, among other potential prognostic factors and found similar results. Use of cognitive enhancers did not significantly affect rate of decline in cognition; no details on mortality impact were provided. No consistent prognostic factors were found across MMSE, neuropsychiatric symptoms, or dementia severity. With regard to disease progression, women declined in cognition more rapidly than men and patients who were diagnosed at a younger age declined faster than those diagnosed at an older age. These latter factors would be important to be explored in other cohort studies to see if they can be validated.

In the *ACP Journal Club* study, multivariate analysis showed functional impairment and older age were associated with higher risk for mortality, and men had a higher risk for mortality compared with women. Investigators did not mention potential prognostic factors, such as the presence of comorbid conditions, different types of dementia, or the effect of cognitive enhancers. This latter issue is a weakness of this study given the growing proportion of patients with Alzheimer dementia who are prescribed these medications.

If the evidence about prognosis appears valid after considering the above guides, we can turn to examining its importance and applicability. But if we answered no to the questions above, we'd be better off searching for other evidence. For the studies we found, although we identified some concerns, we believe that they are sufficiently valid to allow us to proceed. We should also note that sometimes we are left with evidence that might be at high risk of bias but is the best that we have available, and some evidence is better than no evidence to guide clinical decision making.

Is this valid evidence about prognosis important? (Box 6.2)

1. How likely are the outcomes over time?

Once we're satisfied that an article's conclusions are valid, we can examine it further to see how likely each outcome is over time. Typically results from prognosis studies are reported in one of three ways: (1) as a percentage of survival at a particular point in time (e.g., 1-year or 5-year survival rates); (2) as median survival (the length of follow-up by which 50% of study patients have died); or (3) as survival curves that depict, at each point in time, the proportion (expressed as a percentage) of the original study sample who have *not* yet had a specified outcome. In prognosis studies, we often find results presented as Kaplan-Meier curves, which are a type of survival curve. For more information about Kaplan-Meier curves, we suggest you refer to a recent article and tutorial in the *BMJ* (http://www.bmj.com/content/347/bmj.f7118 and http://www.bmj.com/about-bmj/resources-readers/publications/statistics-square-one/12-survival-analysis).

Fig. 6.1 shows four survival curves, each leading to a different conclusion. In Fig. 6.1A, virtually no patients had events by the end of the study, which could mean that either prognosis is very good for this target disorder (in which case the study is very useful to us) or the study is too short (in which case this study isn't very helpful). In panels B, C, and D, the proportion of patients surviving to 1 year (20%) is the same in all three graphs. We could tell our patients that their chances of surviving for a year are 20%. However, the median survival (point at which half will have died) is very different—3 months for panel B, versus 9 months for the disorder in panel C. The survival pattern is a steady, uniform decline in panel D, and the median survival in this panel is approximately 7.5 months. These examples highlight the importance of considering median survival and survival curves to fully inform our patient about prognosis.

> **Box 6.2** Is this valid evidence about prognosis important?
>
> 1. How likely are the outcomes over time?
> 2. How precise are the prognostic estimates?

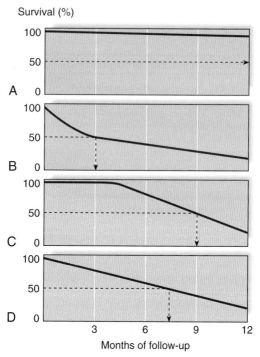

Survival (%)

Fig. 6.1 Prognosis shown as survival curves. **A,** Good prognosis (or too short a study!). **B,** Poor prognosis early, then slower increase in mortality, median survival of 3 months. **C,** Good prognosis early, then worsening, with median survival of 9 months. **D,** Steady prognosis.

2. How precise are the prognostic estimates?

As we pointed out earlier in this chapter, investigators study prognosis in a sample of diseased patients, not the whole population of everyone who has ever had the disease. Thus, purely by chance, a study repeated 100 times among different groups of patients (even with identical entry characteristics) is bound to generate different estimates of prognosis. In deciding whether a given set of prognostic results is important, we need some means of judging just how much the results could vary by chance alone. The confidence interval (CI) provides the range of values that are likely to include the true estimate and quantifies the uncertainty in measurement. By convention, the 95% CI is used and it represents the range of values within which we can be 95% sure that the population value lies. The narrower the CI, the more assured we can feel about the result. Note that if survival over time is the outcome of interest, earlier follow-up periods usually include results from more patients than later periods, so that survival curves are more precise (they provide narrower confidence intervals) earlier in the follow-up. The text, tables, or graphs of a good prognostic study include the CIs for its estimates of prognosis. If they don't, the calculators available at http://ktclearinghouse.ca/cebm/toolbox/statscalc can do this calculation for you.

In our more recent dementia study, the median time from diagnosis to death was 5.7 years (95% CI 5.4–6.1); survival estimates for women versus men were not provided. The median time to severe dementia was 8.4 years (95% CI 7.6–9.2).

From the *ACP Journal Club* study, we found that age, male gender (hazard ratio 1.4), and functional impairment (2.1 [95% CI 1.6–3.3]) were predictors of mortality. Education, social class, and self-reported health didn't predict mortality. Median survival of female patients aged 70 to 79 years was 5.8 years (95% CI 3.6–8.3).

Can we apply this valid, important evidence about prognosis to our patient? (Box 6.3)

1. Is our patient so different from those in the study that its results cannot apply?

This guide asks us to compare our patients with those in the article, using descriptions of the study sample's demographic and clinical characteristics. Inevitably, some differences will turn up, so how similar is similar enough? We recommend framing the question another way: Are the study patients so different from ours that we should not use the

---

Box 6.3 Can we apply this valid, important evidence about prognosis to our patient?

---

1. Is our patient so different from those in the study that its results cannot apply?
2. Will this evidence make a clinically important impact on our conclusions about what to offer or tell our patient?

results at all in making predictions for our patients? For most differences, the answer to this question is no, and thus, we can use the study results to inform our prognostic conclusions.

2. Will this evidence make a clinically important impact on our conclusions about what to offer or tell our patient?

Evidence regarding a person's prognosis is clearly useful for deciding whether or not to initiate therapy, for monitoring therapy that has been initiated, and for deciding which diagnostic tests to order. If, for example, the study suggests an excellent prognosis for patients with a particular target disorder who didn't receive treatment, our discussions with patients would reflect these facts and would focus on whether any treatment should be started. If, however, the evidence suggests that the prognosis is poor without treatment (and if there are treatments that can make a meaningful difference), then our conversations with patients would reflect these facts and more likely lead us to treatment. Even when the prognostic evidence does not lead to a treat/don't treat decision, valid evidence can be useful in providing patients and families with the information they want about what the future is likely to hold for them and their illness.

The patients in the more recent study are from a single setting in Utah; this county was selected because its inhabitants are known for their longevity. And, this population is 99% Caucasian, with a mean of 13.2 (standard deviation [SD] 3.0) years of education. Our patient is Caucasian and was recently diagnosed with dementia, like those in this study. However, she had a grade 8 education, and this may impact her risk of progression. Her functional status is good, and she is able to do most of her activities of daily living. She has no neuropsychiatric symptoms currently.

The patients in this *ACP Journal Club* study are similar to our patient.

Based on the results of both studies, we can provide an estimate of median survival to be approximately 5.5 years for our patient. It is reassuring that both studies showed similar results.

Practising evidence-based medicine in real time

Sometimes, we can't find the answers to our questions in high-quality, preappraised evidence resources and we must appraise the primary literature ourselves, such as with the more recent dementia study we discussed in this chapter. After we've done this, it's useful to keep a copy of the appraisal in case the same question arises again. We developed an app that allows us to quickly record our question, the main study details, the results and any comments/concerns about the study. We can save this as a "Word" file for our computer or smartphone. Using this tool, we can develop our own database of topics that we encounter in our own practice. We've provided this clinical question (CQ) log at http://ktclearinghouse.ca/cebm/toolbox/cqlogbook; you can use it to log your CQs and the answers to those you've managed to track down. However, keep in mind that these should have an expiry date on them! If we have colleagues close by, we can even share the work and collaborate on these.

References

1. Age, sex and functional impairment predicted risk for mortality in incident dementia at 14 year follow-up. ACP J Club 2008;149(1):13.

2. Xie J, Brayne C, Matthews FE, and the MRC Cognitive Function and Ageing Study Collaborators. BMJ 2008;336:258–62.

3. Neale R, Brayne C, Johnson AL. Cognition and survival: an exploration in a large multicentre study of the population aged 65 years and over. Int J Epidemiol 2001;30:1383–8.

4. Peters ME, Schwartz S, Han D, et al. Neuropsychiatric symptoms as predictors of progression to severe Alzheimer's dementia and death: The Cache County Dementia Progression Study. Am J Psychiatry 2015; 172:460–5.

5. Tschanz JT, Corcora CD, Schwartz S, et al. Progression of cognitive, functional and neuropsychiatric symptom domains in a population cohort with Alzheimer's dementia: The Cache County Dementia Progression Study. Am J Geriatr Psych 2011;19:532–42.

6. Mettauer B, Rouleau JL, Bichet D, et al. Sodium and water excretion abnormalities in congestive heart failure: determinant factors and clinical implications. Ann Intern Med 1986;105:161–7.

6

Further reading

Guyatt G, Rennie D, Meade M, Cook DJ, editors. Users' guides to the medical literature. A manual for evidence-based clinical practice. 3rd ed. Chicago, IL: AMA Press; 2015.

Haynes RB, Sackett DL, Guyatt G, Tugwell P. Clinical epidemiology: how to do clinical practice research. Philadelphia, PA: Lippincott Williams & Wilkins; 2006.

7 Harm

The media constantly bombard us with concerns about potentially harmful interventions, leading to questions by us and our patients, such as "Does living close to hydroelectric power lines or wind mills increase the risk of cancer?," "Do statins cause cancer or dementia?," and "Does the MMR (measles–mumps–rubella) vaccine cause autism?" Along with our patients, we often need to make judgements about whether these medical interventions and environmental agents could be harmful.

To make these judgements, we need to be able to evaluate evidence about causation for its validity, importance, and relevance to our patients. Assessing the validity of the evidence is crucial if we are to avoid drawing the false-positive conclusion that an agent does cause an adverse event when, in truth, it does not or the false-negative conclusion that an agent does not cause an adverse event when, in truth, it does. Clinical disagreements about whether a patient has had an adverse drug reaction are not uncommon—and just because an adverse event occurred during treatment, it does not inevitably follow that the adverse event occurred because of that treatment.

The guides in Box 7.1 can help us to appraise the validity of an article about a putative harmful agent. We'll consider the following clinical scenario to illustrate our discussion.

Clinical scenario

A 31-year-old woman with a 15-year history of epilepsy (treated with valproic acid) is considering pregnancy. She saw a news item about the association between valproic acid use by pregnant women and autism in their children. She wants to know if this risk is true and whether she should continue with valproic acid or change to another agent.

In response to this scenario, we posed the question, "In a pregnant woman with epilepsy, is use of valproic acid associated with an increased risk of autism in her children?" Using OVID EBM Reviews and the terms "autism" and "antiepileptics," we found a systematic review (SR) and a single study that look of interest (Fig. 7.1).[1-3] The SR is limited to randomized trials on the use of antiepileptics, and knowing that observational

Box 7.1 Is this evidence about harm valid?

1. Were there clearly defined groups of patients, similar in all important ways other than exposure to the treatment or other cause?
2. Were treatments/exposures and clinical outcomes measured in the same ways in both groups? (Was the assessment of outcomes either objective or blinded to exposure?)
3. Was the follow-up of the study patients sufficiently long (for the outcome to occur in a large enough number of patients) and complete (so that no or very few patients were lost to follow-up)?
4. Do the results of the harm study fulfill some of the diagnostic tests for causation?
   - Is it clear that the exposure preceded the onset of the outcome?
   - Is there a dose–response gradient?
   - Is there any positive evidence from a "dechallenge–rechallenge" study?
   - Is the association consistent from study to study?
   - Does the association make biological sense?

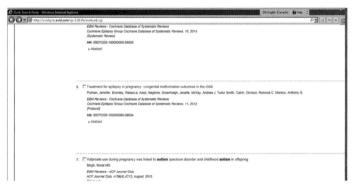

Fig. 7.1 Screenshot from OVID showing results of our search. © Wolters Kluwer, with permission.

study designs would provide important information on the risk of adverse events with these agents, we decide to focus on the single study, which was selected for inclusion in the *ACP Journal Club*.[2,3]

Types of reports on harm/etiology

As we discovered on pages in Chapter 2, ideally, the best evidence that we can find about the effects of therapy (and putative harmful agents) comes from SRs. Individual randomized trials are seldom large enough to detect rare adverse events with precision or have sufficient follow-up duration—emphasizing the need to search for an SR.[4] An SR that combines all relevant randomized trials or cohort studies might provide us with sufficiently large numbers of patients to detect even rare adverse events. When assessing the validity of such an SR, we need to consider the guides in Box 7.1 as well as those in Box 4.6. The discussion in this chapter will focus on randomized trials, cohort studies, case-control studies, and cross-sectional studies.

Are the results of this harm/etiology study valid?

1. Were there clearly defined groups of patients, similar in all important ways other than exposure to the treatment or other cause?

Ideally, our search would yield an SR or a randomized trial in which pregnant women with epilepsy had been allocated, by a system analogous to tossing a coin, to valproic acid (the top row in Table 7.1, whose total is a + b), or some comparison intervention (i.e., another antiepileptic agent; the middle row in Table 7.1, whose total is c + d), and then their offspring are followed up over time for the diagnosis of autism. Randomization would tend to make the two treatment groups identical for all other causes of autism (and we'd look for baseline differences in other putative causal agents between the groups), so we'd likely consider any statistically significant increase in autism (adjusted for any important baseline differences) in the intervention group to be valid. Randomized controlled trials (RCTs), however, are ill-suited (in size, duration, and ethics) for evaluating most harmful exposures, and we often have to

7

Table 7.1 Studies of whether valproic acid exposure causes autism

	Adverse outcome		
	Present (Case)	Absent (Controls)	Totals
Exposed to treatment (randomized controlled trial [RCT] or cohort)	a	b	a + b
Not exposed to treatment (RCT or cohort)	c	d	c + d
Totals	a + c	b + d	a + b + c + d

make do with evidence from other types of studies.[a] For example, we may have to follow up participants for years to monitor development of outcomes, which is costly. Returning to the questions posed at the beginning of this chapter, it would be impossible to randomize families to live in a house either close to or at a distance from power lines to determine the impact on cancer development! Unfortunately, the validity of the study designs used to detect harm is inversely proportional to their feasibility.

In the first of these alternatives, a cohort study, a group of participants who are exposed (a + b) to the treatment (or putative harmful agent) and a group or participants who aren't exposed (c + d) to it are followed up for the development of the outcome of interest (a or c). Returning to our example, a cohort study would include a group of children of mothers who used valproic acid while pregnant and a group of children without this exposure, and then the risk of autism would be determined in each. As we discussed on pages in Chapter 6 in observational studies such as cohort studies, the decision to prescribe and accept exposure is based on the patient's and/or physician's preferences, and it is not randomized. As a result, "exposed" patients may differ from "nonexposed" patients in important determinants of the outcome (such determinants are called *confounders*).[b] For example, other maternal factors may be associated with increased risk of autism; in the paper that we identified, more children with maternal exposure to valproic acid also had a parental history of a psychiatric diagnosis compared with children without maternal exposure to valproic acid; a parental psychiatric diagnosis has been associated with autism in children in other studies, and therefore, it is a potential confounder. Investigators must document the characteristics of both cohorts of patients and either demonstrate their comparability or adjust for the confounders they identify (using, for example, statistical techniques, such as multivariable analysis). Of course, adjustments can only be made for confounders that are already known and have been measured, so we have to be careful when interpreting cohort

---

[a]There are many examples of misleading observational studies whose results were found to be proved wrong when these ideas were tested in randomized trials. Consider the data from observational studies that showed the benefits of hormone replacement therapy (HRT) in women, particularly a decreased risk of cardiovascular mortality. It was only when the Women's Health Initiative was completed that we had cause for concern that we were, in fact, *increasing* the risk of cardiovascular mortality with HRT!! Similarly, we were misled by the observational studies on antioxidants and cardiovascular disease.
[b]Confounders have the following three properties: They are extraneous to the question posed, determinants of the outcome, and unequally distributed between exposed and nonexposed participants.

studies.[c] This is a particularly important issue in autism where there is an evolving body of knowledge around potential confounders.

Cohort studies can be based on existing (sometimes called *retrospective*) data or on newly collected (sometimes called *prospective*) data. The logic in both circumstances is the same: At the time of the first observation, all participants must be known to be free of the outcome of interest (autism in the offspring in our example). During the period of observation, there must be a reliable way to determine which participants were exposed to the putative risk (i.e., valproic acid in our example) and who also experienced the outcome of interest. In this era of large population-based data collection ("big data") associated with health systems, it is common to have complete medication, pregnancy, and child health records, so creating a credible cohort study based on existing data is plausible and efficient. However, for many exposures and outcomes, using existing data won't work well as the data may be incomplete, missing, or poorly standardized. For example, the diagnosis of autism has changed substantively over the past 10 years and has lacked standardization.

There are limitations to many administrative databases (e.g., medical claims databases) that we need to consider when we're reading research studies that have used these resources. First, these databases were not developed for research use and thus often don't contain all the information that would be useful, such as data on severity of illness or dosage of the medication.[5] Second, coding of information is often inaccurate and incomplete because there may be limited space for secondary diagnoses in these databases.[6] Third, we can only find events for which there are codes.[6] Fourth, the databases may not include the entire population. For example, the Medicare files in the United States include only those patients eligible to receive Medicare, which includes people 65 years of age and older, some people under 65 years of age with disabilities, and all people with end-stage renal disease requiring renal replacement therapy.

In 1950, Doll and Hill highlighted the importance of completing prospective cohort studies when they were looking at the possible association between smoking and lung cancer. Several retrospective (case-control) studies found an association between smoking and lung cancer, but the size of the association varied across the studies. There was much discussion around the association, but it was not extended

7

---

[c]As we mentioned on page 75, this is another great thing about randomization—it balances the groups for confounders that we haven't identified yet!

to causation, and they determined that this debate would not be advanced by yet another retrospective study. Instead, they advocated for a prospective approach whereby the development of the disease could be determined over time in people whose smoking habits were already known. This led to their landmark study published in 1951 showing the mortality rates among male physicians in relation to their smoking habits.[7] Remarkably, Doll continued this work for more than 50 years and published an update to the paper in 2004.[8]

If the outcome of interest is rare or takes a long time to develop (e.g., the development of cancer or asbestosis), even large cohort studies may not be feasible and we will have to look for alternatives, such as case-control studies. In this study design, people with the outcome of interest (a + c) are identified as "cases," and those without it (b + d) are selected as controls; the proportion of each group of individuals who were exposed to the putative agent [a/(a + c) or b/(b + d)] is assessed retrospectively. There is even more potential for confounding with case-control studies than with cohort studies because confounders that are transient or lead to early death cannot be measured. For example, if patients are selected from hospital sources, the relationship between outcome and exposure will be distorted if patients who are exposed are more likely to be admitted to the hospital than are the unexposed. This was illustrated nicely in a SR that looked at the association between vasectomy and prostate cancer—the relative risk (RR) of prostate cancer following vasectomy was significantly elevated in hospital-based studies (1.98 [95% confidence interval (CI) 1.37–2.86]) but not in population-based ones (1.12 [95% CI 0.96–1.32]).[9]

Inappropriate selection of control participants can lead to false associations, and "control" participants should have the same opportunity for exposure to the putative agent as the "case" participants. For example, if we found a case-control study evaluating the association between maternal exposure to valproic acid and autism in children that assembled children with autism born of mothers with epilepsy but excluded children born of mothers with epilepsy (or migraine or pain disorders) from the control group (who might be at increased risk of exposure to valproic acid), we would wonder whether an observed association was spurious.

We can see that a case-control study design easily lends itself to the exploration of possible relationships between many exposures and the outcome of interest (especially with the common usage and availability of administrative databases). Therefore, we must bear in mind that if a large number of potential associations were explored, a statistically significant finding could be based on chance alone. This is a similar issue to what we described on page 192 on identification of prognostic factors and the need for validation of these factors in an independent data set.

When we're searching for an answer to an etiology question, the articles that we find most commonly (because they're cheaper and easier to do!) describe cross-sectional studies, and unfortunately, these studies are susceptible to even more bias than case-control studies. In a cross-sectional study, the authors look at a group of children with autism (a + c) and a group without (b + d) and assess exposure to valproic acid (a or b) in both. Exposure and outcomes are measured at the same time, and this highlights one of the major problems with this study type: Which came first? This isn't as difficult an issue to sort through in our current example (it should be reasonably straightforward to find out if mothers used valproic acid in pregnancy if this information is available in a database) because the maternal exposure should precede the diagnosis of autism in the child. However, this is more challenging in situations when there is less clarity on the timing between exposure and outcome. Additionally, as with cohort and case-control studies, adjustment must be made for confounders. These studies may be helpful for hypothesis generation.

Finally, we may only find case reports of one patient (or a case series of a few patients) who developed an adverse event while receiving the suspected exposure (cell *a*). If the outcome is unusual and dramatic enough (phocomelia in children born to women who took thalidomide), such case reports and case series may be enough to answer our question. But because these studies lack comparison groups, they are usually only sufficient for hypothesis generation and thus highlight the need for other studies.

We usually find information about the study type and how participants were selected in the "abstract" and "methods" sections of the article. Information describing participants is often found in the "results" section.

7

We quickly see in the *ACP Journal Club* abstract that this is a population-based cohort with individual-level linkage of several national registries.[2,3] Children born at 37 weeks' gestation or more between 1996 and 2006 were included. The investigators identified those children with valproic acid exposure in utero and those without. There were some differences between those exposed to valproic acid and those who weren't; for example, children exposed to valproic acid in utero were more likely to have parents with a psychiatric diagnosis. The investigators adjusted for these differences.

2. Were treatments/exposures and clinical outcomes measured in the same ways in both groups? (Was the assessment of outcomes either objective or blinded to exposure?)

We should place greater confidence in studies in which treatment exposures and clinical outcomes were measured in the same way in both groups. Moreover, we would prefer that the outcomes assessors were blinded to the exposure in cohort studies and to the outcome and study hypothesis in case-control studies. Consider a report describing a cohort study looking at the association between valproic acid exposure in utero and autism. We'd be concerned if the investigator searched more aggressively for autism in children who were known to have in utero exposure to valproic acid, perhaps picking up very mild cases, for example. Indeed, when the outcomes assessors aren't blinded to the exposure, they may search harder for the disease in the exposed group and identify disease that might otherwise have been unnoticed. Now, consider a case-control study evaluating the same potential association—if the investigator is not blinded to the outcome or study hypothesis, he or she might look harder for a history of in utero exposure to valproic acid in children whom he or she knows to have autism. Similarly, mothers of children with autism might have considered their situation more carefully and may have greater ability or incentive to recall possible exposure (of even a single dose) that may have occurred during pregnancy. Thus, we'd feel more reassured about the study if the report described that the patients (and their interviewers) were blinded to the study hypothesis.

This discussion raises another, finer point regarding the source of the information about the outcome or exposure of interest. In some articles, we find that the investigators used health records to seek information about the exposure or outcome retrospectively, and as clinicians who complete these records (and often have to use them at a later date to dictate a discharge summary!), we have to ask ourselves if we consider this method sufficiently accurate. Consider for example, the impact on a study's results if the likelihood of the data being recorded differs between the groups. Similarly, information from some administrative databases might not be as accurate as that collected prospectively (although for certain types of information, such as drug usage, a drug claims database will provide more accurate information than patient or physician recall).

Information about measurement of the exposure or outcome is usually included in the "methods" and "results" sections.

In the study that we found, information on how the exposure and outcomes were determined is available in the full article rather than the *ACP Journal Club* abstract. The investigators used the Danish Prescription Registry for identifying maternal use of valproic acid and defined exposure as the period from 30 days before the estimated date of conception to the date of birth. Drug use while in hospital was not available in this registry. The outcomes of childhood autism and autism spectrum disorder where identified from the Psychiatric Central Registry, which is known to be very accurate with regard to these diagnoses. This latter registry was also used to obtain information about potential confounders including parental psychiatric history. Detailed information on other potential confounders, such as maternal smoking and actual dose of drugs used by the mothers, was not available.

3. Was the follow-up of the study patients sufficiently long (for the outcome to occur) and complete?

Ideally, we'd like to see that no patients were lost to follow-up, because lost patients may have had outcomes that would affect the conclusions of the study. For example, in a cohort study looking at the association between in utero exposure to valproic acid and autism in children, imagine the impact on its results if a large number of women and children in the valproic acid cohort left the study—we wouldn't know if it was because the children developed autism and left the study to seek treatment or because their mothers became frustrated with the study or moved to a different region. As mentioned on page in Chapter 4, evidence-based journals of secondary publication like the *ACP Journal Club* use a 20% loss to follow-up as an exclusion criterion because it would be rare for a study to suffer such a loss and not have its results affected. We'd like to see that the patients were followed up for an appropriate period. For example, if we found a study on the association between cancer and living close to hydroelectric wires that followed up people for only a few weeks, we wouldn't be able to distinguish a true-negative from a false-negative association.

7

In our study, national registries were used and children were followed up to 14 years of age.

4. Do the results of the harm study satisfy some of the diagnostic tests for causation?

Investigators may identify an association between an exposure and outcome, but is the exposure causative? "Diagnostic tests for causation" can help us with this concern as discussed below.

Is it clear that the exposure preceded the onset of the outcome?

We'd want to make sure that the exposure (e.g., valproic acid) occurred before the development of the adverse outcome (e.g., autism). When Doll and Hill were doing their work on smoking and lung cancer, this was a key issue they identified in their rationale for the prospective study—did the smoking exposure happen before the development of lung cancer? As noted above, this issue is easier to address in our study of children with autism because the registries are able to identify maternal exposure to these agents, which preceded the diagnosis of autism in children.

Is there a dose–response gradient?

The demonstration of an increasing risk (or severity) of the adverse event with increasing exposure (increased dose and/or duration) to the putative causal agent strengthens the association. For example, heavy smokers are at a greater risk of cancer than occasional/light smokers.[9] In the study that we found, the risk of autism appears similar for high-dose and low-dose valproic acid (dose range is provided), but the registry does not provide specific information on the dose the mother actually used. A related factor is duration and timing of use; for example, in the study we found, the adjusted hazard ratio for childhood autism was 4.7 in those children whose mothers filled the prescription in the first trimester of pregnancy versus 8.3 in those whose mothers only filled it later in pregnancy.

Is there any positive evidence from a "dechallenge–rechallenge" study?

We'd like to see that the adverse outcome decreases or disappears when the treatment is withdrawn and worsens or reappears when it is reintroduced. In the 2004 study on tobacco use and mortality, Doll et al. were able to show that smoking cessation leads to a survival benefit. Stopping smoking at age 60, 50, 40, or 30 years lead to a gain of approximately 3, 6, 9, or 10 years, respectively.[8] This criteria isn't relevant to our study because the exposure was in utero and the autism was diagnosed after the child was born.

Is the association consistent from study to study?

If we were able to find multiple studies or, better yet, an SR of the question, we could determine whether the association between exposure and the adverse event is consistent from study to study. We identified some case series that raise awareness of a potential association between autism and in utero exposure to valproic acid.[10,11] There are also a couple of SRs supporting an association between valproic acid and child neurodevelopment outcomes.[12,13]

Does the association make biological sense?

If the association between exposure and outcome makes biological sense (in terms of pathophysiology, etc.), a causal interpretation becomes more plausible. The authors of our study state that although animal models have also shown an association between valproic acid and autistic-like behaviour in offspring, the potential mechanism isn't clear although numerous theories have been postulated.

Are the valid results of this harm study important?

If the study we find fails to satisfy the first three minimum standards in Box 7.1, we'd probably be better off abandoning it and continuing our search. But if we are satisfied that it meets these minimum guides, we need to decide if the association between exposure and outcome is sufficiently strong and convincing for us to do something about it. By this, we mean looking at the risk or odds of the adverse effect with (as opposed to without) exposure to the treatment; the higher the risk or odds, the stronger the association and the more we should be impressed by it. We can use the guides in Box 7.2 to determine whether the valid results of the study are important.

1. What is the magnitude of the association between the exposure and outcome?

As noted above, questions of etiology can be answered by several different study designs. Different study designs require different methods for

Box 7.2 Are the valid results of this harm study important?

1. What is the magnitude of the association between the exposure and outcome?
2. What is the precision of the estimate of the association between the exposure and the outcome?

estimating the strength of association between exposure to the putative cause and the outcome of interest. In randomized trials and cohort studies, this association is often described by calculating the risk (or incidence) of the adverse event in the exposed (or treated) patients relative to that in the unexposed (or untreated) patients. This RR is calculated as: $[a/(a + b)]/[c/(c + d)]$ (from Table 7.1). For example, if 1000 patients receive a treatment and 20 of them develop the outcome of interest:

$a \equiv 20$ and $a/(a + b) \equiv 2\%$ (the risk of experiencing the outcome with treatment is 2%)

If 1000 patients didn't receive the treatment and two experienced the outcome:

$c \equiv 2$ and $c/(c + d) \equiv 0.2\%$ (the risk of experiencing the outcome in the absence of treatment is 0.2%)

Therefore, the RR becomes:

$$2\%/0.2\% \equiv 10$$

This means that patients receiving the treatment are 10 times as likely to experience the outcome as patients not receiving the treatment.

From the preceding example, we can see that to calculate the RR we needed a group of treated participants and a group who didn't receive treatment and then we determined the proportion with the outcome in each group. But, in case-control studies, we can't calculate the RR because the investigator selects the people with the outcomes (rather than those with the exposure) and, therefore, we can't calculate the "incidence." Instead, we look to an indirect estimate of the strength of association in a case-control study, and this is called an odds ratio (OR; or relative odds). Referring to Table 7.1, it is calculated as "ad/bc." The odds of experiencing the outcome in exposed patients is a/b. The odds of experiencing the outcome in those not exposed are c/d. We can then compare the odds of experiencing the outcome in those who are exposed, with the odds of experiencing the outcome in those who are not exposed: (a/b)/(c/d) or ad/bc.

If, for example, 100 cases of children with autism are identified and it's found that 90 of them had a history of valproic acid exposure in utero, a $\equiv$ 90 and c $\equiv$ 10. If 100 patients without the outcome are assembled and it is found that 45 of them received the exposure, b $\equiv$ 45 and d $\equiv$ 55 and the OR becomes:

$$(90/45)/(10/55)$$
$$\equiv 90 \times 55/45 \times 10$$
$$\equiv 11$$

This means that the odds of experiencing the adverse event for children who had a history of valproic acid exposure in utero was 11 times that of those who didn't have the same exposure.

Note that risks $\equiv$ odds/(1 + odds) and odds $\equiv$ [risk/(1 − risk)]. We did this same calculation on page 173 when we were converting pretest probabilities to pretest odds to allow us to multiply this by the likelihood ratio. We then used the second equation to convert from posttest odds to posttest probability.

ORs and RRs that are less than 1 indicate that there is an increased risk of the adverse outcome associated with the exposure. When the RR or the OR $\equiv$ 1, the adverse event is no more likely to occur with than without the exposure to the suspected agent.[d] Conversely, when the ORs and RRs are less than 1, the adverse event is less likely to occur with the exposure to the putative agent than without. It should also be noted that when event rates are very low, the RR and OR approximate each other. They are close when the treatment effect is small. This is sometimes a cause for confusion because often in articles we find ORs have been calculated but the authors report and discuss them as RRs.

How big should the RR or the OR be for us to be impressed? This brings us back to issues of validity because we have to consider the strength of the study design when we're evaluating the strength of the association. As we discussed earlier in this chapter, a well-done randomized trial is susceptible to less bias compared with either a cohort or case-control study. Therefore, we'd be satisfied with a smaller increase in risk from a randomized trial than from a cohort or case-control study. Because cohort studies and, even more so, case-control studies are susceptible

7

---

[d]Remember that a ratio is just a numerator and a denominator. When the numerator is the same as the denominator the ratio is 1 (i.e., there is no difference between the numerator and denominator, or between the risk and odds of events).

to many biases, we want to ensure that the OR is greater than that which would result from bias alone. As rules of thumb, and taking into account the features of one or more individual studies, we might not want to label an odds ratio from a case-control study as impressive unless it is greater than 4 for minor adverse events, and we'd set this value at progressively lower levels as the severity of the adverse event increases. There is less potential bias in cohort studies, and, therefore, we might regard a relative risk of greater than 3 as convincing for more severe adverse events.

Professor Les Irwig has provided another useful tip when looking at the strength of the association. It requires us to find a report that includes some adjustment for potential confounders. He suggested that we compare the unadjusted measure of association with one in which at least one known confounder has been adjusted out. If this adjustment produces a large decline in the RR or the OR, we should be suspicious of a spurious association. If, in contrast, the adjusted OR or RR is stable with this adjustment, or if it rises rather than falls, our confidence in the validity of the association would be greater.

> In our study, in utero exposure to valproic acid was associated with childhood autism (hazard ratio [HR] 5.2; 95% CI 2.7–10) and autism spectrum disorder (2.9; 95% CI 1.7–4.9); these HRs were adjusted for parent (age at conception, psychiatric history, and maternal parity) and child (gender, gestational age, birthweight, and congenital malformation).

Although the OR and the RR tell us about the strength of the association, we need to translate this into some measure that is useful and intelligible both to us and our patient. This is of particular importance when the discussion concerns a medication or some other medical intervention we and our patient are considering. For this, we can turn to the number needed to harm (NNH), which tells us the "number of patients who need to be exposed to the putative causal agent to produce one additional harmful event." The NNH can be calculated directly from trials and cohort studies in a fashion analogous to the NNT, but this time as the reciprocal of the difference in adverse event rates:

$$\equiv 1/[a/(a+b)] - [c/(c+d)]$$

For an OR derived from a case-control study, the calculation is more complex (remember, we can't determine "incidence" directly in a case-control study). Its formula reads (if the OR < 1) (don't worry, we won't test you on this!):

$$1 - [PEER (1 - OR)]/PEER (1 - PEER) (1 - OR)$$

and if the OR > 1:

$$1 + [PEER \times (OR - 1)]/PEER (1 - PEER) (OR - 1)$$

where PEER is the patient expected event rate (the adverse event rate among individuals who are not exposed to the putative cause).

We've made this a bit easier by providing some typical PEERs and ORs and summarizing them in Tables 7.2a and 7.2b. As you can see from the table, for different PEERs, the same OR can lead to different NNHs/NNTs, and it is therefore important that we do our best to estimate our patient's expected event rate when calculating the NNH/NNT. For example, if the OR was 2.9 and the PEER was 0.005, the NNH would be 107, but if the PEER was 0.40 (and the OR was 2.90), the NNH would be 4. We'll consider individual patients in further detail in the next section.

Practising and teaching EBM in real time

The above formula is complex and we rarely use it. If the answer we're looking for isn't in Table 7.2, we use the EBM calculator to quickly

Table 7.2a Translating odds ratios (ORs) to numbers needed to harm (NNHs) when OR < 1*

Patient expected event rate (PEER)	For odds ratio < 1						
	0.9	0.8	0.7	0.6	0.5	0.4	0.3
0.05	209[a]	104	69	52	41	34	29[b]
0.10	110	54	36	27	21	18	15
0.20	61	30	20	14	11	10	8
0.30	46	22	14	10	8	7	5
0.40	40	19	12	9	7	6	4
0.50	38	18	11	8	6	5	4
0.70	44	20	13	9	6	5	4
0.90	101[c]	46	27	18	12	9	4[d]

[a]The relative risk reduction (RRR) here is 10%.
[b]The RRR here is 49%.
[c]The RRR here is 1%.
[d]The RRR here is 9%.
*Adapted from John Geddes, 1999.

7

Table 7.2b Translating odds ratios (ORs) to numbers needed to harm (NNHs) when OR > 1

Patient expected event rate (PEER)	For odds ratio > 1						
	1.1	1.25	1.5	1.75	2	2.25	2.5
0.05	212	86	44	30	23	18	16
0.10	113	46	24	16	13	10	9
0.20	64	27	14	10	8	7	6
0.30	50	21	11	8	7	6	5
0.40	44	19	10	8	6	5	5
0.50	42	18	10	8	6	6	5
0.70	51	23	13	10	9	8	7
0.90	121	55	33	25	22	19	18

The numbers in the body of the table are the NNHs for the corresponding ORs at that particular PEER. Adapted from John Geddes, 1999.

convert an OR to an NNH. You can try the calculation by using our calculator (https://ebm-tools.knowledgetranslation.net/calculator/converter/); we can insert our OR of 0.90 and our PEER of 0.005 and at the click of a button, the NNH is calculated. You can download this to your smartphone for quick use (http://ebm-tools.knowledgetranslation.net/clinical-question).

When teaching, we find it much easier to use NNTs/NNHs than ORs. We also use these as an opportunity to teach how to communicate this information about risk to our patient or a colleague. We've found it fun to give each trainee 1 minute to explain the results/bottom line to a colleague. Other members of the team then give feedback to the trainee.

2. What is the precision of the estimate of the association between the exposure and outcome?

In addition to looking at the magnitude of the RR or the OR, we need to look at its precision by examining the CI around it (for more information on CIs, see Appendix 2, available online). Credibility is highest when the entire CI is narrow and remains within a clinically importantly increased (or decreased) risk. For example, imagine a CI that is statistically significant, but the upper limit of the CI for the OR is 0.96 (i.e., close to 1); this is the smallest estimate of the strength of the association, and it approximates 1, indicating there could be, at worst, a very tiny association! If the CI of the OR overlaps 1, the adverse event is no more likely to occur with than without the exposure to the suspected agent. Similarly, if a study finds no association, the limits of the CI could tell us if a potentially important positive result (indicating an association) has been excluded.

In the study that we found, the CIs for the adjusted HRs for both childhood autism (HR 5.2; 95% CI 2.7–10) and autism spectrum disorder (2.9; 95% CI 1.7–4.9) were statistically significant. Looking at the CIs, the lower limit of each estimate does not approach 1. The upper limits of the CIs (of a 10-fold increase in childhood autism and a fivefold increase in autism spectrum disorder) are clinically important.

Once we have decided that the evidence we have found is both valid and important, we need to consider if it can be applied to our patient (Box 7.3).

Can this valid and important evidence about harm be applied to our patient?

1. Is our patient so different from those included in the study that its results cannot apply?

As emphasized in previous chapters, the issue is not whether our patient fulfills all the inclusion criteria for the study we found but whether our patient is so different from those in the study that its results are of no help to us. See page 102 (in the Therapy section) for further discussion of this issue.

7

Box 7.3 Guides for deciding whether valid important evidence about harm can be applied to our patient

1. Is our patient so different from those included in the study that its results cannot apply?
2. What are our patient's risks of benefit and harm from the agent?
3. What are our patient's preferences, concerns, and expectations from this treatment?
4. What alternative treatments are available?

2. What are our patient's risks of benefit and harm from the agent?

We need to consider both the potential benefits and harms from the agent. In the particular example we've outlined in this chapter, there are benefits and risk for both the mother and the child that should be considered. For the mother, there are risks and benefits of using automated external defibrillators (AEDs) (e.g., risk of seizures during pregnancy). For the child, there is the risk of being exposed to the AED among others. We will focus on the specific risk of the AED to the child in this discussion.

For each patient, we need to individualize these risks. To apply the results of a study to an individual patient, we need to estimate our patient's risk of the adverse event if she were not exposed to the putative cause. There's a hard way and an easy way to tackle this. The hard way requires searching for good evidence on prognosis, and the much easier way requires estimating the risk relative to that of unexposed individuals in the study. Just as with NNTs on page 105, we can express this as a decimal fraction (f): If our patient is at half the risk of study patients, $f \equiv 0.5$; if our patient is at 3 times the risk, $f \equiv 3$. The study NNH can then be divided by f to produce the NNH for our individual patient. For example, suppose a study found we'd only need to treat 150 people with a statin to cause one additional person to experience myalgias. But if we think our patient is at twice the risk of the study patients, $f \equiv 2$ and 150/2 generates an NNH of 75. If, however, we thought our patient was at one-third the risk ($f \equiv 0.33$), the NNH for patients like ours becomes 455.

In situations such as this, when we're considering the use of a medication, the NNH needs to be balanced against the corresponding NNT summarizing the benefit of this treatment. The resulting crude "likelihood of being helped versus harmed" (LHH, see p. 110) by this treatment can provide the starting point for the last step, described in the next section.

3. What are our patient's preferences, concerns, and expectations from this treatment?

It is vital that our patient's unique concerns and preferences are incorporated into any shared decision-making process. In the case of potentially harmful therapy, and just as on page 111, we can ask our patient to quantify her values for both the potential adverse event(s) and the target event(s) we hope to prevent with the proposed therapy. In the current example, we'd need to consider the effectiveness of valproic acid in reducing risk of seizures as well as its safety (i.e., risk of autism in her offspring). The result is a values-adjusted likelihood of being helped or harmed by the therapy. Similarly, we can adjust for her baseline risk of the outcomes if we estimate they are different from those in the study. If we are unsure of our patient's baseline risk, or if she is unsure about her values for the outcomes, a sensitivity analysis can be done. That is, different values for relative severity could be inserted and our patient could determine at which point her decision would change. The challenge occurs when there is more than one outcome to be considered; for example, our patient may be interested in considering not just the risk of autism, but also other outcomes such as major and minor congenital malformations. When all of these various outcomes need to be considered, we need to use a more formal shared decision-making tool, such as a decision aid. We refer you to the Ottawa decision aid database at https:// decisionaid.ohri.ca/ for a more complete discussion of these useful tools.

4. What alternative treatments are available?

If this is a therapy under discussion, we and our patient could explore alternative management options. Is there another medication we could consider? Is there any effective nonpharmacologic therapy available?

Returning to our patient and the article we identified, other antiepileptic drugs used as monotherapy during pregnancy were not associated with increased risk for autism spectrum disorder or childhood autism in offspring compared with no use of the specific monotherapy. For example, we could consider using lamotrigine (adjusted HR 1.7 [95% CI 0.8–3.5] for autism spectrum disorder and 1.7 [95% CI 0.5–5.2] for childhood autism) as an alternative therapy. Note that these estimates don't exclude the possibility of adverse events with lamotrigine, and indeed, the upper limit of the CI indicates a considerable risk.

Practising and teaching EBM in real time

Formulating a question, and then retrieving, appraising, and applying relevant evidence from the primary literature will usually take longer than the average clinical appointment. There are several ways to tackle the time constraints, focusing on finding shortcuts to facilitate practising EBM. As we've already mentioned (in Chapter 2), if we can find our answer in a high-quality preappraised resource, we're ahead in the game—especially with an evidence-based "metasearch." If we're lucky enough to have a local librarian or consultant pharmacist who can help us track down the evidence, we'd ask him or her for some help. (Although this requires that these team members have access to the evidence available online, which isn't always the case in places where we've practised!) Alternatively, we can share tasks with other colleagues, either locally or virtually using e-mail discussion groups or social networking sites. Some regions and countries have formal question answering services; for example, Clinical Enquiry and Response Service (CLEAR) is a question answering service provided by the National Health Services (NHS) in Scotland (http://www.knowledge.scot.nhs.uk/clear/ask-a-question.aspx). This service not only provides the opportunity to have your literature search done but also provides access to the database of previously asked questions and their bottom line answers (http://www.knowledge.scot.nhs.uk/clear/answers/cardiovascular/are-medical-emergency-teams-(met)-effective-in-reducing-mortality-from-cardiac-arrests.aspx). Note that with services like these, it is important to find out about their search process (e.g., do they focus on identifying SRs as a starting point or individual studies? Do they use validated search filters? Do they provide a "best by" date on the search?).

What is their approach for appraising the evidence once it is identified—or do they provide the search results that the user has to appraise?

We'd also consider asking our patient to book a return visit in a week to review the evidence with them at that time, giving us some time to review the evidence between visits. If the same clinical issues arise commonly, we could find (e.g., in texts, such as *DynaMed* or *Clinical Evidence*, or in noncommercial online services, such as Medlineplus [http://medlineplus.gov/]) or develop our own patient information leaflets briefly summarizing some of the evidence.

One resource that we've found useful in shared decision making is (www.healthtalk.org). It is a unique database of patient experiences that has been created through qualitative research. There is material on more than 90 conditions, including epilepsy (http://www.healthtalk.org/peoples-experiences/nerves-brain/epilepsy/topics). This website also has information about patient engagement in research, including stories told by patients about their experiences and their descriptions of study design. This latter resource is tremendously useful in teaching about patient engagement in randomized trials, for example. A sibling site for adolescents is also available (www.youthhealthtalk.org).

Finally, we've found the James Lind Library (http://www.jameslindlibrary.org/) to be a useful resource when we're teaching people to

Address ⬛ http://www.jameslindlibrary.org/trial_records/20th_Century/1960s/mcbride/mcbride_whole.html

Thalidomide and congenital abnormalities

Sir, — Congenital abnormalities are present in approximately 1.5% of babies. In recent months I have observed that the incidence of multiple severe abnormalities in babies delivered of women who were given the drug thalidomide ('Distaval') during pregnancy, as an antiemetic or as a sedative, to be almost 20%.

These abnormalities are present in structures developed from mesenchyme– i.e., the bones and the musculature of the gut. Bony development seems to be affected in a very striking manner, resulting in polydactyly, syndactyly, and failure of development of long bones (abnormally short femora and radii).

Have any of your readers seen similar abnormalities in babies delivered of women who have taken this drug during pregnancy?

Hurstville, New South Wales   W.G McBride

In our issue of Dec. 2 we included a statement from the Distillers Company (Biochemicals) Ltd. referring to "reports from two overseas sources possibly associating thalidomide ('Distaval') with harmful effects on the foetus in early pregnancy". Pending further investigation, the company decided to withdraw from the market all its preparations containing thalidomide. – ED.L.

Fig. 7.2 James Lind Library screenshot.

understand fair tests of treatments in health care (Fig. 7.2). It is fun and useful because it provides examples of how a fair assessment should occur and how these evaluations (randomized trials and SRs) have evolved over time. It includes a "timeline" of various events in evidence-based health care with examples that can be used in teaching; for example, we often use the material describing the randomized trial of streptomycin for tuberculosis to discuss randomized trial design. Some material on this site relates to assessing benefits and harms including examples of "dramatic results," often about putative harm, such as the one in Figure 7.2.

References

1. Hirota T, Veenstra-Vanderweele J, Hollander E, Kishi T. Antiepileptic medications in autism spectrum disorder: a systematic review and meta-analysis. J Autism Dev Disord 2014;44(4):948–57.

2. Valproate use during pregnancy was linked to autism spectrum disorder and childhood autism in offspring. ACP J Club 2013;159:13.

3. Christensen J, Gronborg TK, Soernsen MJ, et al. Prenatal valproate exposure and risk of autism spectrum disorders and childhood autism. JAMA 2013;309:1696–730.

4. Papanikolaou PN, Ioannidis HP. Availability of large-scale evidence on specific harms from systematic reviews of randomized trials. Am J Med 2004;117:582–9.

5. Feinstein AR. ICD, POR, and DRG: Unsolved scientific problems in the nosology of clinical medicine. Arch Intern Med 1988;148: 2269–74.

6. Zhan C, Miller MR. Administrative data based patient safety research: a critical review. Qual Saf Health Care 2003;12(Suppl.II):ii58–63.

7. Doll R, Hill AB. The mortality of doctors in relation to their smoking habits. BMJ 1954;ii:1451–5.

8. Doll R, Peto R, Boreham J, Sutherland I. Mortality in relation to smoking: 50 years' observations on male British doctors. BMJ 2004;doi:10.1136/bmj.38142.554479.AE.

9. Bernal-Delgado F, et al. The association between vasectomy and prostate cancer: a systematic review of the literature. Fertil Steril 1998;70:191–200.

10. Rasalam AD, Hailey H, Williams H, et al. Characteristics of fetal anticonvulsant syndrome associated autism disorder. Dev Med Child Neurol 2005;47:551–5.

11. Bromley RL, Mawer G, Clayton-Smith J, et al. Autism spectrum disorders following in utero exposure to antiepileptic drugs. Neurology 2008;71:1923–4.

12. Galbally M, Roberts M, Buist A. Mood stabilizers in pregnancy: a systematic review. Aust N Z J Psychiatry 2010;44:967–77.

13. Banach R, Boskovic R, Einarson T, Koren G. Long-term developmental outcome of children with epilepsy, unexposed or exposed prenatally to antiepileptic drugs. Drug Saf 2010;33:73–9.

Further reading

Guyatt G, Rennie D, Meade M, Cook DJ, editors. Users' guides to the medical literature. A manual for evidence-based clinical practice. 3rd ed. Chicago, IL: AMA Press; 2015.

Haynes RB, Sackett DL, Guyatt GH, Tugwell P. Clinical epidemiology: how to do clinical practice research. Philadelphia, PA: Lippincott Williams & Wilkins; 2006.

8 Evaluation

The fifth step in practising evidence-based medicine (EBM) is self-evaluation, and we'll suggest some approaches for doing that here. This book is geared to help individual clinicians learn how to practise EBM, so this section will mainly focus on how we can reflect on our own practice. However, some of us are also involved in teaching EBM, and we've provided some tips on how to evaluate our teaching. Some clinicians, managers, and policymakers might be interested in evaluating how evidence-based practice is being implemented at a local, regional, or national level, and although this is not the aim of this book, we'll introduce this topic and point you to some useful resources for further information.

How am I doing?

This part of the chapter will describe the domains in which you might want to evaluate your performance.

Evaluating our performance in asking answerable questions

Box 8.1 suggests some initial questions to consider about our own question asking in practising EBM. First, are we asking any questions at all? As our experience grows, are we using a map of where most questions come from (Box 1.2 is our version) to locate our knowledge gaps and help us articulate questions? When we get stuck, are we increasingly able to get "unstuck" using the map or other devices? On a practical level, have we devised a method to note our questions as they occur, for later retrieval and answering when time permits? There are low-tech and high-tech options for this—some of us keep a logbook in our pocket to record our questions and the answers when we've had a chance to retrieve them. Alternatively, we could go for the high-tech option and use the smartphone clinical questions (CQ) log <https://ebm-tools. knowledgetranslation.net/clinical-question> that allows us to record our questions and answers. In some countries, this type of practice reflection is essential for maintaining certification from professional organizations, with higher level credits given if the questions are answered and then used to change practice.

Box 8.1 Self-evaluation in asking answerable questions

---

1. Am I asking any clinical questions at all?
2. Am I asking focused questions?
3. Am I using a "map" to locate my knowledge gaps and articulate questions?
4. Can I get myself "unstuck" when asking questions?
5. Do I have a working method to save my questions for later answering?

Box 8.2 A self-evaluation in finding the best external evidence

---

1. Am I searching at all?
2. Do I know the best sources of current evidence for my clinical discipline?
3. Do I have easy access to the best evidence for my clinical discipline?
4. Am I becoming more efficient in my searching?
5. Am I using truncations, Booleans, MeSH headings, a thesaurus, limiters, and intelligent free text when searching MEDLINE?
6. How do my searches compare with those of research librarians or other respected colleagues who have a passion for providing best current patient care?

Evaluating our performance in searching

Box 8.2 lists some questions we might want to ask ourselves about our performance in searching for the best evidence. Are we searching at all? Are we trying to find the highest quality evidence, aiming for the top of the "Pyramid 5.0," as described on page 41? Do we have access to the best evidence for our clinical discipline? You might wish to try timing the steps in your search process: locating a resource, starting up the resource, typing in a question, getting the response, and so on. Which of these can you speed up to become more efficient with this process? If we have started searching on our own, are we finding useful external evidence from a widening array of sources, and are we becoming more efficient in our searching? Are we using validated search filters when using MEDLINE? Are we using meta-search engines (i.e., those that search across more than one database)?

An efficient way of evaluating our searching skills is to ask research librarians or other respected colleagues to repeat a search that we've already done and then compare notes on both the search strategy and the usefulness of the evidence we both found. Done this way, we benefit in three ways: (1) from the evaluation itself, (2) from the opportunity to learn how to do it better, and (3) from the yield of additional external evidence on the clinical question that prompted our search. If you don't have access to a local librarian, you can compare your search to one that has been done by a publicly available question answering service, such as the Clinical Enquiry and Response (CLEAR) service from the National Health Services (NHS) in Scotland (http://www.knowledge.scot.nhs.uk/clear.aspx). One thing we've found useful to do during journal club is to search in "real time" and limit ourselves to 2 minutes for finding an answer to a clinical question. We then elicit feedback from colleagues on how we could improve the search the next time. This also provides an opportunity to role model efficient searching for learners.

It might be wise to consult the nearest health sciences library about taking a course (in person or online) or personal tutorial, to get the level of expertise needed to carry out this second step in practising EBM. If a librarian can be persuaded to join the clinical team, it is an extraordinary way to increase proficiency! We have found it very helpful to have a librarian join us (even occasionally) on clinical rounds; it's an opportunity for them to teach us searching tips as we try to become more efficient and effective searchers.

Evaluating our performance in critical appraisal

Box 8.3 lists some questions to examine how we're doing in critically appraising external evidence. Are we doing it at all? If not, can we identify the barriers to our performance and remove them? Once again, we might find that working as a member of a group (e.g., the journal club we describe in chapter 9) could not only help us get going but also give us feedback about our performance.

Most clinicians find that critical appraisal of most types of articles becomes easier with time but find one or two study designs to be more challenging than others. Again, this is a situation in which working in

8

Box 8.3 A self-evaluation in critically appraising the evidence for its validity and potential usefulness

1. Am I critically appraising external evidence at all?
2. Are the critical appraisal guides becoming easier for me to apply?
3. Am I becoming more accurate and efficient in applying some of the critical appraisal measures (e.g., likelihood ratios, numbers needed to treat [NNTs], and the like)?
4. Am I creating any appraisal summaries?

---

a group (even "virtual" groups) can quickly identify and resolve such confusion. Often, in journal clubs, we find that the focus is on therapy articles (we're often in our comfort zone with these articles!), but one strategy we've found useful is to encourage participants to consider other study types and to engage in team learning. With team learning, the journal club is not resting on a single person appraising the article, but instead, it becomes a group activity. We can then proceed to consider whether we are becoming more accurate and efficient in applying some of the measures of effect (e.g., likelihood ratios, numbers needed to treat [NNTs], and the like). This could be done by comparing our results with those of colleagues who are appraising the same evidence (this is made even simpler with the advent of online and Twitter journal clubs that link clinicians and learners worldwide) or by taking the raw data from an article abstracted in one of the journals of secondary publication, completing the calculations, and then comparing them with the abstract's conclusions. Another strategy to facilitate team-based appraisal is to provide half of the participants with an article that has found a positive result to an evaluation of a therapy and the other half of the participants with an article that has found a different result from an evaluation of the same therapy. The two teams then discuss why such different results were obtained from the studies.

Finally, at the most advanced level, are we creating summaries of our appraisals? We could use formal CATMaker (http://www.cebm.net/catmaker-ebm-calculators/) or GATE software (https://www.fmhs.auckland.ac.nz/en/soph/about/our-departments/epidemiology-and-biostatistics/research/epiq/evidence-based-practice-and-cats.html) to create these summaries, or we could develop our own template for storing appraisals. We find CATMaker a useful teaching tool, but often it is too cumbersome for daily use in our clinical practice; instead, we keep abbreviated versions of our appraisals by using a simple template, including the study citation, clinical bottom line, a two-line description of the study methods, and a brief table or summary of results in the CQ log.

Evaluating our performance in integrating evidence and patients' values

Box 8.4 lists some elements of a self-evaluation of our skills in integrating our critical appraisals with our clinical expertise and applying the results in clinical practice. We ask ourselves whether we are integrating our critical appraisals into our practice at all. Because the efforts we've expended in the previous three steps are largely wasted if we can't execute

---

Box 8.4 A self-evaluation in integrating the critical appraisal with clinical expertise and applying the result in clinical practice

---

1. Am I integrating my critical appraisals into my practice at all?
2. Am I becoming more accurate and efficient in adjusting some of the critical appraisal measures to fit my individual patients (pretest probabilities, number needed to treat [NNT]/f, etc.)?
3. Can I explain (and resolve) disagreements about management decisions in terms of this integration?
4. Am I eliciting patient values and preferences?
5. Am I integrating the evidence with my clinical expertise and my patient's values and preferences?

---

this fourth one, we'd need to do some soul searching and carry out some major adjustments of how we spend our time and energy if we're not following through on it. Once again, talking with a mentor or working as a member of a group might help overcome this failure, as might attending one of the EBM workshops. Once we are on track, we could ask ourselves whether we are becoming more accurate and efficient in adjusting some of the critical appraisal measures to fit our individual patients. Have we been able to find or otherwise establish pretest probabilities that are appropriate to our patients and the disorders we commonly seek in them?

Are we becoming more adept at modifying measures like the NNT to take into account the "f" for our patient? One way to test our growing skills in this integration is to see whether we can use them to explain (and maybe even resolve!) disagreements about management decisions. We can do this among our colleagues in our practice or our residents on the teaching service.

Finally, are we eliciting patients' values and circumstances? Are they engaged in shared decision making? How are we prioritizing their concerns?

8

Is our practice improving?

Although a self-evaluation showing success at the foregoing level should bring enormous satisfaction and pride to any clinician, we might want to proceed even further and ask ourselves whether what we have learned has been translated into better clinical practice (Box 8.5). Although there are many, many frameworks that can be used to guide evidence

---

Box 8.5 A self-evaluation of changing practice behaviour

1. When evidence suggests a change in practice, am I identifying barriers and facilitators to this change?
2. Have I identified a strategy to implement this change, targeted to the barriers I've identified?
3. Have I carried out any check, such as audits of my diagnostic, therapeutic, or other evidence-based medicine (EBM) performance, including evidence use as well as impact on clinical outcomes?
4. Am I considering sustainability of this change?

---

implementation, we find the Knowledge to Action Framework is helpful when we are trying to implement evidence in our own practice.[1] This framework was based on a review of more than 30 theories of planned action (which focus on deliberately engineering behaviour change) and includes their common elements. Specifically, the framework includes assessing the gap in care (e.g., performing a chart audit to see if bone mineral density [BMD] tests are being ordered appropriately in our patients at high risk for osteoporotic fractures); adapting the evidence to the local context (e.g., determining what effective osteoporosis medications are available in our setting, at low/no cost to my patients); assessing the barriers and facilitators to evidence use (e.g., are BMD tests readily available? Do we need help in interpreting the results of BMD tests? Are our patients interested in considering osteoporosis medications? In some health care settings, can our patients afford the test, and can our patients afford the medication(s)?); selecting an implementation strategy targeted to these barriers and facilitators (e.g., electronic reminders for physicians; patient information leaflet and web-based educational tool; insurance coverage for medications); evaluating evidence use (e.g., are BMDs being ordered appropriately following the implementation of our strategy? Are we prescribing osteoporosis medications for high-risk patients?); monitoring outcomes (e.g., what is the fracture risk in our patients? What is their quality of life?); and assessing sustainability of evidence use (e.g., are we continuing to order BMD tests and osteoporosis medications in relevant patients at 1 year, at 2 years, etc.?).

We think one of the most important steps in this process is to consider the barriers and facilitators to evidence use in our practice. Failing to do this step often results in failure of evidence implementation. In a systematic review (SR) of barriers to guideline implementation, more than 250 barriers were identified at the level of the physician alone.[2] Do we need new skills, equipment, organizational processes, or a reminder system? For example, in one of our practices, we decided that patients with diabetes should get annual foot checkups, including monofilament testing. To implement this, we needed monofilaments, the skills to use them reliably, and a data entry field added to our annual checkup form as a reminder to test (and the result was a 50% reduction in unnecessary podiatry referrals).

Another important (but time-consuming!) piece in this process is to audit evidence uptake and its impact on clinical outcomes. Audits can tell us how we're doing as clinicians, and if we incorporate individualized feedback, they can have a positive impact on our clinical performance. A bonus for completion is that many professional organizations provide continuing medical education (CME) credits for conducting them (although we don't see this as a reason to complete them!). Audits are much easier to perform if we have an electronic health record, which allows us to capture the relevant data.

Audits can occur at various levels of complexity, and many hospitals have well-developed audit (or quality improvement) committees with full-time staff. Because this book is directed to individual clinicians, we won't devote space to audits carried out at these higher levels of organization. Practice audits are often carried out at the local, regional, or national level, and attempts can be focused on how to change physician behaviour at these levels. Several methods have been found to be effective, including academic detailing, opinion leaders, and electronic reminders, among many others. (For more details on these interventions, we suggest you look at the Cochrane EPOC reviews [http://epoc.cochrane.org/] and the Rx for Change Database [https://www.cadth.ca/resources/rx-for-change/database/browse]. These resources identify SRs of various behaviour change interventions). As we've mentioned before, this is not the focus of this book, and we refer you to some other resources that address this topic that are listed at the end of this chapter. Specifically, these resources focus on knowledge translation or implementation science, which is about putting evidence into practice at various levels within the health care system and not just at the level of the individual clinician–patient dyad, which is the focus of this book.

If the audit shows that we've implemented the evidence, then we can celebrate and then perhaps consider how to sustain this change and improve further. If we haven't changed, rather than self-recriminations, we should ask what were the problems and barriers to change. Perhaps new barriers arose that require us to change our implementation strategy—in the complex health care environment, it is not unusual for this to happen! Thus, we re-enter the "Knowledge-to-Action Cycle."

8

How much of our practice is evidence based?

A number of clinical teams have looked at the extent to which practice is evidence based. The impetus for their work was the "conventional wisdom" that only about 20% of clinical care was based in solid scientific evidence.[a] One of the first studies was performed on David Sackett's clinical service in Oxford, in the United Kingdom, where at the time of discharge, death, or retention in hospital at the end of the audited month, every patient was discussed at a team meeting and consensus reached on his or her primary diagnosis (the disease, syndrome, or condition entirely or, in the case of multiple diagnoses, most responsible for the patient's admission to hospital) and his or her primary intervention (the treatment or other manoeuvre that represented the most important attempt to cure, alleviate, or care for the primary diagnosis).[3] The primary intervention was then traced either into an "instant resource book of evidence-based medicine" maintained by the consultant or to other sources (via computerized bibliographic database searching, into the published literature) and classified into one of three categories: (1) interventions whose value (or nonvalue) is established in one or more randomized controlled trials (RCTs) or, better yet, systematic reviews of RCTs; (2) interventions whose face-validity is so great that randomized trials assessing their value were unanimously judged by the team to be both unnecessary and, if they involved placebo treatments, unethical; and (3) interventions in common use but failing to meet either of the preceding two criteria. Of the 109 patients diagnosed that month, 90 (82%) were judged by preset criteria to have received evidence-based interventions. The primary interventions for 53% of patients were based on one or more randomized trials or SRs of trials. An additional 29% of patients received interventions unanimously judged to be based on convincing nonexperimental evidence, and 18% received specific symptomatic and supportive care without substantial evidence that it was superior to some other intervention or to no intervention at all.

This audit confirmed that inpatient general medicine could be evidence based, and similar audits since then have been conducted in various settings around the world and in many different clinical disciplines, including general surgery, hematology, child health, primary care, anesthesia, and psychiatry. The truth is that most patients we encounter have one of just a few common problems, whereas the rare problems

---

[a]In 1963, the estimate was 9.3%. Forsyth G. an enquiry into the drug bill. *Med Care.* 1963;1:10–16.

are thinly spread among many patients. As a result, searching for the evidence that underpins the common problems provides a greater and more useful reward for our effort than quests for evidence about problems we might encounter once a decade. That these studies have found evidence for the most common interventions has validated the feasibility of practising EBM. The key point for readers of this book is to recognize how such audits not only focus on clinical issues that are central to providing high-quality evidence-based care but also provide a natural focus for day-to-day education, helping every member of the team keep up to date.

Evaluating our performance as teachers[b]

We may be interested in evaluating our own EBM teaching skills or in evaluating an EBM workshop or course. Box 8.6 lists some ways of evaluating how we're doing as teachers of EBM. When did we last issue an Educational Prescription (or have one issued to us)? If not recently, why not? Are we helping our trainees learn how to ask focused questions? Are we teaching and modelling searching skills? Our time may be far too limited to provide this training ourselves, but we should be able to find some help for our learners, and we should try to link them with our local librarians (again, if a librarian can join our clinical team, we

---

Box 8.6 A self-evaluation in teaching evidence-based medicine (EBM)

1. When did I last issue an Educational Prescription?
2. Am I helping my trainees learn how to ask focused questions?
3. Are we incorporating question asking and answering into everyday activities?
4. Are my learners writing Educational Prescriptions for me?
5. Am I teaching and modelling searching skills (and making sure that my trainees learn them)?
6. Am I teaching and modelling critical appraisal skills?
7. Am I teaching and modelling the generation of appraisal summaries?
8. Am I teaching and modelling the integration of best evidence with my clinical expertise and my patients' preferences?
9. Am I developing new ways of evaluating the effectiveness of my teaching?
10. Am I developing, sharing, and/or evaluating EBM educational materials?
11. Am I teaching and modelling behaviour change?

8

---

[b]Note that we have placed this evaluation chapter before the chapter on teaching (Chapter 9) because evaluation is the fifth step of practicing EBM. You may want to read Chapter 9 before you read this section on evaluating our performance as teachers.

can share the teaching). Are we teaching and modelling critical appraisal skills, and are we teaching and modelling the generation of appraisal summaries? Are we teaching and modelling the integration of best evidence with our clinical expertise and our patients' preferences? Are we developing new ways of evaluating the effectiveness of our teaching? Particularly important here are the development and use of strategies for obtaining feedback from our students and trainees about our skills and performance in practising and modelling EBM. Finally, are we developing, sharing, and/or evaluating EBM educational materials?

A very useful way of evaluating our performance is to ask our respected colleagues and mentors for feedback. We can invite our colleagues to join our clinical team or to view a video of our teaching performance and to discuss it with us afterward, giving us and them a chance to learn together. At some institutions, a teaching consultation service is available to observe our teaching and to provide us with constructive feedback. We might also seek out a workshop on practicing or teaching EBM to refine our skills further.

Evaluations of strategies for teaching the steps of evidence-based medicine

Up to this point in this chapter, the focus has been on how to evaluate our own practice of evidence-based medicine (EBM). Sometimes, we might be interested in evaluating how EBM is taught in a course or at a workshop. The next section will summarize evidence on strategies for teaching the elements of EBM. We'll use the "PICO" (population/intervention/comparison/outcome) format for our discussion. Note that when we develop our teaching strategies, it is also critical to understand the context in which our learners will be practising EBM and the barriers/facilitators to its practice. There have been several systematic reviews of barriers to EBM practice by clinicians.[4-6] The common barriers that were identified at the level of the clinician include lack of skills in the EBM competencies and lack of access to evidence resources. These are just at the level of the clinician and don't include barriers to its practice at the patient or health care organization levels.

Who are the "patients"?

Who are the targets for our clinical questions? Two groups can be readily identified—the clinicians who practise EBM and the patients they care for. There is an accumulating body of evidence relating to the impact of EBM on undergraduate students and health care providers.

This ranges from SRs of training in the skills of EBM to qualitative research describing the experience of EBM practitioners and barriers they've encountered to implementation. There is a relatively smaller body of evidence about the effect of EBM on patient care or patients' perceptions of their care. We are also starting to see more educational interventions targeting the public and policymakers, highlighting the "spread" of EBM.

What is the intervention (and the control manoeuvre)?

Studies of the effect of teaching EBM are challenging to conduct because not only would they require large sample sizes and lengthy follow-up periods, but it's unethical to generate a comparison group of clinicians who'd be allowed to become out of date and ignorant of life-saving evidence accessible to and known by the evidence-based clinicians in the experimental group. Similarly, it would be tough to get clinicians to agree to an evidence-poor teaching intervention!

In many studies of the impact of EBM, the intervention has proven difficult to define. It's unclear what the appropriate "dose" or "formulation" should be. Some studies use a comprehensive approach to clinical practice while others use training in one of the discrete "microskills" of EBM, such as performing a search of MEDLINE or a critical appraisal. A recent overview of systematic reviews about the effects of teaching EBM identified 16 systematic reviews and 81 individual studies.[7] In the studies included in these reviews, a variety of multicomponent and single-component interventions, including lecturers, online webinars, and journal clubs, were used. Indeed, over the past 10 years, there has been more work done on blended learning approaches including in-person as well as online materials. Some of these interventions were "one off," and some lasted weeks to months. These interventions targeted undergraduates, postgraduates, and various health care providers, including nurses, pharmacists, occupational therapists, and physicians. There were few studies that assessed the entire process of practising EBM and its impact on practice change.[8] It is not clear if developers of the interventions considered barriers to EBM and targeted their interventions to those identified.

What are the relevant outcomes?

Effective EBM interventions will produce a wide range of outcomes. Changes in clinicians' knowledge, attitudes, and skills are relatively easy

8

to detect and demonstrate. Changes in their behaviours may be harder to confirm. As mentioned previously, changes in clinical outcomes are even more challenging to detect. Accordingly, studies demonstrating better patient survival when practice is evidence based (and worse when it is not) are at present limited to the cohort "outcomes research" studies described in this book's Introduction.

As discussed above, the intervention has proven difficult to define, and as a result, the evaluation of whether the intervention has met its goals has been challenging. In the Introduction, we outlined that not all clinicians want or need to learn how to practise all five steps of EBM. We discussed three potential methods for practising EBM, including the doing, using, and replicating modes. "Doers" of EBM practise steps 1 to 5, whereas "users" focus on searching for and applying preappraised evidence. "Replicators" seek advice from colleagues who practise EBM. Although all of us practise in these different modes at various times in our clinical work, our activity will likely fall predominantly into one of these categories. Most clinicians consider themselves users of EBM, and surveys of clinicians show that only approximately 5% believe that learning the five steps of EBM was the most appropriate method for moving from opinion-based medicine to evidence-based medicine.[6,9] The various EBM courses and workshops must therefore address the needs of these different learners. One size cannot fit all! Similarly, if a formal evaluation of the educational activity is required, the instruments used to evaluate whether we've helped our learners reach their goals should reflect the different learners and their goals. Although many questionnaires have been shown to be useful in assessing EBM knowledge and skills, we must remember that the learners, the knowledge, and the skills targeted by these tools may not be similar to our own. For those of you who are interested, we point you to the SR of instruments for evaluating education in evidence-based practice.[10] More than 104 evaluation instruments were identified, with many of these having reasonable validity. The overview of SRs of teaching EBM identified even more outcomes![7] Both reviews highlighted gaps in the field of evaluation, with most tools focusing on EBM knowledge and skills and few tools focusing on assessing behaviours.

It should be noted that innovative methods of evaluation are being used as attention is moving from assessing not just EBM knowledge and skills but to behaviours, attitudes, and clinical outcomes as well. For example, in a study evaluating an EBM curriculum in a family medicine training program, resident–patient interactions were videotaped and analyzed for EBM content.[11] EBM-OSCE (Objective Structured Clinical

Exam) stations have become standard in many medical schools and residency programs. In a high-stakes certification examination in Canada, postgraduate trainees are tested on their ability to practise EBM with standardized patients and with clinical scenarios. More recent studies have also explored the cost effectiveness of various ways to teach EBM, a much needed area of research.[12]

In the previously mentioned overview of SRs of teaching EBM,[7] because of the heterogeneity in outcomes, interventions, and design, a meta-analysis was not done. We summarize the results of the overview briefly here:

- For undergraduate learners, multicomponent interventions increased knowledge, skills, and attitudes toward EBM compared with single-component interventions.

- For postgraduate learners, multicomponent interventions increased critical appraisal skills and integration of evidence into patient decision making.

- For health care providers, multicomponent interventions increased knowledge, skills, attitudes, and behaviours.

- Journal clubs increased knowledge of clinical epidemiology but did not increase critical appraisal skills.

- Seminars/EBM courses increased critical appraisal skills and knowledge.

Although not mentioned in the overview of reviews, qualitative research has confirmed that teaching and learning critical appraisal are enjoyable, and this should not be underestimated in one's working life!!

Some gaps in the literature:

- We haven't been able to identify any studies that looked at sustained use of medical literature over time.

- We haven't found literature on how teaching strategies could be optimized to overcome barriers to the practice of EBM.

- Although we don't expect to find the "magic bullet" for teaching EBM, it would be useful to understand how to optimize the "dose" and "formulation" for different learners.

References

1. Graham ID, Logan J, Harrison MB, Straus SE, Tetroe J, Caswell W, et al. Lost in knowledge translation: time for a map? J Contin Ed Health Prof 2006;26(1):13–24.

2. Cabana MD, Rand CS, Powe NR, Wu AW, Wilson MH, Abboud PA, et al. Why don't physicians follow clinical practice guidelines? A framework for improvement. JAMA 1999;282(15):1458–65.

3. Ellis J, Mulligan I, Rowe J, Sackett DL. Inpatient general medicine is evidence-based. Lancet 1995;346(8972):407–10.

4. Zwolsman S, te Pas E, Hooft L, et al. Barriers to GPs' use of evidence-based medicine: a systematic review. Br J Gen Pract 2012;doi:10.3399/bjgp12x6s2382.

5. Swennen MHJ, van der Heijden GJMG, Boeije HR, et al. Doctors' perceptions and use of evidence-based medicine: a systematic review and thematic synthesis of qualitative studies. Acad Med 2013;88: 1384–96.

6. Ubbink DT, Guyatt GH, Vermeulen H. Framework of policy recommendations for implementation of evidence-based practice: a systematic scoping review. BMJ Open 2013;3:e001881.

7. Young T, Rohwer A, Volmink J, Clarke M. What are the effects of teaching evidence-based health care? Overview of systematic reviews. PLoS ONE 2014;9:e86706.

8. Straus SE, Ball C, McAlister FA, et al. Teaching evidence-based medicine skills can change practice in a community hospital. JGIM 2005;20:340–3.

9. McColl A, Smith H, White P, Field J. General practitioner's perceptions of the route to evidence-based medicine: a questionnaire survey. BMJ 1998;315:361–5.

10. Shaneyfelt T, Baum KD, Bell D, et al. Instruments for evaluating education in evidence-based practice. JAMA 2006;296:1116–27.

11. Ross R, Verdieck A. Introducing an evidence-based medicine curriculum into a family practice residency – is it effective? Acad Med 2003;78:412–17.

12. Maloney S, Nicklen P, Rivers G, et al. A cost-effectiveness analysis of blended versus face-to-face delivery of evidence-based medicine to medical students. J Med Internet Res 2015;17:e182.

Further reading

Straus SE, Tetroe J, Graham ID. Knowledge translation in health care. 2nd ed. Oxford, UK: Wiley Blackwell BMJ; 2013.

9 Teaching evidence-based medicine

Throughout the book, we've provided ideas for teaching methods when they fit with the themes of previous chapters (e.g., the Educational Prescription in Chapter 1, pp. 29 to 32), and you can find them in the index or by scanning the page margins for the Teaching Moments (TM) icon ◑. In this chapter, we've collected other ideas for teaching learners how to practise evidence-based medicine (EBM). We'll describe three main modes for teaching EBM, consider some successes and failures with various teaching methods, and then examine some specific teaching situations.

We are clinical teachers and collectors of teaching methods, not educational theorists. From what we've learned so far about theories of learning, we find ourselves using ideas and methods from several schools of thought, rather than adhering strictly to one theory, such as either cognitive or social constructivism. We present here a collection of the lessons we've gathered from many sources about how to put these principles into practice, focusing on the pragmatics of implementation. In developing ourselves as teachers, we've studied works on teaching,[1-11] yet we have learned more from observing those who taught us, most especially from David Sackett. Dave's generosity of spirit and humanity, his broad and keen intellect, his clear and memorable communication style, and the irreverent enthusiasm with which he pursued rigorous science, compassionate patient care, and learner-centred teaching, all contributed to the ethos of EBM and inspired each of us to follow our career trajectories and to grow as teachers.[12-14] We are grateful to have had his mentorship and dedicate this book and this chapter to passing onto others lessons that he passed onto us.

Three modes of teaching EBM

Although we reckon there may be as many ways to teach EBM as there are teachers, we suggest most of these methods fall into one of three categories or teaching modes: (1) role modelling evidence-based practice, (2) weaving evidence into teaching clinical medicine, and (3) targeting specific EBM skills (Box 9.1).[15]

Box 9.1 Three modes of teaching evidence-based medicine (EBM)

1. Role modelling evidence-based practice:
   a. Learners see evidence as part of good patient care.
   b. Teaching by example—"actions speak louder than words."
   c. Learners see us use judgement in integrating evidence into decisions.
2. Weaving evidence into clinical teaching:
   a. Learners see evidence as part of good clinical learning.
   b. Teaching by weaving—evidence is taught along with other knowledge.
   c. Learners see us use judgement in integrating evidence with other knowledge.
3. Targeting specific skills of evidence-based practice:
   a. Learners learn how to understand evidence and use it wisely.
   b. Teaching by coaching—learners get explicitly coached as they develop.
   c. Learners see us use judgement as we carry out the five EBM steps with them.

The first teaching mode involves role modelling the practice of EBM. For example, when you and a learner see together an ambulatory patient with asymptomatic, microscopic hematuria, you might ask yourself aloud a question about the frequency of underlying causes of this disorder, admit aloud you don't know the full answer, then find and appraise evidence about this topic, and discuss aloud how you'll use the evidence in planning your diagnostic strategy. When we role model evidence-based practice, our learners see us incorporating evidence with other knowledge into clinical decisions, in the authentic context of providing kind and careful care of the whole person.[16] Learners come to see the use of evidence as part of good practice, not something separate from it. We show by our example that we really do it, when we really do it, and how we really do it. Because actions speak louder than words, we might expect role modelling to be among the more effective ways of teaching EBM, although as far as we know this hasn't been studied.

The second teaching mode involves weaving the results of clinical research with other knowledge you teach about a clinical topic. For instance, when you and a learner examine a patient with dyspnea, after teaching how to do percussion of the posterior thorax, you can summarize research results about this finding's accuracy and precision as a test for pleural effusion. When we include research evidence into what we teach about clinical medicine, our learners see us integrating evidence with knowledge from other sources—the biology of human health and disease, the medical humanities, the understanding of systems of health care, the values and preferences of patients, and our clinical expertise, to name a few. Thus, trainees come to see the use of evidence as part of good clinical learning, not something separate from it, all in the context of making real clinical decisions. We might expect this integration and vivid realism would make weaving evidence into clinical teaching to be another very effective teaching mode, although we haven't seen this studied either.

The third mode involves targeted teaching of the skills of evidence-based practice. For instance, when learning about the care of a patient facing newly diagnosed lymphoma, in addition to teaching the "content" of this cancer's prognosis, you can also teach your team members the "process" of how to find and critically appraise studies of prognosis. When we target the skills of EBM, we help our learners build their capacity to independently develop and maintain their clinical competence. Learners come to see using EBM skills as part of lifelong professional development, not an isolated classroom exercise. It is for this third, targeting mode that an increasing number of studies of the effectiveness of educational interventions have been published. Systematic reviews (SRs) of these data have found that while the overall quality of the evidence varies, a variety of teaching interventions have been associated with increases in EBM knowledge and skill; nevertheless, as of yet, no specific intervention has emerged as consistently superior.[17-23] These reviewers and others have recommended that future research provide more detailed descriptions on interventions, provide more explicit grounding of interventions in the learning sciences, and concentrate on multifaceted interventions that use validated assessments and that are genuinely and longitudinally integrated into the curriculum, including the clinical experiences.[24-26]

We use all three modes of teaching EBM, moving from one to another to fit the clinical and teaching circumstances. Each mode requires different preparation and skills, so we may begin our teaching careers feeling more comfortable with one mode than the others. And because good teachers of EBM (or anything else for that matter) are made, not born, with deliberate practice of and purposeful reflection on each mode, we can refine both our skills with each mode and in blending all three.[11] We find that conscientiously using evidence in our practice and teaching (modes 1 and 2) gives us more authenticity to our learners when we teach them about specifically targeted EBM skills (mode 3).

9

Teaching EBM—top 10 successes

Reflecting on what worked well can help us refine our teaching.[27] Here, we collect 10 characteristics about when teaching EBM has worked well.

1. When it centres on real clinical decisions and actions

Since practising EBM begins and ends with patients, it shouldn't surprise you that our most enduring and successful efforts in teaching EBM have been those that centred on the illnesses of patients directly under the care of our learners. The clinical needs of these patients serve as the starting point for identifying our knowledge needs and asking answerable clinical questions that are directly relevant to those needs. By returning to our patients' problems after searching and appraising evidence about them, we can demonstrate how to integrate evidence with other knowledge and our patients' preferences and unique circumstances. When targeting EBM skills in mode 3, if the learning group members are not on the same clinical service and don't share responsibility for the same patients, we can still engage the group in discussing one or more real clinical decisions they've either faced already or expect to face in the future. By centring our teaching on the care of either current or future patients, our trainees learn how to use evidence in its natural context—informing real decisions and actions.

2. When it focuses on learners' actual learning needs

We think teaching means helping learners learn, so we have become students of our students and their ways of learning. Since our learners can vary widely in their motivations, their starting knowledge, their learning prowess and skills, their learning contexts, and available time for learning, we may need to employ a variety of teaching strategies and tactics. One size does not fit all, so in our teaching practices, we need the skills to accurately assess our learners' developmental stage, diagnose their learning needs, and select appropriate teaching interventions. We need to be patient with our learners, adjusting our teaching to match their developmental stage and the pace of their understanding. Since many of our learners will also have externally imposed demands they must satisfy, such as passing written examinations, we need to acknowledge these conflicting demands, help learners cope with them, and adjust our teaching to fit the circumstances.

3. When it balances passive ("diastolic") with active ("systolic") learning

Learning clinical medicine has been described using the analogy of the cardiac cycle, with passive learning devices, such as listening to a lecture, compared with diastolic filling, and active learning devices compared with systolic pumping.[28] Similar to the phases of the cardiac cycle, both kinds of learning are useful, and both work best when used in balance with each other. Passive techniques may be effective for learning some kinds of knowledge (the "know what"), yet only through active methods can we learn how to put this knowledge into action (the "know how"). Reviews of comparative studies in science curricula suggest that using active and inductive learning strategies helps students achieve higher test scores and other improvements and experience lower failure rates compared with students using passive approaches.[29-31] Because most trainees come into our clinical teams having had much more experience in passive learning than in active learning,[32] we find ourselves strongly emphasizing active learning strategies to help restore balance.

4. When it connects "new" knowledge to "old" (what learners already know)

By the time they come into our clinical teams, most of our learners have very large funds of knowledge from both experiential and book learning. Whether teaching in modes 1, 2, or 3, we can stimulate learners with questions to recall knowledge from their memories, which activates this knowledge for use and helps us identify any knowledge gaps or misunderstandings. By connecting the new information we teach to their existing knowledge networks, we help learners comprehend the new lessons better and put them in context. We also help learners reorganize their knowledge into schemes more useful for clinical decision making.[33]

5. When it involves everyone on the team

When learners join our clinical teams, they join two coexisting communities.[9] They share the responsibility for the care of the team's patients, so they join a "community of practice" that faces the same clinical problems and works together toward their solutions. They also share the responsibility to learn whatever is needed for sound clinical decisions, so they join a "community of learning" that faces common learning challenges and works together to meet them. These two communities

241

don't just coexist, they interact—the shared work makes the learning necessary and useful, and the shared learning informs the team's clinical decisions and actions.[9] Beginning students may be unfamiliar with working in these communities, so their seniors need to orient them when they join. When we as teachers divide the work of learning into chunks so that everyone can be involved, we help the team in four ways. First, a broader range of questions can be asked and answered because the work can be shared by several people. Second, when seniors pair up with juniors to help them track down and appraise answers, their capacity for teamwork is reinforced. Third, because every team member can benefit from each team member's efforts, sharing lessons across the team multiplies the learning yields. Fourth, the team's interactive discussions as they learn can help individual team members clarify misconceptions, consolidate the lessons learned, and consider their implications for decision and action. Involving everyone needn't mean that all are assigned equal amounts of work—"Educational Prescriptions" can be handed out in differing amounts, depending on workloads.

6. When it attends to all four domains of learning—affective, cognitive, conative, and psychomotor

First, as we mentioned on pages 23–24, learning can involve strong emotions, whether "positive," such as the joy of discovery or the fun of learning with others, or "negative," such as the fear of being asked a question, the shame of not knowing the answer, or the anger when learning time is squandered. We can help learners grow in the affective domain of learning by helping them acknowledge the feelings of learning and developing appropriate, rather than maladaptive, responses (modes 2 and 3). We can also help learners by showing some of our own feelings, such as our enthusiasm for learning (mode 1).

Second, recall that making sound clinical decisions requires us to recall, think with, and make judgements about several different kinds of knowledge, developed through different ways of knowing—we develop clinical expertise through experience with patient care and with coaching; we develop knowledge of our patients' perspectives and preferences through conversation and working with them; and we develop knowledge of research results through reading and critical appraisal. We can help our learners grow in the cognitive domain of learning by identifying these different sources of knowledge as we teach (mode 2), and by coaching them to refine their abilities to know and learn in each way (mode 3).

Third, learning evidence-based practice involves translating knowledge into action, and the commitment and drive to perform these actions to the best of our abilities. This disposition to act for the benefit of others, combining ethical principles with the striving for excellence and pride in our work, has been termed the "conative domain of learning."[34] We can help our learners grow in this conative domain by our actions, wherein we show our own striving to improve and demonstrate the pragmatics of how to turn new learning into better doing (mode 1). We can also coach our learners on such things as assessing their own performance and developing plans for change (mode 3).

Fourth, learning EBM involves some physical actions, including practical tasks, such as capturing our questions to answer, using search interfaces, and so forth. We can help our learners grow in this psychomotor domain both by role modelling (mode 1) so that our learners see what the actions look like when done well and by explicit coaching (mode 3) so that they get feedback on how they are doing and how to improve.

7. When it matches, and takes advantage of, the clinical setting, available time, and other circumstances

Each patient situation and clinical setting define a different learning context, where things like the severity of illness, the pace of the work, and the available time and person-power all combine to determine what can be learned and when, where, how, and by whom it is learned. Teaching tactics that work well in one setting (e.g., the outpatient clinic) may not fit at all in other settings (e.g., the intensive care unit). We can improve patient- and learner-centred learning by capitalizing on opportunities that present themselves in these different settings *as they occur,* using a mix of modes 1 and 2.

8. When it balances preparedness with opportunism

Just because teaching EBM in modes 1 or 2 may start and end with today's patient, that doesn't mean it can't be well prepared. Instead, we can anticipate many of the questions our learners will ask because they'll arise from the patients, health states, and clinical decisions we encounter frequently in our practice and teaching settings. To prepare for these opportunities, we can gather, appraise, and summarize the evidence we'll use to inform those decisions and then place these summaries at or near the sites of care. By being well prepared, we need only recognize the clinical situations *when* (not *if*) they occur, seize the

9

teaching moment, and guide the learners in understanding and using the evidence. This kind of opportunism can be supplemented by another kind—recognizing teaching opportunities among questions for which we haven't prepared ahead, modeling and involving learners in the steps of asking questions, finding and appraising evidence, and integrating it into our clinical decisions.

9. When it makes explicit how to make judgements, whether about the evidence itself or about how to integrate evidence with other knowledge, clinical expertise, and patient preferences and circumstances

Practising EBM requires us to use judgement when choosing questions, when selecting knowledge resources, when appraising evidence critically, and when integrating the evidence into clinical decisions. Using judgement requires not only that we be able to sort, weigh, and integrate knowledge of different kinds but also that we reflect on the underlying values made visible by our choices. Learning to make these judgements wisely takes time and practice, so it seems sensible to have our learners spend this time well by making this practice deliberate and these discussions explicit. Although medical educational research may not yet have confirmed the value of such an explicit, reflective (also termed "metacognitive") approach, we reckon that the opposite strategy, that of ignoring judgement and abandoning our learners in their quest to develop it, is both ineffective and irresponsible. Thus, when we're teaching in modes 1, 2, or 3, we use an explicit approach in guiding learners through clinical decisions.

10. When it builds learners' lifelong learning abilities

Clinical practice can be thought of as the ultimate open-book test, occurring daily over a lifetime of practice, with the entire world's knowledge potentially available as "the book" for clinicians to use. To develop and sustain the skills to use this knowledge wisely, learners need hard work and coaching—concentrating on such things as reflection, to recognize their own learning needs; resilience, to respond adaptively to their cognitive dissonance; and resourcefulness, to know how to carry out learning on their own.[6] One method to stimulate this process is to make learning multistaged. When we divide the learning into manageable chunks and plan its achievement over several stages, we allow learners to try their hands at each stage, coming to the next encounter both with the learning yield and with experiences that can guide new learning objectives. Multistaged learning also helps with managing time well because on busy clinical services, it is usually easier to schedule several short appointments for learning rather than one large block. Multistaged learning allows learning to be "vertically aligned"—that is, when we return later to the same material, we can reinforce what was learned before and then add new material appropriate to our learners' advancing skills.

Teaching EBM—top 10 failures

To compare with these successes, we present here a collection of 10 mistakes we've either made or seen in the teaching of EBM because reflecting on failures can also help refine one's teaching.[35]

1. When learning how to do research is emphasized over how to use it

2. When learning how to do statistics is emphasized over how to interpret them

These first two mistakes happen when experts in any field of basic science hold the notion that to pragmatically apply the fruits of a science, learners have to master its methods of inquiry. This is demonstrably untrue (doctors save the lives of patients who have suffered a heart attack by prescribing them beta blockers, not by learning how to measure the number of beta receptors in cardiac muscle cells). It is also counter-productive because it requires learners who want to become clinicians to learn the skills of transparently foreign careers, and we shouldn't be surprised by learners' indifference and hostility to courses in statistics and epidemiology. Our recognition of these mistakes explains why there is so little about statistics in this book and why our emphasis throughout is on how to *use* research reports, not how to *generate* them.

3. When teaching EBM is limited only to finding flaws in published research

4. When teaching portrays EBM as substituting research evidence for, rather than adding it to, clinical expertise and patient values and circumstances

These mistakes can occur when any narrow portion of a complex undertaking is inappropriately emphasized to the exclusion of all other

9

portions. In response, learners may develop skills in one step of EBM, such as the ability to find study flaws in critical appraisal, but don't develop any other skills. This hurts learners in two ways. First, by seeing an unbalanced approach to appraising evidence, learners can develop protracted nihilism, a powerful *de*-motivator of evidence-based learning. Second, without learning to follow critical appraisal by integrating evidence sensibly into clinical decisions, learners aren't prepared to act independently on evidence in the future (when their teachers are gone), so they remain dependent on others to interpret evidence for them and tell them how to act.

5. When teaching with or about evidence is disconnected from the team's learning needs about either their patients' illnesses or their own clinical skills

This mistake can happen in several ways, such as when we fail to begin and end our teaching sessions with the learners' patients, when we fail to diagnose either the patients' clinical needs or our learners' resulting learning needs, or when we fail to connect our teaching to our learners' motivations, career plans, or stage of development as clinicians. The resulting disconnect between what we teach and what the learners need to learn usually means not only that the learners won't retain anything we do cover but also that we consume the available learning time before they can learn what they really needed. As such forgone learning opportunities accumulate, our learners fall behind their peers in developing clinical excellence and lifelong learning skills.

6. When the amount of teaching exceeds the available time or the learners' attention

7. When teaching occurs at the speed of the teacher's speech or mouse clicks, rather than at the pace of the learners' understanding

These two mistakes occur when the teacher overestimates the amount that should be covered in the available time. Although teachers' motives needn't be evil—these mistakes can arise simply out of enthusiasm for the subject—the resulting overly long and/or overly fast presentation taxes the learners' abilities to register, comprehend, or retain the material covered. For example, at a recent lecture the speaker showed 96 visually complex slides while talking rapidly during all of the allotted 30 minutes, leaving listeners unable to decode the graphs on one slide before the next was shown, resulting in more of a "shock-and-awe campaign" than a useful learning experience.

8. When the teacher strives for full educational closure by the end of each session, rather than leaving plenty to think about and learn between sessions

The eighth mistake happens when we behave as if learning only occurs during formal teaching sessions. This behaviour is harmful in two ways. First, it cuts off problem solving during the sessions themselves ("We're running out of time, so I want to stop this discussion and give you the right answers."). Second, it prevents or impairs the development of the self-directed learning skills that will be essential for our learners' continuing professional development.

9. When it humiliates learners for not already knowing the "right" fact or answer

10. When it bullies learners to decide or act based on fear of others' authority or power, rather than based on authoritative evidence and rational argument

These entries are included here because they are still commonplace among medical education programs, and at some of these institutions, they remain a source of twisted pride. Such treatment of learners by their teachers is not simply wrong in human terms, it is counterproductive. First, the resulting shame and humiliation learners feel will strongly discourage the very learning that the teacher's ridicule was meant to stimulate.[36-38] Second, in adapting to the rapid loss of trust and safety in the learning climate, learners will start employing strategies to hide their true learning needs and protect themselves from their teachers, undermining future learning and teaching efforts. Understandably, learners with prior experiences of these behaviours may be very reluctant to even start the practice of EBM by asking a question because it could expose them to the potential threat of repeated abuse. Contrast this with the actions of our colleague David Pencheon, who asks new medical students questions of increasing difficulty until they respond with "I don't know." Upon hearing these words, he rewards them with a box of candy and tells them that these are the three most important words in medicine.[39]

9

Having considered these successes and failures, we'll turn next to ways to incorporate teaching of EBM into some learning encounters that are commonly present in the education of clinicians in many countries. We'll then take two examples of these opportunities to explore in more detail.

Teaching and learning EBM on an inpatient service

Hospitals comprise several different clinical settings, such as general or specialty wards, intensive care units and emergency departments, each with their own opportunities and challenges for learning and teaching.[40] Yet, across hospital settings, there are several common types of teaching rounds, seven of which we've summarized in Table 9.1. Although they differ, these rounds share several features, including severe constraints on learners' time and the innumerable interruptions. Little surprise, then, that for most of these types of rounds, much of our EBM teaching is by modes 1 and 2, modelling evidence-based practice and weaving evidence into teaching clinical topics, rather than by mode 3.

We hope that Table 9.1 is self-explanatory, so we will confine this text to describing the EBM strategies and resources that we use during them. During rounds on newly admitted patients ("posttake" or "admission" rounds), there is usually time only for quick demonstrations of evidence-based bits of the clinical examination and how to get from pretest to posttest probabilities of the leading diagnosis (in about 2–5 minutes), or for introducing concise (one page or two to four smartphone screens) and instantly available (within <15 seconds) synopses of evidence about the key diagnostic and treatment decisions that have been, are being, or ought to be carried out.

Can synopses of evidence really get there that fast? Yes, by using either or both of two strategies: First, anticipate the clinical decisions you're likely to encounter, then find (or make) concise synopses of the evidence that can inform those decisions and carry them with you. We've seen several formats used, including structured synopses on paper in a binder (Dave Sackett always carried along his "Big Red Book"),[41] on notebook computer carried by a cart,[42,43] in concise summaries carried on a tablet or smartphone,[44] and both summaries and articles stored on a portable USB (universal serial bus) flash drive. Second, as information technology advances, more of us may find ourselves working in health systems that provide instant electronic access to evidence resources as outlined in Ch. 2. When the evidence isn't so quickly to hand, we can write

Table 9.1 Incorporating evidence-based medicine (EBM) into inpatient rounds

Type of round	Objectives*	Evidence of highest relevance	Restrictions†	Strategies
"Posttake" or admission rounds (after every period on call, all over the hospital, by postcall team and consultant)	Decide on working diagnosis and initial therapy of newly admitted patients	Accuracy and precision of the clinical examination and other diagnostic tests; efficacy and safety of initial therapy	Time, motion (can't stay in one spot), and fatigue of team after call	Demonstrate evidence-based (EB) examination and getting from pretest to posttest probability; carry a personal digital assistant (PDA) or a loose-leaf book with synopses of evidence; write Educational Prescriptions; add a clinical librarian to the team
Morning report (every day, sitting down, by entire medical service)	Briefly review new patients and discuss and debate the process of evaluating and managing one or more of them	Accuracy and precision of the clinical examination and other diagnostic tests; efficacy and safety of initial therapy	Time	Educational Prescriptions for foreground questions (and fact follow-ups for background questions); give 1–2 minute summaries of critical appraisal topics
Work rounds (every day, on one or several wards, by trainees)	Examine every patient and determine their current clinical state; review and (re)order tests and treatments	Accuracy and precision of diagnostic tests; efficacy and safety of ongoing prescriptions (Rx), and interactions	Time and motion	In electronic records, create links between test results or Rx orders and the relevant evidence

Continued

9

Table 9.1 Incorporating evidence-based medicine (EBM) into inpatient rounds—cont'd

Type of round	Objectives*	Evidence of highest relevance	Restrictions†	Strategies
Consultant walking rounds (one to three times a week, on one or several wards, by trainees and consultant)	As in work rounds, but objectives vary widely by consultant	As in work rounds, plus those resulting from individual consultant's objectives	Time, relevance to junior members ("shifting dullness")	Model how to explain evidence to patients and incorporate into decisions (e.g., likelihood of being helped versus harmed [LHH])
Review rounds (or "card flip") (every day, sitting down and at the bedside, by trainees and consultants)	Forty-five-second reviews of each patient's diagnosis, Rx, progress, and discharge plans; identification of complicated patients who require bedside examination and more discussion	Wherever the Educational Prescriptions have led the learners	Time	Educational Prescriptions for foreground questions (and fact follow-ups for background questions); give 1- to 2-minute summaries of critical appraisal; audit whether you are following through on EB care
Social issues rounds (periodically, by trainees and a host of other professionals)	Review of each patient's status, discharge plan, referral, and posthospital follow-up	Efficacy and safety of community services and social interventions	Time, availability of relevant participants, and enormous burden of paperwork	Ask other health care providers to provide synopses of evidence for what they routinely propose

Preceptor rounds ("pure education") (one or two times a week, by learners [often stratified] and teacher)	Develop and improve skills for clinical examination and presentation	Accuracy and precision of the clinical examination	Time, teacher's energy and other commitments	Practise presentations and feedback; use evidence about clinical examination; Educational Prescriptions for foreground questions (and fact follow-ups for background questions); give concise summaries on critical appraisal
"Down time" or "dead space" during any round	Wait for the elevator or for a report or for a team member to show up, catch up, answer a page, get off the phone, find a chart, etc.	No limit	Imagination and ingenuity	Insert synopses of evidence, either from recent Educational Prescriptions (and fact follow-ups) or from preappraised evidence resources

*Increasingly, all rounds include the objective of discharging patients as soon as possible.
†All rounds require confidentiality when discussions of individual patients occur in public areas.

9

"Educational Prescriptions" to be filled after admission rounds, as we described on pages 29–32. In many centres, the individual teams' posttake rounds are supplemented by a service-wide, sit-down "morning report." Since not every admission needs to be discussed, this round can focus on patients who have the most to teach us.

"Work rounds," during which the team's trainees carry out the rapid, detailed, bedside review of patients' problems and progress and the review and ordering of their diagnostic tests and treatments, provide a challenging yet fruitful setting for teaching in mode 1 or 2. Most challenging perhaps is that the consultant/attending teacher is not present, and yet the teacher can still influence the team's learning during these rounds by using the following three strategies: First, once the team has adopted the approach of integrating evidence into decisions when the attending is present, we can encourage its continued use by debriefing them on their successes and failures in applying evidence to decisions and on questions they had posed during work rounds and by helping them to find evidence-based answers the whole team can use. Second, we can help our entire team get access to the evidence synopses we use when we are there, either by sharing them (e.g., handing them a one-page paper synopsis, or texting the weblink to their smartphones) or by showing them how to access the resources themselves (e.g., providing URLs for filtered resources). Third, in some centres the information systems that record patients' clinical, laboratory, and treatment data are being linked to electronic "pop up" guidelines or summaries of evidence that can help team members take appropriate action.

"Consultant walking rounds" provide an excellent opportunity for the consultant to model how to combine evidence with patients' values and expectations in making management decisions. For example, the consultant might take 5 to 10 minutes to demonstrate how to use the likelihood of being helped versus harmed (LHH) by a treatment under consideration that we showed you in Chapter 4. These rounds also provide great opportunities to teach in mode 2, for example, by incorporating evidence about the accuracy of findings of volume depletion along with teaching how to choose the initial intravenous fluid for a patient with hypovolemia.

Many consultants (some of whom still keep note cards on each patient) lead short (<1 hour), frequent (e.g., daily, when not "on take") "review rounds" (sometimes called the *card flip*) of all patients on the service. This has been most fruitful for us when we held it in a work/seminar room right on or near the wards. Patients are summarized in four quick phrases (what they've got, what we're doing about it, how they are doing, when and where they are going), and this quick review is interrupted for only two reasons. The first reason is when a patient is so sick or his or her condition is so unstable or problematic that he or she needs to be examined by the whole team. The second interruption is for evidence-based learning. These may be precipitated by any team member and are of three types: first, challenges to provide evidence that the evaluation or management decisions being made for a patient are valid and appropriate; second, quick responses, usually with evidence synopses, to earlier challenges from previous rounds; and third, very brief demonstrations of the critical appraisal or application of evidence to specific patients.

" 'Pure' education rounds" are conducted after the patients have been cared for, and the luxuries of relaxed time and choice of topic are then enjoyed. Topics of relevance to EBM include thorough bedside evaluations of the techniques, accuracy, and precision of the clinical examination; detailed learner-led discussions of how they found and appraised evidence; and detailed explanation and practice of skills, such as generating patient-specific numbers needed to treat (NNTs) and numbers needed to harm (NNHs). When these rounds are directed to new clinical clerks, they can include mastery of the orderly, thorough presentation of patients on the service, along the lines shown in Box 9.2.

Finally, all rounds of teams of size n are peppered with "down times" or "dead spaces" that interrupt the learning process and annoy at least $(n - 1)$ of its members. Rather than permitting learning to decelerate or be replaced by thoughts of lunch and sore backs, teachers can seize the moment and insert narrow "slices" of evidence, instead of the "whole pie,"[45] from a recent evidence-based journal or website visit or perhaps from a previously prepared evidence synopsis. Because no learner wants to be excluded from receiving these learning slices, this tactic encourages team members to avoid causing future down time.

Teaching and learning EBM in the outpatient clinic

Time both hampers and favours teaching in the outpatient setting. On the one hand, individual outpatient appointments are short, constraining both the number and breadth of clinical and learning issues that can be addressed during any single visit.[46] On the other hand, outpatient illnesses and their care typically occur over more than one visit, often over months or even years, thereby providing lengthy interludes for extensive learning.[47] Just as with inpatient services, the outpatient setting is particularly well suited to teaching in modes 1 and 2, role modelling,

9

Box 9.2 A guide for learners presenting an "old" patient at follow-up rounds

The presentation should summarize the following in 2 minutes:
1. The patient's name
2. The patient's age
3. The patient's gender
4. The patient's occupation/social role
5. When the patient was admitted (or transferred) to the service
6. The clinical problem(s) that led to admission (or transfer) (A clinical problem can be a symptom, a sign, a cluster of symptoms and signs, a clinical syndrome, an event, an injury, a test result, a diagnosis, a psychological state, a social predicament, etc.)
7. The number of active problems the patient has at present:
8. Its most important symptoms, if any
9. Its most important signs, if any
10. The results of diagnostic tests or other evaluations
11. The explanation (diagnosis or health state) for the problem
12. The treatment plan instituted for the problem
13. The response to this treatment plan
14. The future and contingency plans for this problem
(Repeat 8 to 14 for each active problem.)
15. Your plans for discharge, posthospital care, and follow-up
16. Whether you've filled the fact follow-up or educational prescription that you requested when this patient was admitted (to better understand the background of this patient's condition or the foreground of how best to care for this patient, respectively). If so:
17. How you found the relevant evidence
18. What you found—the clinical bottom line from that evidence
19. Your critical appraisal of that evidence for its validity, importance, and applicability
20. How that critically appraised evidence will alter your care of that (or the next similar) patient; if not, when you are going to fill it.

---

and interweaving evidence with other topics. The types of rounds that occur in outpatient areas are summarized in Table 9.2.

The "clinic conferences," typically devoted to reviewing the diagnosis and management of common outpatient disorders, can abandon passive annual lectures and devote themselves to reviewing and discussing new evidence that guides key clinical decisions for these conditions, emphasizing the use of preappraised or filtered resources. Participants can make concise summaries of the evidence, or review and update the prior years' versions, then store these summaries nearby for ongoing use in their practices. Active learning occurs, and senior trainees can be asked to

Table 9.2 Incorporating evidence-based medicine (EBM) into outpatient rounds

Type of round	Objectives	Evidence of highest relevance	Restrictions*	Strategies
Clinic conference (before or after each half-day session, by small groups of learners and attendings)	Review the diagnosis and management of common outpatient disorders	Manifestations of disease, differential diagnosis, pretest probability, accuracy and precision of diagnostic tests, efficacy and safety of prescriptions (Rx)	Time, tardiness, and duties elsewhere	Educational Prescriptions for foreground questions (and fact follow-ups for background questions); use, make, or update concise summaries of evidence, such as critically appraised topics (CATs)
Preceptorship during initial visits	Decide on working diagnosis and therapy	Accuracy and precision of clinical examination and diagnostic tests; efficacy and safety of initial therapy	Time, incomplete information	Demonstrate evidence-based (EB) examination and getting from pretest to posttest probability; provide preassembled evidence summaries on diagnostic tests and initial Rx; write Educational Prescriptions
Preceptorship during follow-up visits	Review current status and adjust ongoing therapy	Long-term prognosis; efficacy and safety of alternative treatment options; harms from treatment	Time and changing patient needs	Model incorporation of patients' values, e.g., using likelihood of being helped versus harmed (LHH); fill Educational Prescriptions
Ambulatory morning report	Review case of particular outpatient(s)	Anything; most common are diagnostic tests and treatment options	Time; interruptions; widely varying levels of experience	Hold session in room with access to evidence resources; write and fill Educational Prescriptions; review old and new evidence summaries; give 1-minute summaries on critical appraisal, number needed to treat (NNT), etc.

*All rounds require confidentiality when discussions of individual patients occur in public areas.

9

help their junior colleagues "learn the ropes" of how to take part in these processes.

Initial outpatient visits share objectives and constraints with "posttake" rounds on new inpatient admissions, so the same strategies apply. These are quick demonstrations of evidence-based bits of the clinical examination and how to get from pretest to posttest probabilities of the initial diagnosis, plus instantly available (<15 seconds) evidence about key diagnostic and treatment decisions that have been, are being, or ought to be carried out.

Follow-up visits usually occur long enough after initial visits to allow learners to accomplish substantial problem-based learning between visits, and this can even be in multiple stages. When the learner first encounters an ambulatory patient, the teacher can coach him or her on the process of asking an answerable clinical question about one of the patient's problems and writing an educational prescription. At subsequent clinic sessions (and before the patient's follow-up visit) the teacher can review the learner's search strategies and critical appraisal of the evidence found. At the time of patient follow-up, the teacher and the learner can discuss how to integrate the evidence into clinical decisions and actions. The learner can be observed having a discussion with the patient around this evidence, with feedback from the teacher on the learner's approach to incorporation of relevant evidence in shared decision making. The learner can then be asked to write a concise summary of the evidence, which the teacher and learner can review at another clinical session. Learning in this way doesn't take long at each stage (usually <5 minutes) and yet, over time, leads to cumulative development of EBM skills.

Finally, some teaching outpatient departments hold "morning reports" similar to those held on the inpatient service. They labour under the same restrictions but also offer the same rich variety of opportunities for teaching and learning.

Writing structured summaries of evidence-based learning episodes

At several points in the above discussion, we've mentioned the idea of writing or using a structured summary of evidence to aid our learning. Over the years, we've used or heard about several different structures, but the one we find ourselves using most often is the critically appraised topic (CAT) (Box 9.3). A CAT is a structured, one-page summary of the results of an evidence-based learning effort, in which a patient's illness

---

Box 9.3 Writing structured summaries of evidence-based learning, or critically appraised topics (CATs)

Why use written summaries or CATs?
1. To summarize and consolidate our learning
2. To make our learning cumulative, not duplicative
3. To share our learning efforts with others on our team
4. To refine our EBM skills

How should we structure evidence summaries or CATs?

Title—declarative sentence that states the clinical bottom line

Clinical Question—four (or three) components of the foreground question that started it all

Clinical Bottom Line—concise statement of best available answer(s) to the question

Evidence Summary—description of methods and/or results in concise form (e.g., table)

Comments—about evidence (e.g., limitations) or how to use it in your own setting

Citation(s)—include evidence appraised and other resources, if appropriate

Appraiser—so you'll know who did the appraising when you return to it later

Date CAT was "born"/Expiration date—so folks will know when to look again

---

stimulates a learner's question, for which the learner finds evidence, appraises the evidence, and decides whether and how to use that evidence in the care of the patient.[48] Because of its "quick and dirty" nature, a CAT may have limitations. The evidence found and selected for use may not be all there is or even the best there is (thus, a CAT is *not* a systematic review). Because the emphasis is on whether and how to use the evidence in one's own practice setting, the CAT may or may not apply to many or even any other settings (therefore, a CAT is *not* a practice guideline). A CAT might contain errors of calculation or appraisal judgements and is, thus, not guaranteed to be error-free or permanent.

Despite these limitations, we find writing CATs helps us in four ways: First, writing down on one page the question, the answer, and the evidence that supports the answer requires us to summarize the key lesson(s) from an episode of evidence-based learning. Writing a concise summary exercises and disciplines our ability to distill the gist of that learning episode, to *consolidate* our learning, helping us get the most out of it.[49] Second, since many important questions are about common disorders and their management, we can expect to need the knowledge more than

9

once. By storing a CAT and retrieving it later, we can make our learning efforts *cumulative* (starting from where we left off last time) rather than *duplicative* (starting all over again). Third, by sharing CATs with others on our clinical team, they can learn from our efforts, too, so learning can multiply. Keep in mind that CATs are most useful to those who make them. Fourth, with repetition and coaching, writing CATs can help us refine our EBM skills.

Incorporating EBM into existing educational sessions

In the foregoing discussion, we've emphasized strategies and tactics for individual clinical teachers who want to add evidence to the mix of what they teach, whether in modes 1, 2, or 3. Some of us have the added responsibility of planning how to introduce EBM into existing educational sessions and conferences, so we address here some of the considerations in doing this, illustrating with two common situations—morning report and journal club.

Morning report

In many centres, the individual team's postcall rounds are supplemented by a service-wide conference called *morning report.* We've witnessed more than 72 variations of this conference in our travels, although most share six characteristics: (1) most of the senior residents on the clinical service are present, including chief resident(s); (2) faculty who come often include the program director and/or departmental chair; (3) from one to a few recent admissions are presented, although they vary in freshness; (4) the cases are selected for their potential educational value; (5) the discussions vary widely, but usually focus on the initial diagnosis and treatment of the presented patients' conditions; and, (6) follow-up on prior discussed cases can be presented, with occasional educational extras.[50]

The morning report has several features that make it uniquely attractive as a place to start integrating EBM into the program's curriculum. Clinical learners present real patients with real illnesses and discuss real clinical decisions that need to be made in real time. If a safe and stimulating learning climate has been established, learners can identify what they do and don't know yet to make these decisions wisely, yielding many questions that could be asked. Because the morning report occurs repeatedly, its multiple sessions allow learning to be multistaged. As evidence and other knowledge are learned and shared among those who attend, the judgements involved in integrating and applying the new knowledge can be explicitly addressed. Given the high visibility of the conference, particularly when it's actively supported by the departmental leadership, learners can see the importance placed on learning clinical medicine in evidence-based ways and the development of lifelong learning skills. Comparing these features to the list of 10 successes in teaching EBM discussed earlier shows how much potential success that the morning report could have.

However, the morning report may also present several challenges to incorporating EBM, including the following five: First, if those who run the morning report have other goals for the session, such as using the time for record keeping duties, these competing objectives can consume learning time, destroy the learning climate, or derail the learning process altogether. Second, if cases are not presented concisely, so much time can be spent sorting through the clinical data that little time is left for learning, including learning how to inform decisions with evidence. Third, if the learning climate is unsafe, or if learners' ability to ask questions is reduced, then few of the learners' actual knowledge gaps may get asked as questions. Fourth, teacher or learner inexperience with EBM may lead some participants to retreat to pathophysiologic rationale or personal experience when deciding between test or treatment strategies, rather than risk exposing their rudimentary EBM skills by considering evidence to inform their decisions. Specifically, poor question formulation may lead the group's learning astray, poor searching may frustrate attempts to find current best evidence, and poor critical appraisal skills may lead to the unwise use of flawed evidence in decisions. Fifth, in some centres, those who attend the morning report change very frequently, which confounds attempts to make learning multistaged, and might require repeated reorientation to how to use EBM in the morning report, as skills can drift between rotations.

Despite these challenges, our own and others' experiences suggest that the morning report can become a popular and enduring conference in which to incorporate EBM.[51,52] Although occasionally we might model evidence-based practice, in mode 1, the morning report is well suited mostly for weaving evidence into teaching clinical medicine (mode 2) and for targeted teaching of EBM skills (mode 3). Reflecting on how we've taught in mode 3 during the morning report, we find that we emphasize some skills (e.g., asking questions and integrating the evidence with other knowledge into decisions) while mentioning but not emphasizing other skills (e.g., searching or critical appraisal), as outlined in Table 9.3. We've seen others put different emphasis on various EBM

9

Table 9.3 Developing evidence-based medicine (EBM) skills in and out of morning report

EBM skill	During morning report	Elsewhere
Asking Questions	In context: cases, decisions; model and see modelled; question drills; practise and provide feedback.	Read materials on how to ask answerable questions; attend how-to sessions; one-on-one coaching; see modelled elsewhere.
Searching for Evidence	Review searches briefly; explain options briefly; invite clinical librarian; refine, not learn anew.	Read about searching; attend how-to sessions; one-on-one coaching; see modelled elsewhere.
Critical Appraisal	Discuss appraisal briefly; use teaching scripts about selected portions; refine, not learn anew.	Read about appraisal; attend how-to sessions; one-on-one coaching; see modelled elsewhere.
Integration into Decisions	In context: cases, decisions; make judgements explicit; integrate values explicitly; identify factors to weigh.	Read about integration; attend how-to sessions; one-on-one coaching; see modelled elsewhere.
Self-Evaluation	Model, esp. at beginning; use checklists; increase reflection, self-awareness, insight; group feedback.	Read about self-evaluation; attend how-to sessions; one-on-one coaching; see modelled elsewhere.

skills, sometimes devoting whole sessions of the morning report to searching or critical appraisal.

To help you prepare to successfully introduce EBM into your morning report, we suggest these following six manoeuvres. First, find and cultivate allies who will work with you, and advocate for an evidence-based approach to learning during the morning report. Some may be in your program, such as chief residents and faculty, and others may be in other disciplines, including librarians, statisticians, and clinical pharmacists. Second, negotiate teaching and learning EBM to be part of the goals and methods of the morning report, by meeting with or becoming the folks who run the conference at your institution. This may take repeated efforts at persuasion, so be persistent. Third, if possible, simultaneously negotiate the use of group learning techniques and the development of a healthy learning climate into your morning report because they are both very important to success.[53] Fourth, help assemble the infrastructure needed to learn, practise, and teach in evidence-based ways, including quick access to evidence resources and opportunities to learn more about EBM skills outside of the morning report. Fifth, prepare some learning materials for EBM, including introductory materials on how to get started, samples of concise evidence summaries, your own CATs or those from evidence-based preappraised sources, and concise explanations of methods underlying the practice of EBM. Sixth, refine your own skills further in facilitating group discussions and in teaching EBM, whether by getting local coaching or by attending a course in how to teach EBM.

On the first day of the new era, use most of the morning report session to get the group off to a great start, using six tactics. First, identify the main learning goals for your morning report and how EBM fits in—ours are "to improve our abilities to think through our cases with explicit clinical reasoning and to learn from our cases with evidence-based medicine." Second, have participants assess their current skills for each main learning goal, both globally and for each skill. Try the "double you" format: "How comfortable do *you* feel with *your* ability to … ?" Don't forget to celebrate learners' courage when they acknowledge they need help. Third, have participants set specific goals for learning EBM during the morning report on this rotation, taking care to help them set specific goals that are realistic and focused on their own learning needs. Fourth, negotiate the specific formats you'll use to achieve those learning goals, including issues about the case discussions (e.g., How detailed should presentations be? How focused should the discussion be?), about the EBM portions (e.g., How many questions should we aim to formulate? How often should each learner present an "educational prescription"?), and about how much time you'll spend on each. Fifth, negotiate the ground rules for the group's learning efforts in the morning report, including both general issues and any specific to the use of evidence. (See suggestions in "Integrating EBM into 4-year medical school curriculum—a worked example" on page 271.) Sixth, plan when in the rotation you'll revisit the group's learning objectives and adjust the group's methods—we usually do it both at midcycle and at the end of the rotation.

Once your morning report is up and running, using a combination of case discussions and Educational Prescriptions (see pages 29–32), you may find the following six tactics useful: First, during the case presentations, listen "with both ears" to diagnose both the case and the learner, staying alert to both verbal and nonverbal cues. We use a list of common types of clinical questions (see pages 24–25) to help us spot clinical issues and learning needs. Second, help the group select one or a few issues of the case to discuss well, rather than aiming to

9

cover the entire case superficially. This allows the group to pool its knowledge and find its knowledge gaps, on the way to making sound and explicitly informed decisions. Third, help learners articulate these knowledge gaps as answerable clinical questions, and guide them explicitly in the selection of which questions to pursue. Fourth, as learners report their Educational Prescriptions, listen carefully to select one (or a very few) teaching point(s) to make about applying this evidence for the decision at hand. Fifth, if needed, be ready to provide a brief (2- to 5-minute) explanation of one aspect of critical appraisal that has special bearing on the evidence at hand, referring those interested in learning more to sources outside of the morning report. Sixth, when debriefing the chief residents after the morning report about their teaching skills, include teaching EBM along with the other topics in your coaching.

Journal club

In many clinical centres, journal clubs run like Cheynes-Stokes breathing, alternating between a few quick gasps and prolonged apneic inactivity. Many seem to confuse newness with importance, so on a rotating schedule, the participants are asked to summarize the latest issues of preassigned journals. This means that the choice of topics is driven not by patients' or learners' needs, but, instead, by the choices made by investors, investigators, and editors regarding which products get studied or which get published or by the postal workers and web servers who determine which journals get delivered. Little wonder, then, that so many learners find their journal clubs suffocating.

Yet some journal clubs are flourishing,[54] and a growing number of them are explicitly designed and conducted along EBM lines.[55-59] In the Introduction, we also mentioned the growth of Twitter journal clubs, which allow shared learning to happen across countries in some cases.[a] In the many variations we've run, seen, or read about, three different learning goals can be identified: (1) learning about the best evidence to inform clinical decisions, (2) learning about important new evidence that should change our practice, and (3) building EBM skills. Although journal clubs can have more than one learning goal, several of the curricular choices made will depend on which goal is

---

[a]Note that technology has impacted teaching opportunities in a variety of ways from promoting sharing of articles electronically to hosting journal clubs via webinars/Skype. We are only limited by our imagination in how we can exploit technology to enhance EBM teaching.

preeminent (Table 9.4). Although departments will vary in the choices they make, many will recognize that taking the "skills-driven" approach first will lead to greater subsequent success with the "needs-driven" or "evidence-driven" versions.

To help you prepare to successfully introduce EBM into your journal club, we suggest the following six manoeuvres: First, find and cultivate the allies, whether in your department or elsewhere, who will help you achieve your aims. Second, negotiate teaching and learning EBM to be one of the main goals of the journal club, either by meeting with or by becoming those who run the conference. While you're at it, try to negotiate departmental consensus on which of the three learning goals listed in Table 9.4 will be preeminent at your institution. Third, negotiate the use of group learning techniques and the development of a healthy learning climate into your journal club. Fourth, help assemble the infrastructure needed to learn, practice, and teach in evidence-based ways, including quick access to evidence resources and opportunities to learn more about EBM skills outside of journal club. Fifth, prepare some learning materials for EBM, including introductory materials on how to get started, samples of concise evidence summaries, your own CATs or those from evidence-based preappraised sources, and even concise explanations of methods underlying the practice of EBM. Sixth, refine further your own skills in facilitating group discussions and in teaching EBM, whether by getting local coaching or by attending a course in how to teach EBM.

No matter how the learning goals in Table 9.4 are balanced, we've noticed that most evidence-based journal clubs appear to be based on either a three-session cycle or a two-session cycle. In the three-session model, each journal club session can be thought of as consisting of three parts, as described below.

In Part 1, journal club members identify some learning needs to be addressed in the future. In the case of a "needs-driven" group, this can take the form of learners presenting cases where they faced uncertainty in clinical decisions, continuing until there is group consensus that a particular problem is worth the time and effort necessary to find its solution. In the case of an "evidence-driven" group, group members can debate which part of their field they most need to update next. In the case of a "skills-driven" group, the members would discuss and decide which skill for evidence-based practice they most need to develop or refine. No matter which of these three approaches is taken, the group poses one or more answerable clinical questions (usually foreground ones, as mentioned on pages 21–23) with which to start the evidence-based

9

Table 9.4 Three (potentially competing) goals for evidence-based journal clubs

	"Needs driven"	"Evidence driven"	"Skills-driven"
What is the main learning goal?	Learn how best to handle patient problems that are common, serious, or vexing.	Learn about advances in medical knowledge that should change our practice.	Learn the skills for evidence-based practice.
What group learning needs are identified?	Group members identify what patient problems they need most help with.	Group members identify in what aspects or field they aim to keep current.	Group members identify what skills for evidence-based practice they need most to refine.
What type of evidence is valued most?	Current best evidence useful for solving problems, of several types (see Box 1.2 on p. 25), even if not brand new or not strong.	Recent advances in the field that are valid, important, and applicable enough to change our practice (i.e., both new and strong).	Evidence that best allows learners to develop the skills they need, of broad range of types (see Box 1.2 on p. 25), even if not brand new or not strong.
Who should select topics and types of evidence?	All participants who share responsibility for solving patient problems.	All participants who share responsibility for staying current.	Members (usually faculty) responsible for finding learning needs and helping learners develop their skills.
Which EBM teaching mode is preeminent?	Mode 2 (learning good clinical practice in evidence-based ways).	Mode 2 (developing current awareness in evidence-based ways).	Mode 3 (learning EBM skills).

learning episode. Group members take responsibility (either voluntarily or on rotation) for performing a search for evidence to be used—whether the best available for the problem, the newest strong evidence for the field segment, or a useful teaching example for the skill. Groups may have members do this in pairs or triads, so more experienced members can teach skills to newer folks.

In Part 2, the results of the evidence search on the previous session's problem, field segment, or skill are electronically shared in the form of the abstracts of four to six SRs, original articles, or other evidence. Club members decide which one or two pieces of evidence are worth studying, and arrangements are made to get copies of the clinical question and evidence to all members well in advance of the next meeting.

Part 3 is the main part of the journal club and it comprises the critical appraisal of the evidence found in response to a clinical question posed two sessions ago and selected for detailed study last session. This segment often begins with the admission that most learners haven't read the articles, so time (6–10 minutes) can be provided for everyone to see if they can determine the validity and clinical applicability of one of the articles, reinforcing rapid critical appraisal. After that interlude, the evidence is critically appraised for its validity, importance, and applicability, and a decision is made about whether and how it could be applied to the patient problems (for "needs-driven" groups), whether and how it should change current practice (for "evidence-driven" groups), or whether and how it can build skills for evidence-based practice (for "skills driven" groups). Because this is the "pay-off" part of the journal club, members may need to be guided to complete Parts 1 and 2 quickly enough so there's time for Part 3. The order of these three parts of the journal club could be reversed, depending on local preferences.

Alternatively, evidence-based journal clubs can be built on a two-session cycle, with only two of the three elements—question development and evidence appraisal.[58] This omits the consideration of and selection from the search output, which may fit learners who have already mastered searching and selecting. The two-session cycle allows more questions to be addressed over a year's calendar, without increasing the duration of each session.

These two conferences—morning report and journal club—illustrate many of the considerations involved when reorienting existing conferences along evidence-based lines. In a more general and explicit form, we've gathered in Box 9.4 our favourite 20 questions to ask when integrating EBM into a conference, grouped into issues of persons, places, times, things, and ideas.

9

Box 9.4 Twenty questions for integrating evidence-based medicine (EBM) into a learning session

---

Persons

Who will be the learners, and what are their learning abilities and needs?
Who will be the teachers, and what are their teaching strengths and passions?
Who will need to serve as allies or permission-givers for this to succeed?
What conversations and relationships need to be developed for this to succeed?

Places

Where will this learning session be held?
How might the physical space help or hinder learning?
How can the physical space be altered to optimize learning?

Times

When and for how long will this learning session be held?
Can the sessions be scheduled to support multiple learning stages?
How much time will teachers and learners need to prepare for this session?
How much time will learners need after this session to receive feedback and to reflect upon, consolidate, clarify, and extend their learning?
How much time will teachers need after this session to give feedback and to reflect upon, cultivate, and refine their teaching?

Things

What resources need to be present during the learning session?
What resources need to be available for teachers and learners before and after the session?
How should participants summarize their evidence-based learning (e.g., critically appraised topics [CATs] or Educational Prescriptions?)
What tools of measurement, assessment, and evaluation will be used for this session?

Ideas

How well does EBM fit with the other goals of this learning session?
How can the learning climate be optimized for an evidence-based approach?
Which modes of teaching EBM should be emphasized in this session?
How many of the 10 features of success in teaching EBM can be included, and how many of the 10 mistakes in teaching EBM can be avoided?

Integrating EBM into a curriculum

Some of us are also responsible for introducing EBM into the curricula of undergraduate or graduate medical educational programs.[60-63] For those who want to learn more about curricula in general and how to develop, implement, and evaluate them, we refer you to other works on these topics.[64-69]

Learners need to learn not only how to practise each EBM step but also when to do each step and how to integrate EBM with the other tasks of clinical work. In this way, learning EBM resembles learning other complex "clinical process" skills, such as the medical interview and the physical examination. Learning such complex undertakings requires not only starting with a good introduction but also revisiting the field numerous times building on those experiences that came before. This learning trajectory describes an ascending and outwardly curving spiral, allowing each return to subjects to be vertically aligned with prior teaching.[70]

How can we start building this vertically aligned spiral trajectory that integrates EBM into a curriculum? We'll illustrate our suggestions using the 4-year undergraduate medical curriculum template found in many North American medical schools. Since Flexner's time, these 4 years have usually comprised 2 years of preclinical study separate from 2 years of clinical rotations.[71]

As you build or revise your curriculum, we suggest paying attention to nine general aspects that can improve the fit of EBM at your institution: First, establish the overall learning goals you want students to achieve and competencies you want students to demonstrate by graduation. For instance, many schools have examined the Accreditation Council for Graduate Medical Education's six core competencies for graduate medical education—medical knowledge, patient care, communication, professionalism, systems-based practice, and practice-based learning and improvement—and are adopting and adapting these for use with for undergraduate learners. Doing so creates some sensible "homes" for student competence in EBM and lifelong learning, as it connects to several of the core competencies, particularly with practice-based learning and improvement. Second, rather than have students study for separate, discipline-based courses, build the curriculum so that students learn the biological sciences, the clinical sciences, and the social sciences relevant to medicine in a fully integrated way.[72-74] Doing so provides them with deliberate practice in integrating the evidence from clinical care research with other knowledge to inform their decisions. Third, identify authentic

9

health care contexts (across the spectrum of care) for the content students are expected to learn, organized around the decisions to make, problems to solve, conversations to hold, and actions to carry out that will be expected of them upon graduation. Doing this helps students find motivation to learn, helps students and teachers select what is relevant to learn, and provides a concrete situation to practise application and transfer of what is learned. This parallels the "real patients, real decisions" advice we mentioned earlier for individual teachers. Fourth, plan how and where in the curriculum to address all four domains of learning— affective, cognitive, conative, and psychomotor.[34] Doing so helps students develop well-rounded skills for clinical practice, into which EBM and lifelong learning can easily fit. Fifth, plan purposefully how you will balance passive learning strategies, such as assigned reading or web modules, with active learning strategies, such as problem-based learning,[75-81] team-based learning,[82,83] or other active methods.[29-31,84] Doing so will ensure that students will have many opportunities to engage with problems or decisions, discover their knowledge gaps and learning needs, and then get coached on asking questions, finding answers, appraising the answers, applying answers to the problem under study, and deciding how to act. Sixth, because these motivated and curious students will want to learn a great deal, it follows they will also need a rich array of learning resources assembled to help them, including not only knowledge collections, such as the medical literature and multimedia learning resources,[85,86] but extensive simulation and skill-building resources as well.[87-90] Seventh, because these engaged learners will want to know how they are progressing in developing competence and because schools and society will be holding students accountable for learning, a robust program of assessments should be planned in the curriculum that aligns both formative and summative assessments with the learning objectives, activities, and so forth.[34,91-94] Doing so creates the context into which assessments of EBM and lifelong learning skills would readily fit. Eighth, recruit, cultivate, and maintain a critical mass of excellent educators,[95,96] who can teach in the several different roles as needed by students in this type of curriculum.[34] Doing so should maximize the students' exposure to excellent role models who teach EBM in all three modes. Ninth, establish a healthy learning climate that balances a high degree of intellectual challenge and engagement with a high degree of personal support and interpersonal collaboration. Doing so won't eliminate students' cognitive dissonance when they encounter the need to learn more but will help them respond to this dissonance in adaptive and constructive fashion, rather than in maladaptive and destructive ways.

With these general curricular issues addressed, you can turn to six aspects specific to EBM and lifelong learning. First, find and cultivate allies who will work with you and advocate for an evidence-based approach to learning throughout the curriculum. Some of these allies may already be in your school, including other faculty, residents, librarians, and others. Others may be closer than you think, such as in nearby colleges of public health or pharmacy. Second, negotiate that learning EBM becomes an important theme of your curriculum, and this too may take persistence. Our experience suggest that this often means you have to become the person or team that builds and runs this theme, so be prepared. Third, adopt an overall curricular schema of EBM to use in planning and sequencing. To help get you started, we include the one we use in Figure 9.1 and in "Integrating EBM into 4-year medical school curriculum—a worked example," on page 271, to find out what our current 4-year EBM curriculum using this approach looks like. This three-dimensional grid shows on its *x* axis the four main categories of clinical decisions (Harm or Risk, Prognosis, Therapy, and Diagnosis), which form separate chapters in this book; its *y* axis shows the five main skills (Asking questions, Acquiring the evidence, Appraising evidence critically, Applying or integrating into clinical decisions, and Assessing the process and impact of acting on the evidence), which form other chapters in this book; and its *z* axis shows the health care context in which these decisions are being made (for individual patients, for groups of patients, for whole populations, or for future patients). Fourth, using this grid, select milestones for each box in the grid that build toward competence and that are developmentally appropriate for each stage of

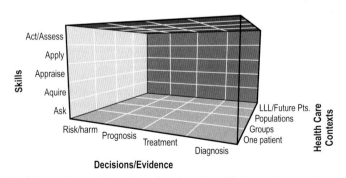

Fig. 9.1 A curricular grid for evidence-based medicine (EBM) in medical education.

the curriculum. For instance, we think that students should be able to ask answerable questions and search for evidence independently by the time they come into their clinical rotations. Fifth, create curricular modules with detailed learning objectives, learning activities, learning resources, and assessment strategies to help students achieve these developmental milestones at the appropriate times. Sixth, embed these curricular modules into the 4-year calendar, and integrate into the relevant workflow, syllabi, and examinations. When considering the cognitive load posed by curricula, commentators recommend sequencing them to start in situations of lower cognitive load, and then progressively increase the fidelity, increase the complexity, and decrease the instructional support, thereby increasing the cognitive load as learners advance through the spiral.[97]

How might such a curriculum look? Although they may not yet be directly responsible for the care of patients, students in the first 2 years can, nonetheless, look ahead and engage with realistic clinical or population health situations. For instance, even on the first day of school, students have all heard that smoking increases the risk of various diseases or that influenza vaccines are recommended annually for many population subgroups. Thus, as the principles of EBM are introduced to them in mode 3 and they encounter the four decision types of the x axis and the five skills of the y axis, students can be actively engaged in addressing authentic health care contexts. Because some of the skills of EBM take time to practise before use in direct patient care, we and others have chosen to introduce the principles of EBM in the first and second pre-clerkship years.[72,98] Several learning approaches, including interactive large groups and team-based learning, can be combined along with small-group and self-directed learning sessions to help students build their fundamental skills on the y axis for the main four decision types on the x axis, with a representative sample of health care contexts on the z axis. Throughout the entire preclerkship curriculum, students could encounter teachers who weave evidence from clinical care research into other knowledge they teach (mode 2) or who role model the practice of EBM (mode 1).

Once in their clinical rotations during years 3 and 4, we expect students to be exposed to the opposite proportions of teaching modes—theoretically, nearly every clinician could model EBM practice and weave evidence into their clinical teaching, although fewer opportunities may be available to teach the fundamental EBM skills. Students who have had a sound introduction to the principles and skills during the first 2 years could be asked to practise these skills deliberately, such as by writing and presenting CATs on each clinical team they join and by taking part in the departmental morning reports and journal clubs, as described above. During elective periods, such as in the final fourth year, students could have the option of taking an advanced course in EBM. Over the period of nearly three decades that we've run these advanced EBM electives for selected learners, we have found the grid shown in Figure 9.1 has helped our students identify the advanced topics they want to learn more about so that we can tailor the elective toward their particular learning needs.

Integrating EBM into 4-year medical school curriculum— a worked example[b,c]

Year 1

1. For "mode 1," exposure to physicians who role model EBM in practice during early clinical experiences, such as at the local student-run free medical clinic

2. For "mode 2," that is, weaving evidence in with other teaching:

   a. Each week's case for small group learning (SGL; variation on problem-based learning [PBL]) has embedded one or more authentic presenting clinical problems and authentic treatment decisions, for both of which evidence can be sought and found to inform these diagnostic and therapeutic decisions.

   b. Selected interactive large group sessions include explicit use of evidence about how well and how safely health care interventions work.

3. For "mode 3," that is, classroom sessions deliberately targeting EBM knowledge and skills:

   a. Questions and Searching, Part 1—background questions and library resources

---

[b]This is a summary of the actual approach to "spiraling through the three-dimensional cube" (see Fig. 9.1) in use during the 2016–2017 academic year at one of our institutions, the AU/UGA Medical Partnership Campus in Athens, Georgia. Each year, we try to advance and refine it further and forge stronger links with the co-occurring science curriculum.
[c]We encourage you to look at some additional references that describe this curriculum: Murrow LB, Crites GE, Goggans DS, Gaines JK, Stowe JM, Richardson WS. Using evidence to inform risk or harm decisions. MedEdPORTAL Publications. 2014;10:9990. Available at: http://dx.doi.org/10.15766/mep_2374-8265.990.

9

b. Introduction to EBCDM—what it is, why we need it, and how we'll learn it

c. Linking Decisions, Knowledge, & Evidence—a worked case example to illustrate

d. Review of Study Designs & Biostatistics—basic study architecture and arithmetic results

e. Questions & Searching, Part II—foreground questions and library resources

f. Harm/Risk—two sessions introduce approach and guide students to practise appraisal

g. Prognosis—two sessions introduce approach and guide students to practise appraisal

h. Treatment—two sessions introduce approach and guide students to practise appraisal

i. Diagnostic Tests—two sessions introduce approach and guide students to practise appraisal

j. Disease Probability—two sessions introduce approach and guide students to practise appraisal

k. Screening—two sessions introduce approach and guide students to practise appraisal

l. Frequencies of Clinical Manifestations of Disease—one session introduction and appraisal

m. Diagnostic Verification—application of explicit diagnostic thinking to reduce diagnostic error

n. Writing CATs and presenting verbal study synopses

Year 2

1. For "mode 1," exposure to physicians who role model EBM in practice during early clinical experiences, such as at the local student-run free medical clinic and the students' hospital medicine experience

2. For "mode 2," that is, weaving evidence in with other teaching:

a. Each week's case for SGL (variation on PBL) has embedded one or more authentic presenting clinical problems and authentic treatment decisions, for both of which evidence can be sought and found to inform these diagnostic and therapeutic decisions.

   b. Selected interactive large group sessions include explicit use of evidence about how well and how safely health care interventions work.

3. For "mode 3," that is, classroom sessions deliberately targeting EBM knowledge and skills:

   a. Treatment—two sessions review and extend randomized trials and adds systematic reviews (SRs)

   b. Practice Guidelines—introduces structure and function, how to appraise and use

   c. Translational and Implementation Research—outlines subsequent steps from evidence to action

   d. Quality Improvement—adds additional dimensions from evidence about quality improvement

   e. Decision Analysis—adds additional dimensions from evidence about decision analyses

   f. Economic Analysis—adds additional dimensions from evidence about economic analyses

   g. Individualizing Decisions—explicit approach to informed, shared decision making is modelled

   h. Diagnostic tests—reviews and extends test accuracy studies and adds SRs

   i. Clinical Prediction Rules—reviews and extends prognosis studies and adds prediction rules

Year 3

1. For "mode 1," exposure to physicians who role model EBM in practice during the clinical clerkships in each of the major disciplines (e.g. Internal Medicine, Surgery, etc.)

2. For "mode 2," that is, weaving evidence in with other teaching:

   a. Selected interactive "Academic Half Day" exercises during the clerkships, including explicit use of evidence when learning about clinical medical topics

3. For "mode 3," that is, classroom sessions deliberately targeting EBM knowledge and skills:

   a. By clerkship group, team CAT assignments—based on a provided scenario, formulate an answerable question, search

9

high-yield resources efficiently, appraise the retrieved evidence critically, derive the main conclusion about whether and how to use this evidence to guide decision making, and summarize this episode of evidence-based learning by writing a CAT

Year 4

1. For "mode 1," exposure to physicians who role model EBM in practice during the clinical clerkships and other clinical experiences of the fourth year

2. For "mode 2," that is, weaving evidence in with other teaching:

   a. Selected interactive "Academic Half Day" exercises during the clerkships, including explicit use of evidence when learning about clinical medical topics

3. For "mode 3," that is, classroom sessions deliberately targeting EBM knowledge and skills:

   a. By clerkship group, team CAT assignments—based on a provided scenario, formulate an answerable question, search high-yield resources efficiently, appraise the retrieved evidence critically, derive the main conclusion about whether and how to use this evidence to guide decision making, and summarize this episode of evidence-based learning by writing a CAT.

   b. "Advanced Evidence-Based Clinical Decision Making" elective—experience is customized for the learners' EBM needs, chosen clinical discipline, and career plans.

Learning more about how to teach EBM

As with any complex craft that's built on experience as well as knowledge, becoming excellent at teaching EBM requires extensive deliberate practice.[11] In addition to trying out the strategies and tactics in this chapter, we suggest five additional ideas: First, keep a teaching journal, in which you record your observations and interpretations of which teaching methods you've tried, what specifically worked, what specifically you'd like to do better, and what you find in watching others teach and in reading about teaching and learning.[99,100] Second, look for excellent teachers in your institution who would be willing to observe your teaching and provide individualized feedback and coaching, and then work with these mentors to develop your skills. Some institutions have formal teaching consultation services available to observe teachers and provide feedback.[101] Third, track down the published series of EBM teaching tips that tackle how to handle teaching difficult material,[102-112] and try your hand at using them in your own teaching practice. Don't forget to record your observations and reflections in your teaching journal. Fourth, attend one of the growing number of workshops on "How to teach EBM" being held around the world, which provide you with time for deliberate practice and the opportunity to gain useful feedback on your teaching methods. Fifth, because learning in small groups is so much a part of clinical learning and teaching and because when group learning works well it can powerfully enhance evidence-based learning, we suggest you devote substantial time and effort to refining your skills for learning and teaching in small groups, starting with the material below, "Tips for teaching EBM in clinical teams," and continuing with additional readings.[113-120] Although connected to teaching, the assessment of learning, practising, and teaching EBM is so important that it deserves its own chapter, and it follows next.

Tips for teaching EBM in clinical teams and other small groups[d]

Help team/group members understand why to learn in small groups

Learners may vary in their prior experiences with learning in groups, so they may benefit from reflecting on why it's worth undertaking. Following are some useful points:

1. Learning in groups allows a broader range of questions about any given topic to be asked and answered because the work is done by several people. As the results of an individual's effort are shared with others, lessons learned have a "multiplier" effect.

2. Learning in groups allows experienced members to pair with inexperienced members during the work, thereby helping novices to learn faster and reinforcing everyone's capacity for teamwork.

3. The interactive discussions groups use as they learn can help individual members clarify their own misconceptions, consolidate

9

---

[d]Thanks again to Martha Gerrity and Valerie Lawrence, who compiled an early version of this list that was published in this book's first edition. Since then, we've kept changing the list as we've gained more experience with small group learning, and because we can't resist the urge to tinker.

the lessons learned by explaining things to others, and hear multiple viewpoints when considering the implications of the new knowledge for decision and action.

4. Learning in groups allows individual participants to practise performance of skills, using other group members within the practice, which helps the individual to learn.

5. Learning in groups also allows individual participants to get feedback on their performance from peers as well as tutors, providing both a "reality check" of their own perceptions and suggestions for further learning.

6. The camaraderie, the interpersonal support, and the cohesion from shared challenges and achievements can make learning in groups more fun than learning in isolation.

7. In many fields of work, leaders spend time building groups of individuals into well-functioning work teams because team performance almost always bests that of individuals.

8. Consider an analogy between group learning and how professional cyclists ride in groups—by riding closely in the peloton to draft and to rotate leading, cyclists can ride faster, longer, and farther than even the best of them can individually.

Help team/group members set sensible ground rules for small group learning

Small groups can succeed in learning EBM (or anything else) if group members establish effective ways of working together. Useful ground rules include the following:

1. Members take responsibility (individually and as a group) for:

   a. Showing up, and on time

   b. Learning each other's names, interests, and objectives

   c. Respecting each other

   d. Removing distractions, such as audible tones, games, or communications on mobile phones and computers

   e. Contributing to, accepting, and supporting individual and group rules of behaviour, including confidentiality

   f. Contributing to, accepting, and supporting both the overall objectives of the group and the detailed plans and assignments for each session

g. Carrying out the agreed-upon plans and assignments, including role playing

h. Listening (concentrating and analyzing), rather than simply preparing your their response to what's being said

i. Talking (including consolidating and summarizing)

2. Members monitor and (by using time in/time out) reinforce positive and correct negative elements of both:

   a. "Process," including:

      i. Educational methods, for example, reinforcing positive contributions and teaching methods, and proposing strategies for improving less effective ones

      ii. Group functioning, for example, identifying behaviours, not motives; encouraging nonparticipants; quieting down overparticipators

   b. "Content," including:

      i. Critical appraisal topics, for example, if unclear, uncertain or incorrect facts or principles, strategies, or tactics about how to carry it out

      ii. Clinical matters, for example, if clinical context or usefulness is unclear

3. Members evaluate self, each other, the group, the session, and the program with candour and respect:

   a. Celebrating what went well and what should be preserved

   b. Identifying what went less well, focusing on strategies for correcting or improving the situation

4. When giving feedback constructively, members do the following:

   a. Give feedback only when asked to do so or when the offer is accepted.

   b. Give feedback as soon after the event as possible.

   c. Focus on the positive; wherever possible, give positive feedback first and last.

   d. Be descriptive (of behaviour), not evaluative (of motives).

   e. Talk about specific behaviours, and give examples, where possible.

   f. Use "I" and give your experience of the behaviour.

9

    g. When giving negative feedback, suggest alternative behaviours.

    h. Confine negative feedback to behaviours that can be changed.

    i. Ask yourself, "Why am I giving this feedback?" (Is it really to help the person concerned?)

    j. Remember that feedback says a lot about its giver as well as its receiver.

5. When receiving feedback constructively, members do the following:

    a. Listen to it (rather than prepare a response or defense).

    b. Ask for it to be repeated if it wasn't easily heard.

    c. Ask for clarification and examples if statements are unclear or unsupported.

    d. Assume it is constructive until proven otherwise; then, use and consider those elements that are constructive.

    e. Pause and think before responding.

    f. Accept it positively (for consideration) rather than dismissively (for self-protection).

    g. Ask for suggestions of specific ways to modify or change the behaviour.

    h. Respect and thank the person giving feedback.

Help team/group members plan the learning activities wisely

During initial introductions, group members should identify their individual learning goals, from which the group can set group learning goals. Tutors and group members should keep these learning goals in mind as they plan the learning objectives for each session, including what to learn, what to emphasize, and how to engage the group in the learning activities. For groups just beginning to learn EBM, consider the following:

1. Plan the session to include a learning situation that is realistic with regard to what group members do in their actual work. For most clinicians, this means using the illnesses of patients actually in their care or using case examples they might encounter frequently.

2. Prepare the question, search, and critical appraisal ahead of time, to be familiar with the teaching challenges that may arise. Of the possible questions this case could generate, select one with a high

yield in terms of learning, which is usually a mix of the following considerations:

a. Relevance to the clinical decision being made

b. Appropriateness to the learners' prior knowledge

c. Availability of good-quality evidence to address the question (so, first experience shows positively how evidence can be used once understood and appraised)

d. Availability of easily understood evidence about the question (so, first experience is not too overwhelming methodologically)

e. Likelihood the question will recur, so learners can benefit more than once

3. As the session begins, engage the group in the clinical situation and have the group focus on the decision to be made. Consider having group members vote on what they would do clinically before the evidence is appraised (if need be, this can be done anonymously).

4. Encourage group members to run the session, yet be prepared to guide them in the early going.

5. As the group works through the critical appraisal portions, emphasize how to understand and use research, rather than how to do research.

6. Summarize important points in the session (if the group is using a scribe, this person could record them for later retrieval).

7. As the session ends, encourage the group to come to closure on how to use the evidence in the clinical decision. Keep in mind that coming to closure needn't require complete agreement; rather, a good airing of the issues that ends in legitimate disagreement can be very instructive.

8. Keep to the time plan overall, but don't worry if the group doesn't cover everything in this one session—if the initial experience goes well, there will be more opportunities.

9. For groups gaining competence and confidence in EBM, the sky is the limit. Encourage the group to invent its own activities, and consider the following:

a. When selecting questions and evidence to appraise, consider using:

i. Flawed evidence so that the group can develop skill in detecting flaws

9

    ii. A pair of articles, one good and one not so good, for the group to compare

    iii. A pair of good articles that reach opposite conclusions

    iv. Controversial evidence so that the group learns to disagree constructively

    v. Evidence that debunks current practice so that the group learns to question carefully

    vi. A systematic review of early small trials, along with a later definitive trial

  b. When selecting learning contexts to employ in the group, encourage group members to try out sessions of increasing difficulty, such as practising teaching jaded senior residents or registrars rather than eager students

  c. When group members disagree, capitalize on the disagreement, by such tactics as:

    i. Trying to sort out whether the disagreement is about the data, the critical appraisal, or the values we use in making the judgements

    ii. Framing the disagreement positively, to give the group a chance to understand more deeply

    iii. Framing the protagonists positively, to give the group a chance to learn by stating the various perspectives on the topic

    iv. Wherever possible, keeping the disagreement from becoming personal, and avoiding trying to defend the article

Help team/group members keep a healthy learning climate

The learning climate is the general tone and atmosphere that pervades the group sessions. Encourage the group to cultivate a safe, positive learning climate, wherein group members feel comfortable identifying their limitations and addressing them. Some tactics include the following:

1. Be honest and open about your own limitations and the things you don't know.

2. Model the behaviour of turning what you don't know into answerable questions and following through on finding answers, using an educational prescription.

3. Show others that finding knowledge gaps and learning can be fun.

4. Encourage all questions, particularly those that aim for deep understanding.

5. Encourage legitimate disagreement, particularly when handled constructively.

6. Encourage group members to use Educational Prescriptions.

7. Provide both intellectual challenge (to stimulate learning) and personal support (to help make learning adaptive).

Help team/group members keep the discussion going

1. Early on, model effective facilitating behaviours that encourage discussion, as follows:

   a. When someone asks a question, turn the question over to the group.

   b. If a group member answers another member's question well, ask others in the group for additional effective ways that they've used to answer the same question.

   c. If a group discussion turns into a debate between two members, ask others to provide additional perspective before the group arrives at a decision.

   d. Don't be afraid of quiet moments and of using silence, when needed.

2. Observe carefully how group members keep discussion moving, and use these observations for feedback and coaching.

3. Encourage group members to reflect on what works well in different teaching situations, and provide each other feedback on this, balancing the desire to move forward with the need to pull everyone along.

Help team/group members keep the discussion on track

1. Early on, model effective facilitating behaviours that help group members to stay focused on the task at hand, as follows:

   a. Break the discussion into observable chunks, and set a short time for each chunk, for example, "For the next 2 minutes, let's

9

brainstorm all the outcomes of clinical interest to us for this condition and its treatment."

b. When someone brings up a tangent, identify it nonjudgementally, and ask group members how they'd like to handle it.

c. Reflect to the group what they seem to be discussing, to inform their choices about how to spend their efforts.

2. Observe carefully how group members keep the discussion on track, and use these observations for feedback and coaching.

3. Encourage group members to reflect on what works well for keeping a discussion focused well, staying alert to recognize good teaching moments that arise spontaneously.

Help team/group members manage time well

To accomplish their group objectives, group members need to manage their time together effectively. This includes spending time on things that are important and avoiding distractions, wherever possible. Some tactics include the following:

1. At the beginning, model effective time management by encouraging the group to set specific plans for how much time to spend on:

    a. Carrying out the learning activities for the present session

    b. Evaluating the present session, including giving feedback

    c. Planning the subsequent session, including revising group objectives

2. As the group takes charge, coach the members on issues of time management, such as:

    a. How to use a "timekeeper," usually a member not leading that session

    b. How to adjust time allotted for various functions, after group negotiation

    c. How to handle new learning issues that arise, which might consume time to address. Here several options exist, including the following:

        i. Address it fully right then (if it's important enough and if the group's work would halt without doing so).

    ii. Address it briefly at the time, and have a group member (or tutor) address it more completely later, either to the group or with the individual.

    iii. Delay addressing the topic; instead, record it for later discussion (in a place sometimes dubbed the "parking lot").

3. Encourage the group to evaluate time management as the members evaluate the group's functioning.

Help team/group members address some common issues in learning EBM jargon

Jargon refers to technical words of any discipline; for EBM, these words can be from epidemiology, biostatistics, decision sciences, economics, and other fields. If unexplained, jargon can be intimidating and might delay learning. Some tactics for dealing with jargon include the following:

1. Introduce and explain the idea first, and then label it with the technical term. In this way, understanding comes before the word can intimidate.

2. If any group member introduces a jargon term, ask him or her to explain the term to others in a concise way. This helps the group's understanding and allows the member to practise giving a brief explanation that can be used in later contexts as well.

3. Consider having the group keep an accumulating glossary of terms covered, for members to refer to during and after the sessions. You can start with the brief glossary provided in Appendix 1 of this book.

Quantitative study results

Most reports contain simple calculations, and many contain complex and intimidating ones. Although most of them don't deserve extensive discussion, others, if left unexplained, can needlessly intimidate some learners. Tactics for dealing with quantitative results include the following:

1. Introduce the concept using real data, and work slowly through the arithmetic so that learners can follow the calculations.

2. Use the word names for the arithmetic functions, rather than "talking in symbols."

9

3. Calculate a result from the study data, and then introduce its name and a general formula. Just as in dealing with jargon, this order helps demystify the terms.

4. To check their understanding, allow group members time to practise the arithmetic until they feel comfortable enough to move on.

5. Consider having the group keep an accumulating glossary of quantitative results, including names, formulae, and uses, for group members to use during the session and later (see Appendix 1).

Statistics

The study's "methods" and "results" sections will usually describe the technical devices of statistics used for the research. Some may be familiar to you and your group members, but many may not be. Groups will need to learn how to handle questions about statistics, epidemiology, or any other methodological issue. Some tactics include the following:

1. Highlight the distinction between statistical significance and clinical significance, and illustrate with evidence being examined.

2. Assuming the group members want to learn how to understand and use research, rather than do research (worth double-checking now and then), consider advising the group to select a few statistical notions to understand well (e.g., confidence intervals [CIs]), and point them to resources that can help them.

3. Ask the group how deeply they'd like to delve into this topic (many will opt for shallow initial treatment, to allow the group's work to continue, followed by provision of resources for deeper learning later). If they choose deeper learning and you cannot provide this on the spot, involve them in choosing among realistic alternatives, including the following:

   a. A single group member (or the tutor, if needed) looks up the statistical measure or test and reports back concisely at a later session.

   b. Pairs or small teams from the group find the needed information outside the session and plan a learning activity around it for a subsequent session.

c. A nearby statistician is persuaded to join the group temporarily to address the topic at a subsequent session.

4. Remind group members that they may face learners with similar questions upon return home. Coach them in developing answers of different lengths and depths, appropriate for different situations:

   a. "One liners"—for when learners want just enough to get back to other work

   b. "One paragraphers"—for when learners want more verbal explanation

   c. "One siders"—one page (or a few) handouts on the topic that might be developed ahead of time, for learners who want a little more depth to read later; this can be coupled with "one citers," that is, a useful citation for even more depth

5. As the group members run sessions themselves, observe carefully how they handle statistical, epidemiologic, or other methodological issues and use these observations in coaching and feedback.

6. Ask the group to assess its handling of methodological topics when they evaluate the session.

7. Consider having the group keep a log of methodological issues covered.

Help team/group members identify and deal with counterproductive behaviours

Nihilism

As learners grow in their ability to detect study flaws, some may go through a period of nihilism ("No study is perfect, so what good is any literature?"). Often, this occurs in those who can find bias but don't yet understand its consequences. This negative imbalance is usually temporary, but it can dampen the spirits of others and impede group function. Some tactics are useful in ameliorating this unease:

1. Select good articles to start with so that early experiences are positive.

2. When using flawed articles, ask the group if something can be learned, even if the study does not provide a definitive answer.

9

3. Help group members put the study in its knowledge context— what else is known about this? Although potentially flawed, a study may be the earliest in a given field, when the state of prior knowledge is low. Thus, the study may represent incomplete knowledge, rather than bad knowledge.

4. Help group members ask whether information was missing because of poor study design and execution or because of editorial decisions about publishing space. Some data missing in the report may be available from the authors of the study.

5. Help group members separate minor problems from major design flaws that seriously affect the likely validity of results.

6. Help group members ask a series of questions:

   a. Do the study methods allow the possibility of bias?

   b. If so, how much distortion of the results might this bias cause?

   c. If so, in which direction might this bias distort the results?

7. Help group members identify what they would find in an ideal study that answers the question. Then, consider how far from ideal is the available evidence.

Discussion tangents

Small group work can stimulate learners, bringing forth not only discussion ideas that would keep the group on its learning spiral but also discussion ideas that could take the group elsewhere (tangents from the spiral). The energy released can be invigorating, yet if every topic were to be discussed, the group would not achieve its objectives. Group members need to learn constructive ways of handling possible discussion tangents, some of which are as follows:

1. Identify to the group that a tangent has arisen, validating it as a possibly productive line of learning.

2. Ask the group to choose how to proceed, based on their overall learning goals, rather than on just the plan for that session. This may mean following the tangent, as it might meet their goals better, or it may mean placing the tangent on a list of topics to address later (the "parking lot"). Either way, encourage group members to decide, letting them know that you'll stick with them on either path.

3. Some tangents can be turned into extended loops of the learning spiral. That is, these topics can be briefly and concisely discussed, enough to inform the original discussion, to which the group then returns. It may help to set a time limit for such a tangent, and have the timekeeper help the group keep to the limit.

4. Observe closely how the group member running the session deals with tangents, and use these observations for feedback and coaching.

5. Encourage the group to assess its management of tangents during its evaluation.

A dominating overparticipator

Some groups may have one or more members whose personality or enthusiasm leads them to contribute a great deal, perhaps to the point of dominating the time and impeding the group's work and the other members' learning. Some tactics for dealing with this include the following:

1. Use nonverbal signals (eye contact, hand gestures, body position, etc.) to encourage this person to talk less and let others contribute more.

2. Seat this person next to one of the tutors, which can encourage moderation.

3. After this person contributes again, ask several others to contribute. This may take reminding the overparticipator to let others have a fair turn to speak.

4. Take a time-out to address the group's process, perhaps by reviewing the group's ground rules about participation, or by asking the group to identify the overparticipation and make adjustments. In doing so, focus on the behaviour (amount and nature of speech), rather than on the person or the motivations for the behaviour.

5. Use a "microphone"—group members can take a simple classroom object, such as white board marker or eraser, and turn it into a pretend microphone. Whoever has this "mic" has permission to speak, and others are to listen. After the speaker is finished, she or he can pass it on to someone else or place it in the middle of the table for anyone to choose. This can be a fun and instructive exercise, through which group members can

9

identify not only underparticipation and overparticipation, but also how many members talk at once.

A quiet nonparticipator

Some group members are quiet initially but soon "warm up" to the others and to the group's activities. Other members may be quiet for a longer period, either because of personal style of participation or for other reasons, such as limited language skills. Still others may be quiet because of lack of preparation, fear of embarrassment, or lack of engagement. Although not always pathologic, quietness can signal individual or group troubles. Groups will need tactics to recognize members who contribute little and address this issue. Some of these tactics are as follows:

1. Be sensitive to the individual's reasons for quietness, and make adjustments accordingly. If needed, approach the group member between sessions to find out why.

2. Use nonverbal signals (eye contact, hand gestures, body position, etc.) to encourage this person to contribute more.

3. Seat this person next to one of the tutors, which can encourage participation.

4. Take a time-out to address the group's process, perhaps by reviewing the group's ground rules about participation or by asking the group to identify underparticipation and make adjustments. In doing so, focus on the behaviour (amount and nature of speech), rather than on the person or the motivations for the behaviour.

5. Consider pairing the quiet person with another group member for an activity so that both can work together on planning and carrying out this activity. Make sure quiet folks (and all group members) feel more supported as they take on challenges in the group.

6. Consider using the "mic" (see above). To help underparticipators, tutors and group members can make it a point to pass the "mic" to them, asking them to contribute at least a little before passing it on to others.

Help team/group members prepare for using EBM skills "back home"

As they grow in competence and confidence in their EBM skills, group members will begin to consider how to start or advance the use of EBM in their daily work. For clinicians and teachers, this may mean facing, for the first time, some of the barriers to incorporating evidence in practice addressed elsewhere in this book. (See also the accompanying CD, which includes more on the limitations of and misunderstandings about EBM.) You can help them prepare to overcome these barriers with a mix of enthusiasm, realism, and practicality. Some tactics include the following:

1. Encourage each group member to select one or a few places to start introducing EBM, rather than trying to start everywhere at once. Consider having them rank three or more candidate activities for introducing EBM, and then discuss in buzz groups the advantages and disadvantages of each.

2. Use the group members' collective experience to brainstorm how to prepare to introduce EBM into a given learning activity. This brainstorming might be usefully organized around five areas—persons, places, times, things, and ideas (see Box 9.4 on p. 268)—that would need to be considered when introducing EBM "back home."

3. Since changes involving only a few may be easier than changes involving many, it may be wise to work toward an early success by introducing EBM in a way that doesn't require massive shifts in institutional culture. Indeed, the simplest may be a change that involves the actions of only the group member, at least at first. Once momentum is gained, more challenging tasks can be tackled.

4. Encourage group members to be realistic in setting expectations for what can be accomplished early and yet optimistic about what can be achieved in the long term.

For those of you who have read this far, that's it, we're done! We hope you have enjoyed this book and its accompanying resources as well as learned from them, and we would appreciate your suggestions on how to make them more useful as well as more enjoyable.

9

References

1. Schon DA. Educating the reflective practitioner. San Francisco, CA: Jossey-Bass; 1987.

2. Candy PC. Self-direction for lifelong learning: A comprehensive guide to theory and practice. San Francisco, CA: Jossey-Bass; 1991.

3. Neighbour R. The inner apprentice. Newbury, UK: Petroc Press; 1996.

4. Davis D, Thomson MA. Continuing medical education as a means of lifelong learning. In: Silagy C, Haines A, editors. Evidence-based practice in primary care. London, UK: BMJ Books; 1998.

5. Palmer PJ. The courage to teach. San Francisco, CA: Jossey-Bass; 1998.

6. Claxton G. Wise up: The challenge of lifelong learning. New York, NY: Bloomsbury; 1999.

7. Davis DA, O'Brien MA, Freemantle NA, et al. Impact of formal continuing medical education: do conferences, workshops, rounds, and other traditional continuing education activities change physician behaviour or health care outcomes? JAMA 1999;282: 867–94.

8. Bransford JD, Brown AL, Cocking RR, editors. How people learn: Brain, mind, experience, and school. Washington, DC: National Academy Press; 2000.

9. Brown JS, Duguid P. The social life of information. Boston, MA: Harvard Business School Press; 2000.

10. Sawyer RK, editor. The Cambridge handbook of the learning sciences. Cambridge, UK: Cambridge University Press; 2006.

11. Ericsson KA, Charness N, Feltovich PJ, Hoffman RR. The Cambridge handbook of expertise and expert performance. Cambridge, UK: Cambridge University Press; 2006.

12. Straus SE, Haynes RB. David Sackett's legacy includes evidence-based mentorship. J Clin Epidemiol 2016;73:61–3.

13. Fletcher RH, Fletcher SW. David Sackett was one of a kind. J Clin Epidemiol 2016;73:67–72.

14. Guyatt GH. Dave Sackett and the ethos of the EBM community. J Clin Epidemiol 2016;73:75–81.

15. Richardson WS. Teaching evidence-based practice on foot. ACP J Club 2005;143:A10–12.

16. Hargraves I, Kunneman M, Brito JP, Montori VM. Caring with evidence based medicine: Using evidence for kind and careful care. BMJ 2016;353:i3530.

17. Parkes J, Hyde C, Deeks J, Milne R. Teaching critical appraisal in health care settings. Cochrane Database Syst Rev 2001;(3): CD001270.

18. Maggio LA, Tannery NH, Chen HC, ten Cate O, O'Brien B. Evidence-based medicine training in undergraduate medical education: A review and critique of the literature published 2006 – 2011. Acad Med 2013;88(7):x–y.

19. Young T, Rohwer A, Volmink J, Clarke M. What are the effects of teaching evidence-based health care (EBHC)? Overview of systematic reviews. PLoS ONE 2014;9(1):e86706.

20. Ahmadi SF, Baradran HR, Ahmadi E. Effectiveness of teaching evidence-based medicine to undergraduate medical students: A BEME systematic review. Med Teacher 2015;37:21–30.

21. Hecht L, Buhse S, Meyer G. Effectiveness of training in evidence-based medicine skills for healthcare professionals: a systematic review. BMC Med Educ 2016;16:103.

22. Hitch D, Nicola-Richmond K. Instructional practices for evidence-based practice with pre-registration allied health students: a review of recent research and developments. Adv Health Sci Ed 2016;doi:10.1007/s10459-016-9702-9.

23. Kyriakoulis K, Patelarou A, Laliotis A, Wan AC, Matalliotakis M, Tsiou C, et al. Educational strategies for teaching evidence-based practice to undergraduate health students: systematic review. J Educ Eval Health Prof 2016;13:34.

24. Phillips AC, Lewis LK, McEvoy MP, Galipeau J, Glasziou P, Hammick M, et al. A systematic review of how studies describe educational interventions for evidence-based practice: stage 1 of the development of a reporting guideline. BMC Med Educ 2014;14:152.

25. Maggio LA, ten Cate O, Irby DM, O'Brien BC. Designing evidence-based medicine training to optimize the transfer of skills from the classroom to clinical practice: Applying the four component instructional design model. Acad Med 2015;90:1457–61.

26. Maggio LA, ten Cate O, Chen C, Irby DM, O'Brien BC. Challenges to learning evidence-based medicine and educational approaches to meet these challenges: A qualitative study of selected EBM curricula in U.S. and Canadian medical schools. Acad Med 2016;91:101–6.

27. Pinsky LE, Monson D, Irby DM. How excellent teachers are made: reflecting on success to improve teaching. Adv Health Sci Ed 1998;3: 207–15.

28. Dodek PM, Sackett DL, Schechter MT. Systolic and diastolic learning: an analogy to the cardiac cycle. CMAJ 1999;160:1475–7.

29. Prince MJ. Does active learning work? A review of the research. J Engr Education 2004;93:223–31.

9

30. Prince MJ, Felder RM. Inductive teaching and learning methods: definitions, comparisons, and research bases. J Engr Education 2006;95:123–38.

31. Freeman S, Eddy SL, McDonough M, Smith MK, Okoroafor N, Jordt H, et al. Active learning increases student performance in science, engineering, and mathematics. Proc Nat Acad Sci USA 2014;111(23): 8410–15.

32. Hurst JW. The over-lecturing and under-teaching of clinical medicine. Arch Intern Med 2004;164:1605–8.

33. Custers EJFM. Thirty years of illness scripts: Theoretical origins and practical applications. Med Teacher 2015;37:457–62.

34. Reeves TC. How do you know they are learning? The importance of alignment in higher education. Int J Learning Technology 2006;2: 294–309.

35. Pinsky LE, Irby DM. If at first you don't succeed: Using failure to improve teaching. Acad Med 1997;72:973–6.

36. LeBlanc VR. The effects of acute stress on performance: implications for health professions education. Acad Med 2009;84(10 Suppl.): S25–33.

37. Artino AR, Holmboe ES, Durning SJ. Control-value theory: Using achievement emotions to improve understanding of motivation, learning, and performance in medical education: AMEE guide number 64. Med Teacher 2012;34:e148–60.

38. McConnell MM, Eva KW. The role of emotion in the learning and transfer of clinical skills and knowledge. Acad Med 2012;87: 1316–22.

39. Smith R. Thoughts for new medical students at a new medical school. BMJ 2003;327:1430–3.

40. Reilly BM. Inconvenient truths about effective clinical teaching. Lancet 2007;370:705–11.

41. Ellis J, Mulligan I, Rowe J, Sackett DL. Inpatient general medicine is evidence-based. Lancet 1995;346:407–10.

42. Sackett DL, Straus SE. Finding and applying evidence during clinical rounds: the evidence cart. JAMA 1998;280:1336–8.

43. Straus SE, Eisinga A, Sackett DL. What drove the Evidence Cart? Bringing the library to the bedside. J Roy Soc Med 2016;109(6): 241–7.

44. Richardson WS, Burdette SD. Practice corner: Taking evidence in hand. ACP J Club 2003;138:A9.

45. Richardson WS. One slice or the whole pie? Evidence-Based Health Care Newsletter 2001;21:17–18.

46. Irby DM, Wilkerson L. Teaching when time is limited. BMJ 2008; 336:384–7.

47. Sprake C, Cantillon P, Metcalf J, Spencer J. Teaching in an ambulatory care setting. BMJ 2008;337:690–2.

48. Sauve S, Lee HN, Meade MO, Lang JD, Farkouh M, Cook DJ, et al. The critically appraised topic: a practical approach to learning critical appraisal. Ann Royal Coll Phys Surg Canada 1995;28:396–8.

49. Lloyd FJ, Reyna VF. Clinical gist and medical education: Connecting the dots. JAMA 2009;302:1332–3.

50. Amin Z, Guajardo J, Wisniewski W, Bordage G, Tekian A, Niederman LG. Morning report: focus and methods over the past three decades. Acad Med 2000;75(Suppl. 1):S1–5.

51. Richardson WS. Teaching evidence-based medicine in morning report. Clin Epidemiol Newsl 1993;13:9.

52. Reilly B, Lemon M. Evidence-based morning report: a popular new format in a large teaching hospital. Am J Med 1997;103:419–26.

53. Stinson L, Pearson D, Lucas B. Developing a learning culture: twelve tips for individuals, teams, and organizations. Med Teacher 2006;28: 309–12.

54. Ebbert JO, Montori VM, Schultz HJ. The journal club in postgraduate medical education: a systematic review. Med Teacher 2001;23:455–61.

55. Dirschl DR, Tornetta P, Bhandari M. Designing, conducting, and evaluating journal clubs in orthopedic surgery. Clin Ortho Rel Res 2003;413:146–57.

56. Forsen JW, Hartman JM, Neely JG. Tutorials in clinical research, part VIII: Creating a journal club. Laryngoscope 2003;113:475–83.

57. Phillips RS, Glasziou PP. What makes evidence-based journal clubs succeed? ACP J Club 2004;140:A11–12.

58. Doust J, Del Mar CB, Montgomery BD, Heal C. EBM journal clubs in general practice. Aust Fam Phys 2008;37:54–6.

59. Deenadayalan Y, Grimmer-Somers K, Prior M, Kumar S. How to run an effective journal club: A systematic review. J Eval Clin Pract 2008;14(5):898–911.

60. Dawes M, Summerskill W, Glasziou P, Cartabellotta A, Martin J, Hopayian K, et al. Sicily statement of evidence-based practice. BMC Med Educ 2005;5:1.

9

61. Hatala R, Keitz SA, Wilson MC, Guyatt G. Beyond journal clubs: Moving toward an integrated evidence-based medicine curriculum. J Gen Intern Med 2006;21:538–41.

62. Glasziou P, Burls A, Gilbert R. Evidence-based medicine and the medical curriculum: The search engine is now as essential as the stethoscope. BMJ 2008;337:704–5.

63. Shaughnessy AF, Torro JR, Frame KA, Bakshi M. Evidence-based medicine and life-long learning competency requirements in new residency teaching standards. J Evid Based Med 2016;21(2): 46–9.

64. Hunter KM. Eating the curriculum. Acad Med 1997;72(3): 167–72.

65. Kern DE, Thomas PA, Howard DM, Bass EB. Curriculum development for medical education: A six-step approach. Baltimore, MD: Johns Hopkins University Press; 1998.

66. Ornstein AC, Hunkins FP, editors. Curriculum: Foundations, principles, and issues. 3rd ed. Boston, MA: Allyn and Bacon; 1998.

67. Green ML. Identifying, appraising, and implementing medical education curricula: a guide for medical educators. Ann Intern Med 2001;135:889–96.

68. Kaufman DM. ABC of learning and teaching in medicine: Applying educational theory in practice. BMJ 2003;326:213–16.

69. Prideaux D. ABC of learning and teaching in medicine: Curriculum design. BMJ 2003;326:268–70.

70. Harden RM, Stamper N. What is a spiral curriculum? Med Teacher 1999;21(2):141–3.

71. Fincher RM, Wallach PM, Richardson WS. Basic science right, not basic science lite: Medical education at a crossroad. J Gen Intern Med 2009;[Epub ahead of print]; PMID: 19774422.

72. Neville AJ, Norman GR. PBL in the undergraduate MD program at McMaster University: Three iterations in three decades. Acad Med 2007;82:370–4.

73. Wilkerson L, Stevens CM, Krasne S. No content without context: Integrating basic, clinical, and social sciences in a pre-clerkship curriculum. Med Teacher 2009;31:812–21.

74. Brauer DG, Ferguson KH. The integrated curriculum in medical education: AMEE Guide No. 96. Med Teacher 2015;37:312–22.

75. Taylor D, Miflin B. Problem-based learning: Where are we now? AMEE Guide No. 36. Med Teacher 2008;30:742–63.

76. Koh GCH, Khoo HE, Wong ML, Koh D. The effects of problem-based learning during medical school on physician competency: a systematic review. CMAJ 2008;178:34–41.

77. Azer SA. Becoming a student in a PBL course: twelve tips for successful group discussion. Med Teacher 2004;26:12–15.

78. Azer SA. Challenges facing PBL tutors: 12 tips for successful group facilitation. Med Teacher 2005;27:676–81.

79. Azer SA. Twelve tips for creating trigger images for problem-based learning cases. Med Teacher 2007;29:93–7.

80. Azer SA. Interactions between students and tutor in problem-based learning: The significance of deep learning. Kaohsiung J Med Sci 2009;25:240–9.

81. Azer SA. What makes a great lecture? Use of lectures in a hybrid PBL curriculum. Kaohsiung J Med Sci 2009;25:109–15.

82. Michaelson LK, Parmelee DX, McMahon KK, Levine RE, editors. Team-based learning for health professions education: A guide to using small groups for improving learning. Stylus Publishing; 2007.

83. Michaelson LK, Sweet M, Parmelee DX. Team-based learning: Small group learning's next big step. San Francisco, CA: Jossey-Bass; 2009.

84. Graffam B. Active learning in medical education: Strategies for beginning implementation. Med Teacher 2007;29:38–42.

85. Mayer RE. Applying the science of learning: evidence-based principles for the design of multimedia instruction. Am Psychol 2008;63:760–9.

86. Means B, Toyama Y, Murphy R, Bakia M, Jones K Evaluation of evidence-based practices in online learning: a meta-analysis and review of online learning studies. US Department of Education, 2009.

87. Issenberg SB, McGaghie WC, Petrusa ER, Gordon DL, Scalese RJ. Features and uses of high-fidelity medical simulations that lead to effective learning: a BEME systematic review. Med Teacher 2005; 27:10–28.

88. Ziv A, Ben-David S, Ziv M. Simulation based medical education: an opportunity to learn from errors. Med Teacher 2005;27:193–9.

89. Ruiz JG, Cook DA, Levinson AJ. Computer animations in medical education: a critical literature review. Med Educ 2009;43:838–46.

90. Kneebone R. Simulation and transformational change: The paradox of expertise. Acad Med 2009;84:954–7.

9

91. Epstein RM. Assessment in medical education. N Engl J Med 2007; 356:387–96.

92. Larsen DP, Butler AC, Roediger HL. Test-enhanced learning in medical education. Med Educ 2008;42:959–66.

93. Hols-Elders W, Bloemendaal P, Bos N, Quaak M, Sijstermans R, De Jong P. Twelve tips for computer-based assessment in medical education. Med Teacher 2008;30:673–8.

94. Kogan JR, Holmboe ES, Hauer KE. Tools for direct observation and assessment of clinical skills of medical trainees: A systematic review. JAMA 2009;302:1316–26.

95. DeAngelis CD. Professors not professing. JAMA 2004;292:1060–1.

96. LaCombe M. High society. CMAJ 2002;166:1044–5.

97. Leppink J, Duvivier R. Twelve tips for medical curriculum design from a cognitive load perspective. Med Teacher 2016;38(7):669–74.

98. Crites GE, Richardson WS, Stolfi A, Sydelko B, Markert RJ. An evidence-based medicine and clinical decision making course was successfully integrated into a medical school's preclinical, systems-based curriculum. Med Sci Educ 2012;22(1):17–23.

99. Richardson WS. A teacher's dozen. Nordic Evidence-Based Health Care Newsletter 2001;5:167.

100. Richardson WS. Using a teaching journal to improve one's teaching of evidence-based practice. International Society for Evidence-Based Health Care Newsletter 2013;11:12–13.

101. Beckman TJ. Lessons learned from a peer review of bedside teaching. Acad Med 2004;79:343–6.

102. Wyer PC, Keitz SA, Hatala RM, Hayward RSA, Barratt A, Montori VM, et al., for the Evidence-Based Medicine Teaching Tips Working Group. Tips for learning and teaching EBM: Introduction to the series [Commentary]. CMAJ 2004;171:347–8.

103. Barratt A, Wyer PC, Hatala RM, McGinn TG, Dans AL, Keitz SA, et al., for the Evidence-Based Medicine Teaching Tips Working Group. Tips for learners of EBM: 1. Relative risk reduction, absolute risk reduction, and number needed to treat. CMAJ 2004;171:353–8.

104. Montori VM, Kleinbart J, Newman TB, Keitz SA, Wyer PC, Moyer VA, et al., for the Evidence-Based Medicine Teaching Tips Working Group. Tips for learners of EBM: 2. Measures of precision (confidence intervals). CMAJ 2004;171:611–15.

105. McGinn TG, Wyer PC, Newman TB, Keitz SA, Leipzig R, Guyatt GH, for the Evidence-Based Medicine Teaching Tips Working Group. Tips

for learners of EBM: 3. Measures of observer variability (kappa statistic). CMAJ 2004;171:1369–73.

106. Hatala RM, Keitz SA, Wyer PC, Guyatt GH, for the Evidence-Based Medicine Teaching Tips Working Group. Tips for learners of EBM: 4. Assessing heterogeneity of primary studies in systematic reviews and whether to combine their results. CMAJ 2005;172:661–5.

107. Montori VM, Wyer PC, Newman TB, Keitz SA, Guyatt GH, for the Evidence-Based Medicine Teaching Tips Working Group. Tips for learners of EBM: 5. The effect of spectrum of disease on the performance of diagnostic tests. CMAJ 2005;173:385–90.

108. Richardson WS, Wilson MC, Keitz SA, Wyer PC, for the EBM Teaching Scripts Working Group. Tips for teachers of evidence-based medicine: Making sense of diagnostic test results using likelihood ratios. J Gen Intern Med 2008;23(1):87–92.

109. Prasad K, Jaeschke R, Wyer P, Keitz SA, Guyatt GH, for the Evidence-Based Medicine Teaching Tips Working Group. Tips for teachers of evidence-based medicine: Understanding odds ratios and their relationship to risk ratios. J Gen Intern Med 2008;23(5): 635–40.

110. Kennedy CC, Jaeschke R, Keitz SA, Newman T, Montori VM, Wyer PC, et al., for the Evidence-Based Medicine Teaching Tips Working Group. Tips for teachers of evidence-based medicine: adjusting for prognostic imbalances (confounding variables) in studies on therapy or harm. J Gen Intern Med 2008;23(3):337–43. PMID: 18175191.

111. McGinn T, Jervis R, Wisnivesky J, Keitz SA, Wyer PC, for the Evidence-Based Medicine Teaching Tips Working Group. Tips for teachers of evidence-based medicine: Clinical prediction rules (CPRs) and estimating pretest probability. J Gen Intern Med 2008;23(8):1261–8.

112. Lee A, Joynt GM, Ho AMH, Keitz S, McGinn T, Wyer PC, for the Evidence-Based Medicine Teaching Tips Working Group. Tips for teachers of evidence-based medicine: Making sense of decision analysis using a decision tree. J Gen Intern Med 2009;24(5):642–8.

113. Tiberius RG. Small group teaching: A trouble-shooting guide. Toronto, ON: OISE Press; 1990.

114. Jason H, Westberg J. Fostering learning in small groups: A practical guide. Philadelphia, PA: Springer; 1996.

115. Brookfield SD, Preskill S. Discussion as a way of teaching: Tools and techniques for democratic classrooms. San Francisco, CA: Jossey-Bass; 1999.

9

116. Maudsley G. Roles and responsibilities of the problem based learning tutor in the undergraduate medical curriculum. BMJ 1999;318:657–61.

117. Jaques D, Salmon G. Learning in groups: A handbook for face-to-face and online environments. 4th ed. Oxford, UK: Routledge; 2007.

118. Elwyn G, Greenhalgh T, Macfarlane F. Groups: a guide to small group work in healthcare, management, education and research. Oxford, UK: Radcliffe Publishing; 2001.

119. Exley K, Dennick R. Small group teaching: Tutorials, seminars, and beyond. London, UK: Routledge Falmer; 2004.

120. McCrorie P. Teaching and leading small groups, Understanding Medical Education Booklet Series. ASME; 2007.

Appendix 1 Glossary

Terms you are likely to encounter in your clinical reading

Absolute risk reduction (ARR). *See* Terms specific to treatment effects.

Allocation concealment. Occurs when the person who is enrolling a participant into a clinical trial is unaware whether the next participant to be enrolled will be allocated to the intervention or control group.

Case-control study. A study that involves identifying patients who have the outcome of interest (cases) and control patients without the same outcome and looking back to see if they had the exposure of interest.

Case series. A report on a series of patients with an outcome of interest. No control group is involved.

Clinical practice guideline. A systematically developed statement (that provides recommendations) designed to assist clinician and patient decisions about appropriate health care for specific clinical circumstances. They are informed by a systematic review of evidence and an assessment of the benefits and harms of alternative care options.

Cohort study. Involves identification of two groups (cohorts) of patients, one that received the exposure of interest, and one that did not, and following these cohorts forward for the outcome of interest.

Confidence interval (CI). Quantifies the uncertainty in measurement. It is usually reported as 95% CI, which is the range of values within which we can be 95% sure that the true value for the whole population lies. For example, for a number needed to treat (NNT) of 10 with a 95% CI of 5 to 15, we would have 95% confidence that the true NNT value lies between 5 and 15.

Control event rate (CER). *See* Terms specific to treatment effects.

Cost–benefit analysis. Assesses whether the cost of an intervention is worth the benefit by measuring both in the same units; monetary units are usually used.

Cost-effectiveness analysis. Measures the net cost of providing an intervention as well as the outcomes obtained. Outcomes are reported in a single unit of measurement.

Cost-minimization analysis. If health effects are known to be equal, only costs are analyzed and the least costly alternative is chosen.

Cost–utility analysis. Converts health effects into personal preferences (or utilities) and describes how much it costs for some additional quality gain (e.g., cost per additional quality-adjusted life-year [QALY]).

Crossover study design. The administration of two or more experimental therapies one after the other in a specified or random order to the same group of patients.

Cross-sectional study. The observation of a defined population at a single point in time or time interval. Exposure and outcome are determined simultaneously.

Decision analysis (or **clinical decision analysis**). The application of explicit, quantitative methods that quantify prognoses, treatment effects, and patient values to analyze a decision under conditions of uncertainty.

Event rate. The proportion of patients in a group in whom the event is observed. Thus, if out of 100 patients, the event is observed in 27, the event rate is 0.27. Control event rate (CER) and experimental event rate (EER) are used to refer to this rate in control and experimental groups of patients, respectively. The patient expected event rate (PEER) refers to the rate of events we'd expect in a patient who received no treatment or conventional treatment. *See* Terms specific to treatment effects.

Evidence-based health care. Extends the application of the principles of evidence-based medicine *(see below)* to all professions associated with health care, including purchasing and management.

Evidence-based medicine (EBM). The conscientious, explicit, and judicious use of current best evidence in making decisions about the care of individual patients. The practice of evidence-based medicine requires the integration of individual clinical expertise with the best available external clinical evidence from systematic research and our patient's unique values and circumstances.

Experimental event rate (EER). *See* Terms specific to treatment effects.

Incidence. The proportion of new cases of the target disorder in the population at risk during a specified time interval.

Inception cohort. A group of patients who are assembled near the onset of the target disorder.

Intention-to-treat (ITT) analysis. A method of analysis for randomized trials in which all patients randomly assigned to one of the treatments are analyzed together, whether or not they completed or received that treatment, to preserve randomization.

Likelihood ratio (LR). The likelihood that a given test result would be expected in a patient with the target disorder compared with the likelihood that that same result would be expected in a patient without the target disorder. *See* Table A1.2 for calculations.

Meta-analysis. The statistical analysis done to pool the results of two or more primary studies.

n-of-1 trials. In such trials, the patient undergoes pairs of treatment periods organized so that one period involves the use of the experimental treatment and the other involves the use of an alternative or placebo therapy. The patient and physician are blinded, if possible, and outcomes are monitored. Treatment periods are replicated until the clinician and patient are convinced that the treatments are definitely different or definitely not different.

Negative predictive value. Proportion of people with a negative test who are free of the target disorder. *See* Likelihood ratio.

Number needed to treat (NNT). The inverse of the absolute risk reduction and the number of patients that need to be treated to prevent one bad outcome. *See* Table A1.1 Terms specific to treatment effects.

Odds. Chances of the number of people incurring an outcome event relative to the number of people who don't have an event.

Odds ratio (OR). The ratio of the odds of having the target disorder in the experimental group relative to the odds in favour of having the target disorder in the control group (in cohort studies or systematic reviews [SRs]) or the odds in favour of being exposed in participants with the target disorder divided by the odds in favour of being exposed in control participants (without the target disorder). *See* Table A1.4 for calculations.

Patient expected event rate. *See* Terms specific to treatment effects.

Overview of reviews. A summary of two or more systematic reviews.

Positive predictive value (PPV). Proportion of people with a positive test who have the target disorder. *See* Likelihood ratio.

Posttest odds. The odds that the patient has the target disorder after the test is carried out (calculated as: pretest odds × likelihood ratio).

Posttest probability. The proportion of patients with that particular test result who have the target disorder [posttest odds/(1 + posttest odds)].

Pretest odds. The odds that the patient has the target disorder before the test is carried out [pretest probability/(1 − pretest probability)].

Pretest probability/prevalence. The proportion of people with the target disorder in the population at risk at a specific time (point prevalence) or time interval (period prevalence). *See* Likelihood ratio.

Randomization (or **random allocation).** Method analogous to tossing a coin to assign patients to treatment groups (the experimental treatment is assigned if the coin lands "heads" and a conventional, "control" or "placebo" treatment is given if the coin lands "tails").

Randomized controlled trial (RCT). Participants are randomly allocated into an experimental group or a control group and followed over time for the variables/outcomes of interest.

Relative risk reduction (RRR). *See* Terms specific to treatment effects.

Risk ratio (RR). The ratio of the risk of the outcome event in the treated group (EER) to the risk of the event in the control group (CER)—used in randomized trials and cohort studies: RR ≡ EER/CER. Also called *relative risk.*

Sensitivity. Proportion of people with the target disorder who have a positive test result. It is used to assist in assessing and selecting a diagnostic test/sign/symptom. *See* Likelihood ratio.

SnNout. When a sign/test/symptom has a high Sensitivity, a Negative result can help rule out the diagnosis. For example, the sensitivity of a history of ankle swelling for diagnosing ascites is 93%; therefore, if a person does not have a history of ankle swelling, it is highly unlikely that the person has ascites.

Specificity. Proportion of people without the target disorder who have a negative test result. It is used to assist in assessing and selecting a diagnostic test/sign/symptom. *See* Likelihood ratio.

SpPin. When a sign/test/symptom has a high Specificity, a Positive result can help to rule in the diagnosis. For example, the specificity of a fluid wave for diagnosing ascites is 92%; therefore, if a person does have a fluid wave, it rules in the diagnosis of ascites.

Systematic review (SR). A summary of the literature that uses explicit methods to perform a comprehensive literature search and critical appraisal of individual studies and that may use appropriate statistical techniques to combine these valid studies, when appropriate. The statistical technique for pooling studies is called a *meta-analysis.*

Terms specific to treatment effects

Journals on EBM (e.g., *ACP Journal Club*) have achieved consensus on some terms they use to describe both good and bad effects of therapy. We will illustrate them by using a synthesis of three randomized trials in diabetes, which individually showed that several years of intensive insulin therapy reduced the proportion of patients with worsening retinopathy to 13% from 38%, raised the proportion of patients with satisfactory hemoglobin A_{1c} levels to 60% from about 30%, and increased the proportion of patients with at least one episode of symptomatic hypoglycemia to 57% from 23%. Note that in each case the first number constitutes the EER and the second number the CER.

We will use the following terms and calculations to describe these effects of treatment.

When the experimental treatment reduces the probability of a bad outcome (worsening diabetic retinopathy)

RRR (relative risk reduction). The proportional reduction in rates of bad outcomes between experimental and control participants in a trial, calculated as $|EER - CER|/CER$, and accompanied by a 95% CI. In the case of worsening diabetic retinopathy, $|EER - CER|/CER \equiv |13\% - 38\%|/38\% \equiv 66\%$.

ARR (absolute risk reduction). The absolute arithmetic difference in rates of bad outcomes between experimental and control participants in a trial, calculated as $|EER - CER|$, and accompanied by a 95% CI. In this case, $|EER - CER| \equiv |13\% - 38\%| \equiv 25\%$. (This is sometimes called the *risk difference.*)

NNT (number needed to treat). The number of patients who need to be treated to achieve one additional favourable outcome, calculated as 1/ARR and accompanied by a 95% CI. In this case, $1/\text{ARR} \equiv 1/25\% \equiv 4$.

When the experimental treatment increases the probability of a good outcome (satisfactory hemoglobin A_{1c} levels)

RBI (relative benefit increase). The proportional increase in rates of good outcomes between experimental and control patients in a trial, calculated as |EER − CER|/CER, and accompanied by a 95% confidence interval (CI). In the case of satisfactory hemoglobin A_{1c} levels, $|\text{EER} - \text{CER}|/\text{CER} \equiv |60\% - 30\%|/30\% \equiv 100\%$.

ABI (absolute benefit increase). The absolute arithmetic difference in rates of good outcomes between experimental and control patients in a trial, calculated as |EER − CER|, and accompanied by a 95% CI. In the case of satisfactory hemoglobin A_{1c} levels, $|\text{EER} - \text{CER}| \equiv |60\% - 30\%| \equiv 30\%$

NNT (number needed to treat). The number of patients who need to be treated to achieve one additional good outcome, calculated as 1/ARR and accompanied by a 95% CI. In this case, $1/\text{ARR} \equiv 1/30\% \equiv 3$.

When the experimental treatment increases the probability of a bad outcome (episodes of hypoglycemia)

RRI (relative risk increase). The proportional increase in rates of bad outcomes between experimental and control patients in a trial, calculated as |EER − CER|/CER, and accompanied by a 95% CI. In the case of hypoglycemic episodes, $|\text{EER} - \text{CER}|/\text{CER} \equiv |57\% - 23\%|/23\% \equiv 148\%$. (RRI is also used in assessing the impact of "risk factors" for disease.)

ARI (absolute risk increase). The absolute arithmetic difference in rates of bad outcomes between experimental and control patients in a trial, calculated as |EER − CER|, and accompanied by a 95% confidence interval (CI). In the case of hypoglycemic episodes, $|\text{EER} - \text{CER}| \equiv |57\% - 23\%| \equiv 34\%$. (ARI is also used in assessing the impact of "risk factors" for disease.)

NNH (number needed to harm). The number of patients who, if they received the experimental treatment, would result in one

Table A1.1 Treatment effects

Occurrence of diabetic retinopathy at 5 years among patients with insulin-dependent diabetes		Relative risk reduction (RRR)	Absolute risk reduction (ARR)	Number needed to treat (NNT)
Usual insulin regimen control event rate (CER)	Intensive insulin regimen experimental event rate (EER)	IEER − CERI/CER	IEER − CERI	1/ARR
38%	13%	I13% − 38%I/38% ≡ 68%	I13% − 38%I ≡ 25%	1/25% ≡ 4 patients

additional patient being harmed, compared with patients who received the control treatment, calculated as 1/ARR and accompanied by a 95% CI. In this case, $1/ARR \equiv 1/34\% \equiv 3$.

How to calculate likelihood ratios (LRs)

We can assume that there are four possible groups of patients, as indicated (**a**, **b**, **c**, **d**) in Table A1.2 below:

Table A1.2 Test annually

Diagnostic test result		Target disorder		
		a	**b**	a + b
	−	**c**	**d**	c + d
		a + c	b + d	a + b + c + d

From these we can determine the *sensitivity* and *specificity* as follows:

$$\text{Sensitivity} \equiv a/(a + c)$$

$$\text{Specificity} \equiv d/(b + d)$$

We can consider the calculation of the LR for a positive test in a couple of ways:

1. We can consider: How likely is a positive test in someone with the disease?

$$\equiv a/(a + c)$$

We also need to consider: How likely is a positive test result in someone without the disease?

$$\equiv b/(b + d)$$

And, how likely is this test result to occur in someone with compared with someone without the disease?

$$\equiv [a/(a + c)]/[b/(b + d)]$$

2. We can use sensitivity and specificity to calculate the LR for a positive test result (LR+):

$$LR+ \equiv sensitivity/(1 - specificity)$$
$$\equiv [a/(a + c)] \div [b/(b + d)]$$

Similarly, we can calculate the LR for a negative test result (LR−):

$$LR- \equiv (1 - sensitivity)/specificity$$
$$\equiv [c/(a + c)] \div [d/(b + d)]$$
$$Positive\ predictive\ value \equiv a/(a + b)$$
$$Negative\ predictive\ value \equiv d/(c + d)$$
$$Pretest\ probability \equiv (a + c)/(a + b + c + d)$$

Sample calculation

Suppose you have a patient with anemia and a serum ferritin of 60 mmol/L. You come across a systematic review* of serum ferritin as a diagnostic test for iron-deficiency anemia, with the results summarized in Table A1.3.

These results indicate that 90% of the patients with iron-deficiency anemia have a positive test result (serum ferritin <65 mmol/L). This is known as *sensitivity*, which is calculated as:

$$Sensitivity \equiv a/(a + c) = 731/809 \equiv 90\%$$

The results also show that 85% of patients who do not have iron-deficiency anemia have a negative test result. This is referred to as *specificity*, which is calculated as:

$$Specificity \equiv d/(b + d) = 1500/1770 \equiv 85\%$$

*(Guyatt GH, Oxman AD, Ali M, et al. Laboratory diagnosis of iron-deficiency anemia: an overview. *J Gen Intern Med.* 1992;7:145–153.)

Table A1.3 Test annually

		Target disorder (iron-deficiency anemia)		
		Present	**Absent**	
Diagnostic test result (serum ferritin)	+ (<65 mmol/L)	731	270	1001
		a	b	a + b
	− (≥65 mmol/L)	c	d	c + d
		78	1500	1578
		a + c	b + d	a + b + c + d
		809	1770	2579

Table A1.4 Odds ratio (OR)/relative risk (RR)

	Adverse event occurs (infectious complication)	Adverse event doesn't occur (no infectious complication)	Totals
Exposed to treatment (experimental event rate [EER])	1	29	30
	a	b	a + b
Not exposed to treatment (control event rate [CER])	9	21	30
	c	d	c + d
Totals	10	50	60
	a + c	b + d	a + b +c + d

$CER \equiv c/(c + d) \equiv 0.30$
$EER \equiv a/(a + b) \equiv 0.033$
Control event odds $\equiv c/d \equiv 0.43$
Experimental event odds $\equiv a/b \equiv 0.034$
$RR \equiv EER/CER \equiv 0.11$
Relative odds $\equiv OR \equiv (a/b)/(c/d) \equiv ad/bc \equiv 0.08$

Note that risks $\equiv$ odds/(1+odds) and odds $\equiv$ risk/(1−risk). We used the second equation in the description of posttest odds and probabilities above. We convert pretest probabilities to pretest odds to multiply this by the likelihood ratio (LR). We then used the first equation to convert from posttest odds to posttest probability.

From these the positive and negative LRs can be determined:

$$LR+ \equiv sensitivity/(1-specificity) \equiv 90\%/15\% \equiv 6$$

$$LR- \equiv (1-sensitivity)/specificity \equiv 10\%/85\% \equiv 0.12$$

Thus, from your calculation of LR+, you determine that your patient's positive test result would be about six times as likely to be seen in someone with iron-deficiency anemia than in someone without the disorder.

Calculation of odds ratio/relative risk

Calculation of OR/RR for the use of trimethoprim-sulfamethoxazole prophylaxis in cirrhosis is performed as shown in Table A1.4.

Index

Page numbers followed by "*f*" indicate figures, "*t*" indicate tables, and "*b*" indicate boxes.

A

Abnormality/normality, 157–158, 157*b*
Absolute benefit increase (ABI), 90
Absolute risk difference, 98*b*
Absolute risk increase (ARI), 94
Absolute risk reduction (ARR), 89*t*, 90
 for individual patients, 104–105
ACC/AHA risk calculator, 56
ACCESSSS, 46, 57, 61
ACP Journal Club, 51, 73
 EBM in real time and, 99–100
 economic analyses in, 134
 prognostic studies in, 185–186, 188
 trial follow-up in, 81
ACP Journal Wise, 45, 50–51
Active learning, in teaching EBM, 241
ADAPTE, 142
Administrative databases, in harm/etiology studies, 205
Admission rounds, 248, 249*t*–250*t*
ADVANCE (Action in Diabetes and Vascular Disease: Preterax and Diamicron MR Controlled Evaluation) trial, 86–87, 88*t*
Adverse effects, 94
 see also Harm; Harm/etiology studies; Number needed to harm

Adverse event, in harm/etiology studies, 207
Affective domain of learning, in teaching EBM, 242–243
"Aggregators," Internet-based, 43
AGREE (Appraisal of Guidelines for Research and Evaluation) Collaboration, 140
Allocation concealment, 78–79
Alzheimer's disease, 188–189
 see also Dementia
Ambulatory Morning Report, 255*t*
Anemia, iron-deficiency, 155, 156*b*, 161–162, 162*t*, 164
Answerable questions, evaluation in asking, 223, 224*b*
Anticoagulation, for atrial fibrillation, 128–130
Antiplatelet therapy, for atrial fibrillation, 128–130
Applicability, of harm/etiology studies, 217–219, 217*b*
 alternative treatments, 219
 patient's preferences, concerns, and expectations in, 218–219
 risks of benefit and harm, 218
Appraiser, in CAT, 257*b*
Atherosclerotic cardiovascular disease (ASCVD), 57
Audit, 229

B

Background questions, 21–22, 22*b*
arising, 24, 25*b*
experience and, 22, 23*f*
formulation of, 27–29
Bargain, in practice guidelines, 144
Barriers, to implementing
guidelines, 144
Bedside patient presentation,
educational prescription in,
32*b*
Behaviour
evaluation of, 227–228, 228*b*
in practice guidelines, 145
Beliefs of patients, 143–144
Best Practice (BP), 57
Bias
in diagnostic tests, 160–161
"5 and 20" rule of losses to,
190
minimization of, 112–113
sources of, 67
Biological sense, of diagnostic tests
for causation, 211
BioMed Central, 48–49
Blinding, 83
in diagnostic tests, 160–161
double, 84
in prognostic studies, 191
qualitative research and, 126
see also Randomization,
concealed
BMC Musculoskeletal Disorders,
124–125
"Born"/expiration date, in CAT,
257*b*
Breast cancer, early detection of,
180
British Medical Journal (BMJ), 44
Best Practice, 57
Bullying, teaching EBM and, 247
Burden of illness, 143

C

Caffeine consumption, urinary
incontinence from, 203*t*
Can-IMPLEMENT groups, 142
Canadian Task Force for Preventive
Health Care, 140–141
Card flip, 249*t*–250*t*, 252–253
Cardiovascular risk calculator, 56
Cardiovascular risk reduction
ACCESSSS for, 57
Dynamed Plus for, 57–58
Case-control studies, prognostic,
186–187
Case finding, 177–182
CAT banks, 112
CATMaker, 226
CATs *see* Critically appraised topics
Causation, 201, 210–211
Citations, in CAT, 257*b*
Clinic conferences, 254–256,
255*t*
Clinical bottom line, in CAT, 257*b*
Clinical decision analyses (CDA),
71–72, 107–108
applicability of, 133, 133*b*
components of, 138–139, 139*t*
importance of, 132–133, 132*b*
reports of, 128–134
validity of, 131–132, 131*b*
Clinical Enquiry and Response
Service (CLEAR), in harm/
etiology studies, 219–220
Clinical Evidence, 47–48, 101, 101*f*
Clinical expertise, in teaching EBM,
245
Clinical findings, as clinical
questions, 25*b*
Clinical manifestations, as clinical
questions, 25*b*
Clinical medicine, weaving
evidence into, in teaching
EBM, 237–239

Clinical practice guidelines (CPGs), 72
  applicability of, 142–145
  defined, 138
  reports of, 138–145
  validity of, 140–142, 140*b*
Clinical prediction guides, 176, 187, 193–194
  examples of, 176*t*
  interactive versions of, 177
  validity of, 176
Clinical Queries (CQ screen), 44–47
Clinical scenarios
  on coronary heart disease, 51*b*–52*b*
  on diagnostic tests, 155, 156*b*
  on harm, 201, 201*b*
Clinical setting, in teaching EBM, 243
Clinical skills, in teaching EBM, 246
Clinical teams, teaching EBM in, 275–289
  with counterproductive behaviours, 285–288
  EBM skills "back home", 288–289
  healthy learning climate, 280–281
  issues in learning EBM jargon, 283–285
  keep the discussion going, 281
  keep the discussion on track, 281–282
  learning activities, 278–280
  sensible ground rules for, 276–278
  time management, 282–283
  understand why to learn, 275–276
Clinical work, central issues in, 25*b*
Clot PLUS, 50–51

Cochrane Collaboration, 44
Cochrane Library, 48
Cognitive dissonance, 23
  learners', 244–245, 267–268
Cognitive domain of learning, in teaching EBM, 242–243
Cognitive resonance, 23
Cohort studies, prognostic, 186–187, 191
Comments, in CAT, 257*b*
"Community of learning", 241–242
"Community of practice", 241–242
Compliance, early diagnosis and, 181
Composite outcomes, 86–87
Conative domain of learning, in teaching EBM, 242–243
Confidence intervals (CIs), 97, 98*b*
  Forest Plot and, 120
  in prognostic studies, 196–197
Confounders, 75–76
  in harm/etiology studies, 204–205
Consensus opinion, 132
Consolidated Standards of Reporting Trials (CONSORT) Guidelines, 73–74
  inclusion of flow diagrams in, 79–80, 80*f*
Consultant walking rounds, 249*t*–250*t*, 252
Control event rate (CER), 89*t*, 90, 93*t*
  estimates of benefits and risks of therapy and, 104
Control manoeuvre, 233
Core competencies, of Accreditation Council for Graduate Medical Education, 267–268
Coronary artery disease, hormone replacement therapy and, 74

Coronary heart disease (CHD), 51b–52b, 56
Cost-benefit analysis, 136
Cost-effectiveness analysis, 136
Cost utility analysis, 136
Courses/workshops, 234
Critical appraisal, 225–226, 225b, 260t
Critically appraised topics (CATs), 112
    in diagnosis, 173
    learning in, 256–257
    limitations of, 256–257
    writing, 257b
Curriculum, integrating EBM into, 267–271, 269f
    4-year medical school, 271–274

D

D-dimer test, 155, 156f
"Dead spaces", 249t–250t, 253
Dechallenge-rechallenge study, 210–211
Decision aids, validated, 107–108
Decision analysis see Clinical decision analyses
Decision making, support for, 107–109
Decision nodes, 128–130
Decision tree, 119f, 128–130
Dementia
    Alzheimer, 185
    in prognostic studies, 185–186, 194, 197
    see also Alzheimer's disease
Diabetes, type 2, 86–87, 88t
Diagnosis, 153–183
    learning and teaching with CATs, 177b
    stages and strategies in, 153b, 154f
    thinking modes in, 153
    see also Early diagnosis

Diagnostic odds ratio, 166
Diagnostic tests, 154–155, 158–161
    applicability of, 166–177, 168b
    availability/affordability of, 167–168
    for causation, 210–211
    clinical prediction guides of, 187
    as clinical questions, 25b
    clinical scenario on, 155, 156b
    evidence-based medicine in real time, 177
    importance of, 161–162
    multilevel likelihood ratios in, 175
    multiple, 172, 176
    normal or abnormal, 157–158, 157b
    patient referral, effects of, 168
    patient willingness to, 181
    posttest probability in, 161, 164, 165f, 170–176
    precision/accuracy of, 167–168
    pretest probability in, 161, 165f
        estimation of, 168–170
    reference standards and, 160–161
        ascertainment of, 160
        measurements compared to, 160–161
    representativeness of, 159–160
    ruling diagnoses in/out, 164–166
    sensitivity, specificity, and likelihood ratios in, 163–177
    teaching tips for, 181b–182b
    test threshold in, 170–171, 171f
    validity of, 158–161, 159b, 166–177

Diastolic learning, in teaching EBM, 241

Differential diagnosis, as clinical questions, 25b

Digital library licenses, 48

Direct oral anticoagulants (DOACs), for atrial fibrillation, 128–130

Discussion tangents, 286–287

Disutility, 110–111

Domains of learning, in teaching EBM, 242–243

Dominating overparticipator, 287–288

Dose-response gradient, 210

Double-blind, 84

"Down times", 249t–250t, 253

DynaMed, 37–38

Dynamed Plus, 57–58

E

Early diagnosis, 155, 178–180
  benefit of
    evidence of, 178–180
    harm *vs.*, 178, 179b, 181
    lead time, 178–180, 179f
    patient willingness, 181
    teaching about, 182

EBM *see* Evidence-based medicine

EBM calculator, 98–99, 99f
  for ORs and RRs conversion, to NNTs or NNHs, 121, 122b, 122t–123t
  via PEER, 104–107

EBM courses/workshops, 234

EBM skills, 237, 239

Economic analyses, 71–72
  applicability of, 135b, 137
  importance of, 135b, 137
  reports of, 134–138
  validity of, 134b, 135–137

Education
  courses and workshops, 234
  evaluation of, 234
  see also Learning; Teaching EBM

Educational prescription, 29, 31
  in bedside patient presentation, 32b
  form, 30f
  in teaching EBM, 248–252
  written by learners, 31

Educational sessions, incorporating EBM into, 258–265
  journal club in, 262–265, 264t, 266b
  Morning Report in, 258–262, 260t

Electronic medical record systems, 42

EMBASE, 44–45

eMedicine, 47

End-stage renal disease, 205

Essential Evidence Plus, 45

Etiology, as clinical questions, 25b

Etiology studies *see* Harm/etiology studies

Evaluation, 223–236
  EBM courses/workshops, 234
  see also Self-evaluation

Evidence
  appraising, 67–69
    PICO format from, 67–68
    racing analogy of, 67–68
  barriers to use, 232b
  in diagnosis, 154–155
  evaluating integration of, 226–227, 227b
  finding current best, 35–65
  see also Preappraised evidence

Evidence Alerts
  screenshot of, 100f
  searchable database within, 100

Evidence-based journal clubs, 265
Evidence-based medicine (EBM)
  incorporating, into existing
      educational sessions,
      258–265
  integrating
    into 4-year medical school
      curriculum, 271–274
    into curriculum, 267–271,
      269f
  practicing, 230–231
  in real-time *see* Real-time, EBM
      in
  teaching, 232b, 237–298
    on an inpatient service,
      248–253, 249t–250t,
      254b
    in clinical teams and other
      small groups, 275–289
    learning more about,
      274–275
    modes of, 237–239, 238b
    in outpatient clinic, 253–256,
      255t
    top 10 failures of, 245–248
    top 10 successes of,
      240–245
    writing structured summaries
      of, 256–258, 257b
Evidence-Based Medicine (EBM)
    Guidelines, 58
Evidence-Based Medicine electronic
    Decision Support
    (EBMeDS), 42
Evidence-Based Medicine Journal,
    160–161
Evidence-Based Medicine Reviews
    (EBMR) service, 44
"Evidence refinery" services, 45
Evidence summary, in CAT, 257b
EvidenceUpdates, 44, 48–51, 56
Existing data, in harm/etiology
    studies, 205

Experience, clinical questions and,
    22, 23f, 25b
Experimental event rate (EER), 89t,
    90, 93t
Experimental studies, 74
Exposure
  in diagnostic tests for causation,
    210
  in harm/etiology studies, 207
Extracranial-intracranial (EC/IC)
    arterial bypass, case series
    and case reports of, 74–75

F

False-positive or false-negative
    outcomes, 173
Feasibility, of treatment, 103
Ferritin, serum, test for, 155, 156b,
    161–162, 162t, 173, 174f
Follow-up rounds, old patient at,
    254b
Follow-up visits, 255t, 256
Foreground questions, 21–22,
    22b
  arising, 24, 25b
  experience and, 22, 23f
  formulation of, 27–29
Forest Plot, 120, 129f
Framingham risk calculator, 56

G

GATE software, 226
Gaussian definition, of normality,
    157, 157b, 158f
Glasziou, Paul, 67
Google, 47, 51, 55–56
GRADE system, 141–142
Grading of Recommendations,
    Assessment, Development,
    and Evaluation (GRADE),
    43

H

Harm, 201–222, 201*b*
Harm/etiology studies
applicability, 217–219, 217*b*
alternative treatments, 219
patient's preferences, concerns,
and expectations in,
218–219
risks of benefit and harm,
218
association consistency, 211
dechallenge-rechallenge study,
210–211
EBM in real-time, 215–217,
219–221
magnitude of association,
211–215
precision of estimate of
association, 216–217
importance of, 211–215, 212*b*
report types, 202–221
systematic reviews in, 201–202,
202*f*
validity, 201, 202*b*, 203–211,
203*t*
assessment, 201
causation tests for, 210–211
feasibility *vs.*, 203–204
follow-up in, 209
patient groups, 203–207
treatments/exposures and
clinical outcomes, 208
Health care professionals,
evidence-based medicine
for, 235
Health Information Research Unit,
50–51
Health Internetwork Access to
Research Information
(HINARI) program, 48
Hormone replacement therapy
(HRT), 74

I

I^2 statistic, 118
Improvement, as clinical questions,
25*b*
"Inception cohort", 187–188
Individual studies *see* Studies,
individual
Information resources
evidence-based, 36–49
application of, 62–63
clinical scenario in, 51*b*–52*b*
examination of, 62
online texts in, guidelines for,
37, 38*t*–39*t*
organize access to, 47–49
"P5" approach to, 40–47,
41*f*
for patient problems,
51–63
"prompt" approach to, 49
"pull" approach to, 49–50
"push" approach to, 49–51
recommendations in, 43–44,
60
references in, 37
screening test for, 37
selection of, 55–57
studies in, 45, 60–61
summaries in, 42–43
synopsis in, 45–47
syntheses in, 44–45
systems in, 40–42
traditional textbooks and,
36–40, 61–62
orientation to, 36–49
see also specific resources
Initial visits, 255*t*, 256
Inpatient service, teaching and
learning EBM in, 248–253,
249*t*–250*t*, 254*b*
Intention-to-treat analysis,
randomization and, 82

Internet
  free, 48–49
  information services in, 47–48
  preappraised studies in, 45
  see also Online evidence services
Intervention, of EBM, 233
Iron-deficiency anemia, 155, 156*b*,
  161–162, 162*t*, 164

J

James Lind Library, 220–221, 221*f*
Jargon, 283–285
Journal clubs
  evidence-based medicine for, 235
  goals of, 262–263, 264*t*
  in incorporating EBM, 262–265
  learning needs, 263–265
  team learning, 225–226
  three-session model in, 263
  two-session cycle in, 265
Journals
  evidence-based, 50–51
  full-text, 50
Judgements, in teaching EBM, 244

K

Killer Bs, 138–139, 139*b*, 143
Knowledge
  background/foreground, 23, 23*f*
  gaps/deficit, 24

L

Labelling, 178, 181
Language, restrictions in, 114–115
Learners' actual learning needs, in
  teaching EBM, 240
Learning
  active, 241
  domains of, 242–243
  follow-up rounds, 254*b*
  in inpatient service, 248–253,
    249*t*–250*t*, 254*b*
  lifelong, 244–245, 267–268
  to make judgements, 244
  multistaged, 244–245
  in outpatient clinic, 253–256,
    255*t*
  passive, 241
  problem-based (by inquiry), 35
  spiral trajectory, 267
  structured summaries in,
    256–258, 257*b*
  systolic, 241
  team learning, 225–226
  see also Teaching EBM
Learning session, integrating EBM
  into, 266*b*
LHH *see* Likelihood of being
  helped *versus* harmed
Librarians
  on clinical rounds, 231–232
  evidence sources from, 35–36
  in teaching EBM, 260–261
Library
  digital license, 48
  public, 48–49
Lifelong learning, teaching EBM in,
  244–245, 267–268
Likelihood of being helped *versus*
  harmed (LHH), 108
  in teaching EBM, 252
Likelihood ratios
  "chain", 172
  in diagnostic tests, 163–177,
    167*t*
  multilevel, 175
  nomogram, 175*f*

M

McMaster PLUS Federated search
  (MPFS), 61–62
Meaning, as clinical questions, 25*b*

MEDLINE, 46–47, 49
Medline Plus, 109–110, 110*f*
Meta-analysis (MAs), 71, 112–113
Meta-search services, evidence-based, 46
Mini Mental State Exam (MMSE), 191
Morning Report
    in incorporating EBM, 258–262, 260*t*
    in inpatient service, 248–252, 249*t*–250*t*
    in outpatient clinic, 255*t*, 256
Multilevel likelihood ratios, 175

N

N-of-1 trials, 72, 78, 145–148
    guides for, 147*b*
    strategies for, 146–147
National Institute for Health and Care Excellence (NICE), 138
Network MA, 123–124
"Network met-analysis", 68
Newly collected data, in harm/etiology studies, 205
Nihilism, 285–286
NNH *see* Number needed to harm
NNT *see* Number needed to treat
Nomogram, 105, 106*f*
Nonrandomized trials, 77–78
Normality/abnormality, 157–158, 157*b*
Number needed to harm (NNH), 214, 215*t*–216*t*
    conversion from ORs and RRs, 121, 122*b*, 122*t*–123*t*
    estimates of benefits and risks of therapy and, 104
    follow-up time, 94–95
    in RCTs, 93*t*, 94

Number needed to treat (NNT), 89*t*
    adjustment for baseline risk of, 96
    confidence intervals and, 97
    control event rate and, 95
    conversion from ORs and RRs, 121, 122*b*, 122*t*–123*t*
    estimates of benefits and risks of therapy and, 104
    in RCTs, 88*t*, 93*t*, 94–95
Nursing PLUS, 50–51

O

Obesity PLUS, 50–51
Observational studies, 74
Odds ratio (OR), 212–213, 215*t*–216*t*
    conversion to NNTs/NNHs, 121, 122*b*, 122*t*–123*t*
    diagnostic, 166
Online evidence services, 50–51
Online links, 55–56
Online texts, guidelines for, 37, 38*t*–39*t*
Opportunism, preparedness with, in teaching EBM, 243–244
Opportunity cost, 134
Optimal Aging Portal, 50–51
Osteoporosis, medications for, experience with initiation of, 127*b*
Outcomes
    assessment, 83–84
    composite, 86–87
    criteria, 191
    in harm/etiology studies, 207
    surrogate, 86
Outpatient clinic, teaching and learning EBM in, 253–256, 255*t*

Index

P

p value, 97–98

Pain PLUS, 50–51

Passive learning, in teaching EBM, 241

Patient values, in teaching EBM, 245

Patients
  appropriate spectrum of, 125
  evaluation of, 232–233
  evidence researched by, 55–56
  individual data for, in systematic reviews, 117
  labelling of, 178, 181
  preappraised literature for, 109–112, 110*f*
  preferences *see* Utilities (patient preferences)
  shared decision-making and, 107–109
  subgroups, 102–103, 103*b*
    in prognostic studies, 192–195
  trial participants *vs.*, 102
  values and expectations of, in treatment effect calculation, 107–109

Patient's expected event rate (PEER), in treatment effect calculation, 104–107

Patients' illnesses, in teaching EBM, 246

Pattern recognition, in diagnosis, 153

PedsCCM Evidence Based Journal Club, 51

PEER *see* Patient's expected event rate

Per protocol (PP) analysis, 83

Percentile, 157, 157*b*, 158*f*

PICO, 22*b*, 67–68, 187
  evaluation of, 232*b*

Placebo, 76–77

Positive predictive value, 161–162

Postgraduate learners, evidence-based medicine for, 235

Posttake rounds, 248, 249*t*–250*t*, 256

Posttest odds, 164

Posttest probability, in diagnostic tests, 161, 164, 165*f*, 170–176

Practising, evaluating changes in, 227–229

Preappraised evidence, 36
  EBM in real-time and, 99–101

Preappraised literature, for patients, 109–112, 110*f*

Preceptor rounds, 249*t*–250*t*

Preceptorship, 255*t*

Preferred Reporting Items for Systematic Reviews and Meta-Analyses (PRISMA) statement, 114–115, 116*f*

Preparedness, with opportunism, in teaching EBM, 243–244

Pretest odds, 164

Pretest probability, in diagnostic tests, 161, 165*f*
  critical appraisal in, 170*b*
  estimation of, 168–170

Prevention, as clinical questions, 25*b*

Printed texts, currency of, 37

Probability revision graph, 155, 156*f*, 165*f*

Prognosis, 185–199
  blinding, 191
    outcome criteria in, 191
  clinical prediction guides of, 187
  as clinical questions, 25*b*
  clinical scenario of, 185
  EBM in real-time of, 198–199
  importance of, 191
  patient subgroups of, 192–195

precision of, 196–197
report types on, 186–187
as survival curves, 195, 196f
systematic reviews of, 186
validity of, 187–195
    evidence, 186b, 195–198,
        195b, 197b
    follow-up of, 189–190
    outcome criteria, 191
    prognostic factors, adjustment
        for, 192–195
    representativeness, 187–188
Prognostic factors
    distribution of, 76
    randomization and, 76–77
PROGRESS trial, 97
Prospective cohort studies, in
        harm/etiology studies,
        205–206
Prospective data, in harm/etiology
        studies, 205
Psychomotor domain of learning,
        in teaching EBM, 242–243
Public Library of Science, 48–49
Publish-ahead-of-print (PAP)
        articles, 46–47
Published research, in teaching
        EBM, 245
PubMed, 44–45
    Clinical Queries, 73
'Pure' education rounds, 249t–
        250t, 253
Purposive sampling, 125

Q

Qualitative literature, 124–128
    evidence for, 125b
Qualitative studies, 71
    applicability of, 127
        phenomena in, patient/
            participant and, 127
    blinding and, 126
    data collection and analysis for,
        methods for, 126
    importance of, 126–127
    impressive, 126–127
    validity of, 125
Quality-adjusted life-years
        (QALYs), 128–130
    average gains in, 132
    in economic analysis, 136
Quantitative study results, 283–284
Questions, clinical, 19–34, 19b, 22b
    background/foreground, 21–22,
        22b
    in CAT, 257b
    components of, 21, 22b
    examples of, 22b
    formulation of, 27–29
    issues in, 24, 25b
    patients involvement in, 25
    saving/recording of, 26
    scheduling, 26–27
    selecting, 27
    teaching
        key steps, 29b
        questions for real-time EBM,
            29–33
Quiet nonparticipator, 288

R

Racing analogy, 67–68
RAM acronym, 160–161
Random error minimization,
        112–113
Randomization, 76–77
    benefits of, preservation of, 82
    concealed, 78–79
        see also Blinding
Randomized controlled trials (RCTs)
    analysis of patients in, 82–83
    blinding in, 83–84
        see also Randomization,
            concealed

Randomized controlled trials
(RCTs) *(Continued)*
follow-up, 79–82
in harm/etiology studies,
203–204
prognostic, 186–187
similarity of groups in, 79
Rating scale, for assessing values,
110–111, 111*f*
"Raw" unappraised evidence
services, 36
RCTs *see* Randomized controlled
trials
Real clinical actions, in teaching
EBM, 240
Real clinical decisions, in teaching
EBM, 240
Real-time, EBM in
calculating measures of
treatment effect, 98–99
in diagnostic tests, 177
in harm/etiology studies,
215–217, 219–221
magnitude of association,
211–215
precision of estimate of
association, 216–217
practising, 26–27
prognostic studies and, 198–199
teaching questions for, 29–33
Reasoning, analytic/non-analytic,
153
References, 37
Rehab PLUS, 45, 50–51
Relative benefit increase (RBI), 90
Relative odds *see* Odds ratio
Relative risk increase (RRI), 104
Relative risk reduction (RRR),
85–86, 88*t*–89*t*
confidence intervals in, 97
disadvantages of, 90
estimates of benefits and risks of
therapy and, 104

Relative risks (RRs), 98*b*
conversion to NNTs/NNHs, 121,
122*b*, 122*t*–123*t*
Forest Plot and, 120
Relevant outcomes, of EBM
interventions, 233–235
Research, in teaching EBM, 245
Retrospective data, in harm/
etiology studies, 205
Review rounds, 249*t*–250*t*,
252–253
Risk, as clinical questions, 25*b*
Risk calculators, 56
Risk difference, 90
Risk factors, 192
in normality/abnormality,
157–158, 157*b*
Risk ratio (RR), 119–120
Role modelling, in teaching EBM,
237–238, 270
Rounds
in inpatient service
admission, 248, 249*t*–250*t*
consultant walking, 249*t*–250*t*,
252
follow-up, 254*b*
posttake, 248, 249*t*–250*t*
preceptor, 249*t*–250*t*
pure' education, 249*t*–250*t*,
253
review, 249*t*–250*t*,
252–253
social issues, 249*t*–250*t*
work, 249*t*–250*t*, 252
in outpatient clinic
clinic conferences, 254–256,
255*t*
follow-up visits, 255*t*, 256
initial visits, 255*t*, 256
Morning Reports, 255*t*,
256
posttake, 256
preceptorship, 255*t*

S

Sampling, purposive, 125
Screening, 155, 177–182
    benefit *vs.* harm, 178, 179*b*, 181
    diagnostic lead-time, 179*f*
    RCTs of
        evidence of benefit, 178–180
        structure for, 180*f*
Search engines
    "federated", 47
    general, 46–47
    meta-search, 46
Searching for evidence
    execution of, 57–62
    in Morning Report, 260*t*
    question formulation in, 54–55
    resource selection in, 55–57
    self-evaluation in, 224–225,
        224*b*
    steps to, 54–63
    strategy, 55*f*
    see also Information resources
Self-evaluation, 223
    in critical appraisal, 225–226,
        225*b*
    in integrating evidence, 226–227,
        227*b*
    in Morning Report, 260*t*
    in patients' values, 226–227
    PICO, 232*b*
    in practice, changes in behavior,
        227–228, 228*b*
    in question asking, 223, 224*b*
    in searching, 224–225, 224*b*
    of teachers, 231–235, 231*b*–232*b*
Seminars, evidence-based medicine
    for, 235
Sensitivity, in diagnostic tests,
    163–177, 167*t*
Sensitivity analysis, 132–133, 190
Significance tests, 98*b*
SnNout, 165–166, 166*f*

Social issues rounds, 249*t*–250*t*
Specificity, in diagnostic tests,
    163–177, 167*t*
Spiral trajectory, 267
SpPin, 165–166
Standard gamble method, 128–130
Statins, 90, 201
Statistics, in teaching EBM, 245,
    284–285
Structured summaries *see* Critically
    appraised topics
Studies, individual, 41–42, 45,
    60–61, 68
    applicability of, 101–109, 102*b*
    assessment of, for validity, 115
    importance of, 85, 85*b*
    potential benefits and harms for,
        104–107
    reports of, 72–112
    treatment effects in
        calculation shortcut, 98–99
        confidence intervals, 97
        estimate of, precision of,
            96–98
        magnitude of, 86–96, 88*t*
        treatment feasibility, 103
        validity of, 74–85
    values expectations of, 107–109
    see also Nonrandomized trials;
        Qualitative studies;
        Randomized controlled
        trials
Subgroups *see* Patients, subgroups
Substituting research evidence, in
    teaching EBM, 245
Summaries, 42–43
    open access, 47
    structured *see* Critically appraised
        topics
Summary publications, 43
SUMSearch, 48–49
Surrogate outcomes, 86
Survival curves, 195, 196*f*

Synopsis, 45–47
  evidence-based meta-search
    services and, 46
  general search engines for, 46–47
Syntheses, 41–42, 44–45
Synthesized summaries, for clinical
    reference, 42–43
Systematic deviation, 67
Systematic reviews (SRs), 44–45, 71
  applicability of, 121–124, 123*b*
  consistency across studies,
    117–118
  definition of, 112–113
  in harm/etiology studies,
    201–202, 202*f*
  importance of, 113*b*
  individual patient data in, 117
  of randomized trials, 114
  relevant trials and search,
    114–115
  reports of, 112–124
  treatment effect in, magnitude
    of, 119–121
  validity of, 68, 113*b*, 114–121,
    186
    of individual studies, 115
Systematically derived
    recommendations, 43–44,
    60
Systems, clinical information,
    40–42
Systolic learning, in teaching EBM,
    241

T

Teachers, evaluation of, 231–235,
    231*b*–232*b*
Teaching EBM, 237–298
  on available time, 243, 246–247
  bullying style, 247
  clinical medicine, weaving
    evidence into, 237–239
  on clinical setting, 243
  in clinical teams and other small
    groups, 275–289
    with counterproductive
      behaviours, 285–288
    EBM skills "back home",
      288–289
    healthy learning climate,
      280–281
    issues in learning EBM jargon,
      283–285
    keep the discussion going, 281
    keep the discussion on track,
      281–282
    learning activities, 278–280
    manage time, 282–283
    sensible ground rules for,
      276–278
    understand why to learn,
      275–276
  core competencies in, 267–268
  diagnostic tests
    with CATs, 177*b*
    tips for, 181*b*–182*b*
  disconnected from the team's
    learning needs, 246
  domains of learning in,
    242–243
  EBM skills, 237, 239
  full educational closure in, 247
  humiliating learners and,
    247–248
  incorporating EBM, into existing
    educational sessions,
    258–265
  in inpatient service, 248–253,
    249*t*–250*t*, 254*b*
  integrating EBM
    into 4-year medical school
      curriculum, 271–274
    into curriculum, 267–271,
      269*f*
  in judgements, 244

on learners' actual learning needs, 240
in learners' lifelong learning abilities, 244–245
learning more about, 274–275
modes of, 237–239, 238b
in "new" knowledge to "old", 241
in outpatient clinic, 253–256, 255t
pace of the learners' understanding, 246
passive with active learning in, 241
preparedness with opportunism, 243–244
in published research, 245
questions asking
    in real-time, 29–33
on real clinical decisions and actions, 240
in research, 245
role modelling in, 237–238, 270
spiral trajectory in, 267
in statistics, 245
structured summaries of, 256–258, 257b
as substituting research evidence, 245
on team, 241–242
top 10 successes of, 240–245
see also Learning
Therapy, 71–152
in abnormality/normality, 157–158, 157b
as clinical questions, 25b
evidence about, validity of, 73–74, 73b
see also Adverse effects; Treatment effects
Three-session model, in journal club, 263

Time, in teaching EBM, 243, 246–247
Time trade-off method, 128–130
Title, in CAT, 257b
Traditional textbooks, 36–40, 61–62
Treatment effects
    calculation shortcut for, 98–99
    confidence intervals, 97
    consistent, from study to study, 117–118
    estimate of, precision of, 96–98
    magnitude of
        in individual studies, 86–96, 88t
        in systematic reviews, 119–121
    patient subgroups and, 102–103, 103b
    see also Number needed to treat
Turning Research Into Practice (TRIP), 48–49
Two-session cycle, in journal club, 265

U

Undergraduate learners, evidence-based medicine for, 235
UpToDate, 37–38, 59
Urinary incontinence, caffeine consumption causing, 203t
Utilities (patient preferences), 128–130, 132
    in economic analysis, 136

V

Validated decision aids, 107–108
Validity
    of harm/etiology studies, 201, 202b, 203–211, 203t
    assessment, 201
    causation tests for, 210–211

Validity *(Continued)*
    feasibility *vs.*, 203–204
    follow-up in, 209
    groups of patients in, 203–207
    treatments/exposures and
      clinical outcomes in,
      measurement of, 208
  in prognostic studies, 187–195
    evidence, 186*b*, 195–198,
      195*b*, 197*b*
    follow-up of, 189–190
    outcome criteria, 191
    prognostic factors, adjustment
      for, 192–195
    representativeness, 187–188

Valproic acid, in harm/etiology
    studies, 203–204, 208–209
Values, evaluation of, 226–227

W

Warfarin, for atrial fibrillation,
    128–130
Women's Health Initiative, 74
Work rounds, 249*t*–250*t*, 252
Workshops/courses, 234

Y

Youden Index, 164–165, 167*t*

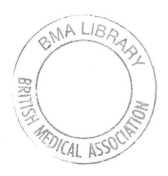